OPERATIVE ORTHOPAEDICS

OPERATIVE ORTHOPAEDICS

THE STANMORE GUIDE

SECOND EDITION

Edited by

Timothy WR Briggs MD MBBS (Hons), MCH (Orth), FRCS (Eng), FRCS (Ed), MD (Res)
Royal National Orthopaedic Hospital Trust, Stanmore, UK

Jonathan Miles MBChB, FRCS (Tr & Orth)
Royal National Orthopaedic Hospital Trust, Stanmore, UK

William Aston BSc, MBBS, FRCS (Tr & Orth) (Edinb)
Royal National Orthopaedic Hospital Trust, Stanmore, UK

Heledd Havard BSc, MBBCh, MSc, FRCS (Tr & Orth)
Royal National Orthopaedic Hospital Trust, Stanmore, UK

Daud TS Chou MBBS, BSc, MSc, FRCS (Tr & Orth)
Cambridge University Hospitals NHS Foundation Trust
Cambridge, UK

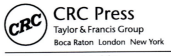

CRC Press is an imprint of the
Taylor & Francis Group, an **informa** business

Second edition published 2020
by CRC Press
6000 Broken Sound Parkway NW, Suite 300
Boca Raton, FL 33487-2742

and by CRC Press
2 Park Square, Milton Park, Abingdon, Oxon, OX14 4RN

© 2021 Taylor & Francis Group, LLC

CRC Press is an imprint of Taylor & Francis Group, LLC

This book contains information obtained from authentic and highly regarded sources. While all reasonable efforts have been made to publish reliable data and information, neither the author[s] nor the publisher can accept any legal responsibility or liability for any errors or omissions that may be made. The publishers wish to make clear that any views or opinions expressed in this book by individual editors, authors or contributors are personal to them and do not necessarily reflect the views/opinions of the publishers. The information or guidance contained in this book is intended for use by medical, scientific or health-care professionals and is provided strictly as a supplement to the medical or other professional's own judgement, their knowledge of the patient's medical history, relevant manufacturer's instructions and the appropriate best practice guidelines. Because of the rapid advances in medical science, any information or advice on dosages, procedures or diagnoses should be independently verified. The reader is strongly urged to consult the relevant national drug formulary and the drug companies' and device or material manufacturers' printed instructions, and their websites, before administering or utilizing any of the drugs, devices or materials mentioned in this book. This book does not indicate whether a particular treatment is appropriate or suitable for a particular individual. Ultimately it is the sole responsibility of the medical professional to make his or her own professional judgements, so as to advise and treat patients appropriately. The authors and publishers have also attempted to trace the copyright holders of all material reproduced in this publication and apologize to copyright holders if permission to publish in this form has not been obtained. If any copyright material has not been acknowledged please write and let us know so we may rectify in any future reprint.

Except as permitted under U.S. Copyright Law, no part of this book may be reprinted, reproduced, transmitted, or utilized in any form by any electronic, mechanical, or other means, now known or hereafter invented, including photocopying, microfilming, and recording, or in any information storage or retrieval system, without written permission from the publishers.

For permission to photocopy or use material electronically from this work, access www.copyright.com or contact the Copyright Clearance Center, Inc. (CCC), 222 Rosewood Drive, Danvers, MA 01923, 978-750-8400. For works that are not available on CCC please contact mpkbookspermissions@tandf.co.uk

Trademark notice: Product or corporate names may be trademarks or registered trademarks, and are used only for identification and explanation without intent to infringe.

ISBN: 978-0-367-47053-1 (hbk)
ISBN: 978-1-138-03176-0 (pbk)
ISBN: 978-1-315-18583-5 (ebk)

Typeset in Utopia Std
by Nova Techset Private Limited, Bengaluru and Chennai, India

Visit the Taylor & Francis Web site at
http://www.taylorandfrancis.com

and the CRC Press Web site at
http://www.crcpress.com

Contents

Preface vii
Acknowledgements ix
Contributors xi

1 **Anaesthesia in Orthopaedic Surgery** 1
   James Cremin and Michael Cooper

2 **Tumours** 11
   Heledd Havard, William Aston and
   Timothy WR Briggs

3 **Surgery of the Cervical Spine** 25
   Julian Leong and Kia Rezajooi

4 **Surgery of the Thoracolumbar
   Spine** 43
   Daniel P Ahern, Joseph S Butler,
   Matthew Shaw and Sean Molloy

5 **Surgery of the Peripheral Nerve** 63
   Ravikiran Shenoy, Gorav Datta,
   Max Horowitz and Mike Fox

6 **Surgery of the Shoulder** 85
   Nick Aresti, Omar Haddo and
   Mark Falworth

7 **Surgery of the Elbow** 113
   Alan Salih, David Butt and
   Deborah Higgs

8 **Surgery of the Wrist** 159
   Ramon Tahmassebi, Sirat Khan and
   Kalpesh R Vaghela

9 **Surgery of the Hand** 193
   Norbert Kang, Ben Miranda and
   Dariush Nikkhah

10 **Surgery of the Hip** 239
   Daud TS Chou, Jonathan Miles and
   John Skinner

11 **Surgery of the Knee** 279
   Alexander D Liddle, Lee A David
   and Timothy WR Briggs

12 **Soft Tissue Surgery of the Knee** 321
   Stephen Key, Jonathan Miles and Richard
   Carrington

13 **Surgery of the Ankle** 367
   Matthew Welck, Laurence James and
   Dishan Singh

14 **Surgery of the Foot** 385
   Yaser Ghani, Simon Clint and
   Nicholas Cullen

15 **Limb Reconstruction** 427
   Robert Jennings and Peter Calder

16 **Paediatric Orthopaedic Surgery** 443
   Jonathan Wright, Russell Hawkins,
   Aresh Hashemi-Nejad and Peter Calder

17 **Amputations** 483
   Heledd Havard, William Aston and
   Rob Pollock

Index 495

Preface

Orthopaedic training and surgical practice have seen significant developments over recent decades and continue to represent some of the most exciting surgical sub-specialities. While the original concept of this book was none other than a 'professorial moment … in the bath', editing the recent edition has been somewhat of a marathon over the past three years. This text is not intended to serve as a complete guide to elective orthopaedics; it is designed to illustrate the basic principles and surgical techniques of common orthopaedic procedures, providing the reader with a solid overview presented in a systematic format.

High-pressure environments are somewhat commonplace in the life of the orthopaedic trainee, not least during preparation for the Fellowship of the Royal College of Surgeons (FRCS) examination – thus the format of this text is set to be utilised both as a learning model and also in structuring answers. Procedures are described in a concise and consistent format to enable the reader to describe and carry out safe, evidence-based approaches while reinforcing the fundamentals of basic principles.

While this text offers a general overview of common procedures and techniques, it certainly should not be used as a substitute for the detailed knowledge required of the senior trainee approaching the exam. Under stressful conditions trainees can find themselves fumbling over answers, and developing strategies to structure answers succinctly is an investment worth making. As in the world of rugby, 'the more you sweat in training, the less you bleed in battle', and in the words of Albert Einstein, 'If you can't explain it simply, you don't understand it well enough'.

To all future trainees, I hope that this book serves as a general guide with solid principles presented in a readable format and will act as a stepping stone in your learning and understanding of the curriculum.

Acknowledgements

1 Anaesthesia in Orthopaedic Surgery contains some material from Anaesthesia in Orthopaedic Surgery by Hui Yin Vivian Ip and Michael Cooper. The material has been revised and updated by the current authors.

3 Surgery of the Cervical Spine contains some material from Surgery of the Cervical Spine by Raman Kalyan and David Harrison. The material has been revised and updated by the current authors.

7 Surgery of the Elbow contains some material from Surgery of the Elbow by Simon Lambert. The material has been revised and updated by the current authors.

8 Surgery of the Wrist contains some material from Surgery of the Wrist by James Donaldson and Nicholas Goddard. The material has been revised and updated by the current authors.

9 Surgery of the Hand contains some material from Surgery of the Hand by Robert Pearl and Lauren Ovens. The material has been revised and updated by the current authors.

Contributors

Daniel P Ahern
Centre for Biomedical Engineering
Trinity College
Dublin, Ireland

Nick Aresti
Barts Health NHS Trust
London, United Kingdom

William Aston
Royal National Orthopaedic Hospital Trust
Stanmore, United Kingdom

Timothy WR Briggs
Royal National Orthopaedic Hospital Trust
Stanmore, United Kingdom

Joseph S Butler
Mater Private Hospital
Dublin, Ireland

David Butt
Royal National Orthopaedic Hospital Trust
Stanmore, United Kingdom

Peter Calder
Royal National Orthopaedic Hospital Trust
Stanmore, United Kingdom

Richard Carrington
Royal National Orthopaedic Hospital Trust
Stanmore, United Kingdom

Daud TS Chou
Cambridge University Hospitals NHS Foundation Trust
Cambridge, United Kingdom

Simon Clint
Royal National Orthopaedic Hospital Trust
Stanmore, United Kingdom

Michael Cooper
Department of Anaesthetics
Royal National Orthopaedic Hospital Trust
Stanmore, United Kingdom

James Cremin
Department of Anaesthetics
Royal National Orthopaedic Hospital Trust
Stanmore, United Kingdom

Nicholas Cullen
Royal National Orthopaedic Hospital Trust
Stanmore, United Kingdom

Gorav Datta
Royal National Orthopaedic Hospital Trust
Stanmore, United Kingdom

Lee A David
Maidstone and Tunbridge Wells NHS Trust
Maidstone, United Kingdom

Mark Falworth
Royal National Orthopaedic Hospital Trust
Stanmore, United Kingdom

Mike Fox
Royal National Orthopaedic Hospital Trust
Stanmore, United Kingdom

Yaser Ghani
Royal National Orthopaedic Hospital Trust
Stanmore, United Kingdom

Omar Haddo
Whittington Hospital
London, United Kingdom

Aresh Hashemi-Nejad
Royal National Orthopaedic Hospital Trust
Stanmore, United Kingdom

and

University College London
London, United Kingdom

Heledd Havard
Royal National Orthopaedic Hospital Trust
Stanmore, United Kingdom

Russell Hawkins
Royal National Orthopaedic Hospital Trust
Stanmore, United Kingdom

Deborah Higgs
Royal National Orthopaedic Hospital Trust
Stanmore, United Kingdom

Max Horowitz
Royal National Orthopaedic Hospital Trust
Stanmore, United Kingdom

Laurence James
Royal National Orthopaedic Hospital Trust
Stanmore, United Kingdom

Robert Jennings
Royal National Orthopaedic Hospital Trust
Stanmore, United Kingdom

Norbert Kang
Royal Free Hospital
London, United Kingdom

Stephen Key
Royal National Orthopaedic
 Hospital Trust
Stanmore, United Kingdom

Sirat Khan
Royal Free London NHS
 Foundation Trust
Stanmore, United Kingdom

Julian Leong
Royal National Orthopaedic
 Hospital Trust
Stanmore, United Kingdom

Alexander D Liddle
Division of Surgery
Imperial College
and
Imperial College Healthcare
 NHS Trust
London, United Kingdom

Jonathan Miles
Royal National Orthopaedic
 Hospital Trust
Stanmore, United Kingdom

Ben Miranda
Andrew's Centre for Plastic
 Surgery and Burns
Essex, United Kingdom

Sean Molloy
Royal National Orthopaedic
 Hospital Trust
Stanmore, United Kingdom

Dariush Nikkhah
Department of Plastic and
 Reconstructive Surgery
Royal Free London NHS
 Foundation Trust
Stanmore, United Kingdom

Rob Pollock
Royal National Orthopaedic
 Hospital Trust
Stanmore, United Kingdom

Kia Rezajooi
Royal National Orthopaedic
 Hospital Trust
Stanmore, United Kingdom

Alan Salih
School of Medicine
King's College London
London, United Kingdom

Matthew Shaw
Royal National Orthopaedic
 Hospital Trust
Stanmore, United Kingdom

Ravikiran Shenoy
Royal Free London NHS
 Foundation Trust
Stanmore, United Kingdom

Dishan Singh
Royal National Orthopaedic
 Hospital Trust
Stanmore, United Kingdom

John Skinner
Royal National Orthopaedic
 Hospital Trust
Stanmore, United Kingdom

Ramon Tahmassebi
King's College Hospital
London, United Kingdom

Kalpesh R Vaghela
Trauma and Orthopaedic
 Registrar
Royal National Orthopaedic
 Hospital
Percivall Pott Rotation
London, United Kingdom

Matthew Welck
Royal National Orthopaedic
 Hospital Trust
Stanmore, United Kingdom

Jonathan Wright
Royal London Hospital
Barts and London NHS Trust
London, United Kingdom

1 Anaesthesia in Orthopaedic Surgery

James Cremin and Michael Cooper

Introduction	1	Postoperative care	6
Preoperative assessment	1	Viva questions	9
Intraoperative techniques	5		

Introduction

The orthopaedic patient population presents many challenges. It includes the extremes of age, comes with a range of embedded medical co-morbidities and presents with diverse surgical pathology requiring varied intervention. Procedures range from day-case minimally invasive arthroscopic procedures to extensive operations that test the physiological reserve of an individual patient. Due to these concerns, an individual anaesthetic is customised to the medical demands of the patient, the requirements for the surgical technique and the limitations of the institution in which the surgery occurs.

Preoperative assessment

This is the process of assessing the relevance, severity and treatment of medical pathologies. This allows referral for better treatment ('optimisation') and quantification of the risk of adverse perioperative events, including death, to be discussed and documented. Factors specific to anaesthesia, such as a possible difficult airway, may also be considered. Guidelines exist to inform the ordering of preoperative laboratory tests. In addition, the optimisation of patients prior to admission for surgery is aimed to reduce cancellations on the day of surgery and to increase the productivity of the theatre suite.

Fasting
In elective surgery, standard local fasting times must be adhered to. A typical regimen is given in *Table 1.1*. Food includes milk and fresh fruit juices. It is safe for patients (including diabetics) to drink specialised carbohydrate-rich (maltodextrins) drinks up to 2 hours before elective surgery as this improves subjective well-being, reduces thirst and hunger and reduces postoperative insulin resistance.

Table 1.1 Fasting times

	\multicolumn{4}{c}{Typical foods}
	Solid food	Water	Breast milk	Formula milk
Fasting time	6 hours	2 hours	4 hours	6 hours

In trauma situations, gastric emptying is affected from the time of injury and is further complicated by the use of opiate analgesics that prolong gastric emptying. Fasting times are difficult to interpret in this situation but can be calculated as the time of intake to time of trauma. In certain situations, the clinical priority for surgical intervention may override fasting policy, and clear discussion between clinicians caring for the patient needs to occur.

Airway

Airway assessment involves both bedside tests and if needed, radiological tests. A range of bedside tests exist that aim to predict difficulties in maintaining an airway or intubating an anaesthetized patient. Used individually, each airway assessment has poor sensitivity and specificity, however when combined can be a useful marker.

Of particular importance in orthopaedic surgery is pathology or trauma to the cervical column. Rigidity of the cervical column (e.g. in ankylosing spondylosis) may cause a problem with maintaining an airway and with difficult laryngoscopy. An unstable cervical column (e.g. trauma or rheumatoid arthritis) can lead to cord injury. Initial radiological assessment is with a plain film in anteroposterior (AP), lateral, flexion and extension views. If there are any concerns, then specialised investigations to delineate pathology include computed tomography (CT) and magnetic resonance imaging (MRI).

Cardiovascular assessment

Cardiovascular assessment is aimed at quantifying the ability of the cardiovascular pump to increase work to match perioperative metabolic demands. This is during both the operative period and rehabilitation. It is an assessment of reserve and a prediction of adverse events such as an acute coronary syndrome. Key clinical markers are described in the following sections.

Exercise tolerance/functional status

For patients having major, non-cardiac surgery, the inability to climb two flights of stairs confers an increased risk of major postoperative complications but is not predictive of mortality. Difficulties in this assessment are common for orthopaedic patients due to their pathology affecting mobility.

Previous myocardial infarction

There is a risk of recurrent perioperative myocardial infarction (MI), which has a 60% mortality rate. The longer surgery can be postponed after an MI, the lower is the rate of recurrent MI (*Table 1.2*).

Table 1.2 Percentage risk of recurrent myocardial infarction (MI) at different times after MI

Time since MI	Risk of recurrent MI (%)
<3 months	5.7
4–6 months	2.3
>6 months	1.5

Investigations

Typical investigations used to quantify cardiac reserve are as follows:

- *Exercise electrocardiogram* (ECG): This helps to determine any coronary flow limitation when cardiac work increases.
- *24-hour ECG recording* (Holter monitor): This involves continuous ECG recording for 24–48 hours to investigate possible arrhythmia.
- *Thallium scintigraphy and dobutamine stress echocardiography*: These dynamic 'stress tests' are especially useful for patients who are unable to perform exercise ECG due to musculoskeletal disease or severe cardiopulmonary disease. Perfusion defects of the myocardium under physiological stress indicate coronary insufficiency.
- *Cardiovascular MRI*: This is a non-invasive assessment of the function and structure of the cardiovascular system. It provides information on cardiac structure, cardiomyopathy and perfusion defects.
- *Cardiopulmonary exercise testing*: This is a dynamic test that predicts the patient's anaerobic threshold. It can indicate the respiratory and cardiac reserve but can be affected by other factors such as motivation, mobility and nutrition. It can be used to predict the risk of surgery and obviate the need for other tests such as angiography or echocardiography.
- *Coronary angiography*: This is used to visualize coronary arterial flow and disease. This is often the end point of coronary investigation and may allow treatment by stenting and angioplasty at the same time.

Hypertension

Hypertensive patients are at a higher risk of labile blood pressures intraoperatively compared to the non-hypertensive population. Blood pressure management is aimed to reduce cardiovascular morbidity over years and decades, but there is no evidence that perioperative blood pressure reduction affects cardiovascular risk.

For elective surgery, if mean blood pressures in primary care in the past 12 months are less than 160 mm Hg systolic and less than 100 mm Hg diastolic (160/100 mm Hg), surgery can proceed.

If there is no evidence of normotension in primary care, then elective surgery should proceed for patients if their blood pressure is less than 180 mm Hg systolic and 110 mm Hg diastolic (180/110 mm Hg) when measured in the hospital setting.

Heart murmurs

The valve pathology underlying murmurs may have significant implications for anaesthetic technique. Lesions that limit the cardiac output (particularly aortic stenosis) can cause profound hypotension as the heart cannot increase cardiac output to maintain blood pressure as peripheral vascular resistance drops. This is most marked with neuraxial anaesthesia and can cause morbidity due to organ hypo-perfusion. For example, coronary perfusion may become critically low resulting in an acute coronary syndrome. Echocardiography is useful to determine the nature and the severity of the valve lesion.

Respiratory assessment

Preoperative assessment determines the severity and potential reversibility of respiratory pathology. Disease states limit gas flow, gas exchange or both. The end point of respiratory disease is hypoxaemia and tissue hypoxia. This can precipitate organ failure with serious adverse outcomes. Common pathologies are described in the following sections.

Asthma

Stable asthma is usually benign, but some anaesthetic agents can trigger bronchospasm and are avoided. Conversely, some anaesthetic agents can result in bronchodilation and are favoured. Assessment should include spirometry and peak flow measurements. Preparation may include bronchodilator premedication, e.g. salbutamol, and some anaesthetists prefer a regional technique to avoid airway instrumentation and opiate use. Elective surgery should not proceed with concurrent upper respiratory tract infection.

Chronic obstructive airways disease

Gas flow and exchange are limited in this disease. These patients are at risk of postoperative respiratory failure due to atelectasis and segmental lung collapse causing hypoxaemia. Assessment includes spirometry (a forced expiratory volume in 1 second greater than 1 L indicates an ability to clear secretions), oximetry (and perhaps arterial blood gas sampling) and an assessment of exercise ability. A baseline chest radiograph may be useful but is by no means mandatory. An ECG may show signs of right heart strain and is also indicated as this group is likely to have co-existent cardiovascular disease. Preoperative and postoperative chest physiotherapy are essential. Anaesthetists will tend towards regional anaesthesia in patients with significant disease burden to minimise the chances of postoperative respiratory failure. Opiates are a potent source of respiratory depression and, coupled to sedation and pain, can be a powerful trigger for respiratory decompensation.

Respiratory tract infection

Respiratory tract infections are often viral, and the most common are located in the upper respiratory tract. Patients with a productive cough or objective symptoms of pyrexia, fatigue, myalgia and/or anorexia should only proceed if emergency surgery is indicated. The risk of laryngospasm and bronchospasm is increased. Viral myocarditis may also occur, leading to cardiac failure or even death in the perioperative period. Guidelines advise a 4- to 6-week delay for elective surgery.

Groups at special risk

Patients with cerebral palsy may have poor bulbar function and weak cough, which puts them at risk of aspiration, and they have a higher incidence of postoperative respiratory tract infection. This is exacerbated by any cognitive impairment that reduces their ability to cooperate with physiotherapy and interventions such as non-invasive ventilation. Patients with low-tone neuromuscular syndrome are at risk of postoperative respiratory failure, and plans will include intensive care, possible postoperative ventilation and tracheostomy requirement. Of note, volatile anaesthesia is usually avoided in this group due to the risk of rhabdomyolysis, renal failure and hyperkalaemic cardiac arrest.

Recommended references

Fischer HBJ, Simanski CJP. A procedure specific and systematic review and consensus recommendations for analgesia after total hip replacement. *Anaesthesia*. 2005;**60**:1189–1202.

Fischer HBJ, Simanski CJP, Sharp C et al. A procedure specific systematic review and consensus recommendations for postoperative analgesia following total knee arthroplasty. *Anaesthesia*. 2008;**63**:1105–1123.

Fowler SJ, Symons J, Sabato S et al. Epidural analgesia compared with peripheral nerve blockade after major knee surgery: A systematic review and meta-analysis of randomized trials. *Br J Anaesth*. 2008;**100**:154–164.

Goodnough LT, Shander A. Patient blood management. *Anesthesiology*. 2012;**116(6)**:1367–1376.

Muñoz M, Acheson AG, Auerbach M et al. International consensus statement on the peri-operative management of anaemia and iron deficiency. *Anaesthesia*. 2017;**72**:233–247.

Simpson JC, Moonesinghe SR, Grocott MP et al. Enhanced recovery from surgery in the UK: An audit of the enhanced recovery partnership programme 2009–2012. *Br J Anaesth*. 2015;**115(4)**:560–568.

Intraoperative techniques

Discussion of the selection and conduct of individual techniques is beyond the scope of this chapter. The technique chosen is multifactorial and is dependent upon the patient, hospital, procedure, surgeon and anaesthetist. There is little conformity of opinion.

General anaesthesia

This is the most common option and is entirely appropriate for most procedures, environments and patients. It is a balanced technique of analgesia, muscle relaxation and sedation. This is confirmed by data review as exemplified by recent publications concerning primary joint replacement.

Peripheral regional anaesthesia

This is the placement of local anaesthetic adjacent to individual nerves or plexus of nerves to produce a zone of sensory and motor block. This may be the only mode of anaesthesia. More commonly, it is a pain-relieving adjunct to general anaesthesia or sedation. The main benefit is to reduce opiate requirement to aid earlier mobilisation but neurological injury may be masked. A prolonged motor block may occur which is to the detriment of the patient. Increasingly this modality is preferred for primary arthroplasty but is increasing into other areas.

Neuroaxial local anaesthesia

For lower limb procedures, spinal, epidural or a combined spinal-epidural block can provide complete analgesia and motor block. As with previous techniques, they may be used alone or in combination with sedation or general anaesthesia. They are often the technique of choice in those with severe respiratory disease burden to reduce the respiratory complications associated with opiate use. Outcome evidence is poor but there is some literature base to support this practice. In addition historical data suggest a lower incidence of deep vein thrombosis and perioperative blood loss. This may no longer be valid in light of new advances in perioperative care and enhanced recovery programmes. These techniques remain an important part of a multimodal approach to fast-track surgery.

Contraindications

Patient refusal.
Local or systemic infection.
Allergy to agents used.
Coagulopathy.
Anticoagulants (relative contraindication) increase the risk of haematoma at the site of infiltration, around nerves or in the epidural space.
Aspirin is not a contraindication.
Chronic neurological diseases (relative contraindication).

Local Anaesthesia

Some body surface procedures are amenable to surgery using local infiltration alone. Maximal dosages and drug information are given in *Table 1.3*.

Postoperative care

Analgesia

The "analgesic ladder" was originally published in 1986 by the World Health Organization (WHO) as a guideline for the use of drugs in the management of pain. Initially intended for the management of cancer pain, it has evolved to be more widely used for the management of all types of pain. The general principle is to start with simple analgesics and to escalate to strong opioids as required. It is advised that medications should be given at regular

Table 1.3 Local anaesthetic drug information

Drug	Maximum dose (mg/kg)	Relative Potency	Onset (minutes)	Duration (hours)
Lidocaine	3	2	5–10	1–2
Lidocaine with adrenaline (1:200 000)	7	2	5–10	2–4
Bupivicaine	2	8	10–15	3–12
Ropivicaine	3	6	10–15	3–12
Prilocaine	6	2	5–10	1–4

intervals so that continuous pain relief occurs, and dosing be directed by relief of pain rather than by fixed dosing guidelines.

Simple analgesics

These can be very effective for mild and moderate pain. Common drugs are paracetamol and non-steroidal anti-inflammatory drugs. Best effect is gained when they are given regularly, ideally after a loading dose in theatre. In more severe pain, they are still useful adjuncts with well-documented opiate-sparing properties. Increasing evidence points to using NSAIDs with care in patients with cardiovascular disease.

Oral opiates

Oral opiates include codeine derivatives, complex agonists such as tramadol and morphine derivatives. These are well recognised for more severe pain and can be used regularly, with stronger alternatives available for breakthrough pain. Newer formulations provide excellent pharmacokinetics with twice daily dosing of modified-release compounds, each providing 12-hour analgesia. These modified-release tablets are supplemented by short-acting versions to treat breakthrough pain.

Intravenous opiates

For severe pain, intravenous opiates may be given as patient-controlled analgesia (PCA). This allows the patient to titrate their own dosing. It is effective, safe and popular. Better pain scores and fewer side effects (nausea, vomiting and sedation) are regularly achieved using this modality of opiate delivery compared with intermittent intramuscular dosing. Once the acute postoperative period has passed, the patient may be stepped down to oral alternatives.

Alternatives

Other routes such as transdermal delivery are available. These take a long time to reach a steady plasma concentration and are similarly slow to decline when discontinued. They are more suited to long- term use in chronic pain syndromes. This inflexibility makes them difficult to use in the perioperative period but consideration should be made preoperatively to existing analgesic requirements.

Local anaesthesia

Local anaesthetic techniques may be continued into the postoperative period. These provide excellent analgesia with minimal side effects. However, immobility may be a problem. In units where utilising local anaesthetic blocks is embedded in practice, they are very successful and do not need to delay mobilisation.

Oxygen

Oxygen therapy should be given to patients with an epidural infusion which contains opiates, or those using a PCA. This supplemental oxygen maintains alveolar oxygen tension longer if respiratory depression and hypoventilation occur. Supplemental oxygen used for the first three days postoperatively can also minimise the risk of perioperative ischaemic events.

Any patient with pre-existing respiratory pathology or acquired (respiratory tract infection, atelectasis, thromboembolism) will be relatively hypoxic, and oxygen therapy is essential.

Fluid management

The goal of intravenous fluid therapy is to maintain normovolaemia. This allows adequate cardiac output and, assuming an appropriate haemoglobin concentration, tissue oxygen delivery. Maintenance water and electrolytes need to be supplied and ongoing blood loss compensated for in the form of blood substitute, or blood itself. Patient blood management has recently been advocated for the perisurgical period to enable treating physicians to have the time and tools to provide patient-centered evidenced-based care to minimise allogeneic blood transfusions. It aims to optimise erythropoiesis, minimise blood loss and manage anaemia.

Triggers for transfusion vary. Blood is expensive, immunosuppressant, associated with worse outcome and a vehicle for disease transmission. However, red cells are vital to oxygen delivery and haemostasis. The trigger will depend on the predicted continuing blood loss, the patient's co-morbidities and symptoms. This haemoglobin concentration trigger can be as low as 7 g/dL.

Disposal

High-dependency care may benefit many orthopaedic patients. Delivery of this will depend on local protocol and infrastructure. Clearly, those at increased risk of organ failure or requiring a higher level of nursing supervision should be placed in an appropriate environment.

Enhanced recovery

Enhanced recovery is the delivery of a consistent, protocolised pathway of care with the aim to minimise perioperative stress and to expedite recovery. The amount of evidence for each individual element of the enhanced recovery bundle is variable. However, good compliance with enhanced recovery protocols (≥80% compliance) is associated with a shorter median length of stay by one day in orthopaedic surgery. In particular, individualised fluid therapy and early mobilisation were the strongest indicators. This reduction in length of stay represents a clinically important reduction in morbidity and significant cost savings.

Recommended references

Association of Anaesthetists of Great Britain and Ireland. The measurement of adult blood pressure and management of hypertension before elective surgery 2016. *Anaesthesia*. 2016;**71**:326–337.

Biccard BM. Relationship between the inability to climb two flights of stairs and outcome after major non-cardiac surgery: Implications for the pre-operative assessment of functional capacity. *Anaesthesia*. 2005;**6**:588–593.

Howell S, Sear J, Foex P. Hypertension, hypertensive heart disease and perioperative cardiac risk. *Br J Anaesth*. 2004;**92**:570–583.

National Institute for Health and Care Excellence. April 2016. Routine preoperative tests for elective surgery. NICE guideline [NG45]. Accessed April 2017. https://www.nice.org.uk/guidance/ng45

Viva questions

1. In patients with hypertension, how would you determine whether elective surgery can proceed?
2. What are the contraindications to neuraxial blockade?
3. Why is a respiratory tract infection a problem?
4. Who should receive oxygen therapy in the postoperative period?
5. What are the postoperative options for analgesia for a primary arthroplasty?

2 Tumours

Heledd Havard, William Aston and Timothy WR Briggs

Principles of biopsy	11	Bone cyst curettage with or without bone graft	17
Needle biopsy of bone	11	Malignant tumour principles	20
Open biopsy of bone	14	Viva questions	22
Excision of benign bone tumour	16		

Sarcomas can broadly be classified into benign or malignant tumours and can be either of soft tissues or of bone. All tumours should be managed via a multidisciplinary team (MDT) approach at an appropriate dedicated tumour unit consisting of specialised oncology surgeons, radiologists, histopathologists, paediatricians and oncologists. Appropriate early referral to a sarcoma unit with careful diagnosis and coordinated management play a fundamental role in achieving the most successful outcome. Careful discussion and planning from time of initial presentation through to postoperative care and surveillance are critical.

Principles of biopsy

All patients presenting with a suspected sarcoma or isolated metastasis should be referred and discussed at a sarcoma MDT. Once appropriate staging investigations have been performed, a tissue diagnosis is required to gain a histological diagnosis and plan subsequent treatment. The biopsy is planned as part of the MDT between the oncology surgeon and the interventional radiologist.

1. Performed at a specialised sarcoma centre with appropriate histopathology support
2. Planned in accordance with the operating oncology surgeon
3. Includes representative tissue – often from the periphery of the lesion or a membrane as the central part is often necrotic and non-diagnostic
4. Should not violate any surrounding compartments
5. Biopsy tract should be marked by tattoo to aid excision at time of definitive surgery

Needle biopsy of bone

Preoperative planning

Indications

To obtain a histological diagnosis so that further treatment can be planned.

Contraindications

Lesions that are closely related to neurovascular structures, where a needle biopsy would put these structures at risk.

Patients should also be warned that a second needle biopsy or open biopsy may be necessary if an inadequate tissue specimen for histological diagnosis is obtained.

> **Consent and risks**
> - Neurovascular injury and infection are the main risks
> - Possible tumour seeding

Templating

The needle entry point and tract need careful thought and should be planned by the surgeon performing the tumour resection, as the biopsy tract will need to be excised if malignancy is found.

Fine needle aspiration (FNA) is not used in sarcoma diagnosis and is largely reserved to diagnosing carcinoma. A thicker-bore needle (11G or 13G), capable of boring through the outside of the lesion and taking core biopsies such as a Jamshidi needle (**Figure 2.1**), is preferable.

For tumours that have a large soft tissue component or that have destroyed the cortex, a Tru-Cut or Temno (preloaded) needle can be used. These take a slice of tissue and come in 11 and 14 gauges. If there is doubt that the tissue obtained at biopsy may not be representative, a smear and/or frozen section can be performed by the histopathologist which may also provide a provisional diagnosis.

Anaesthesia and positioning

Needle biopsy can be done under local, local with sedation or general anaesthesia. For children, hard lesions and lesions that may be difficult to access, a general anaesthetic should be used.

Positioning is dependent on the area to be reached and if necessary the imaging modality being used.

Surgical technique

Landmarks and incision

The line of the biopsy should be sited *in the line of a possible future surgical incision*, so that it can be excised at the time of surgery (**Figure 2.2**). It must pass directly to the site of the tumour

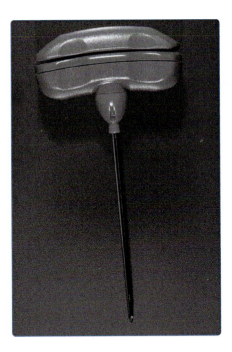

Figure 2.1 Jamshidi needle.

and through only the myofascial compartment in which the tumour is located, preferably through muscle and away from the neurovascular structures at risk. It should aim to take a representative sample of the tumour, which can be identified on pre-biopsy imaging. The needle is passed after a simple stab incision in the skin with a number 15 blade.

Deep dissection
The needle is passed through the stab incision directly into the area being biopsied, under radiological control.

Technical aspects of procedure
Multiple core biopsies are needed, aiming to minimise diversion from the tract. In cases where preoperative imaging is atypical or where infection is suspected, samples should also be sent for microbiology.

The needle should not be passed through the lesion into normal tissue. For lesions close to joints, the needle *must not pass through the capsule* and therefore potentially contaminate the joint. It may be necessary to drill the bone prior to needle insertion in sclerotic lesions. Careful handling of the specimens is important so as not to destroy the microarchitecture. Discussion with the histopathologist will elucidate whether they wish to receive the specimen fresh or fixed in formalin.

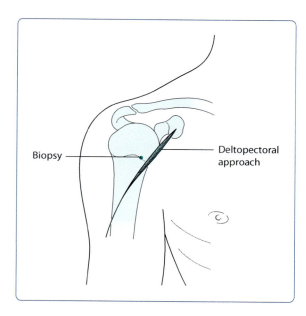

Figure 2.2 Position of biopsy for proximal humeral tumour – in the line of the deltopectoral approach, but slightly lateral so that the needle passes through the deltoid muscle and avoids the cephalic vein.

Closure
Use Steri-Strips.

Postoperative instructions
- Neurovascular and routine observations.
- Local pressure in the case of vascular lesions.

Recommended references
Saifuddin A, Mitchell R, Burnett S et al. Ultrasound guided needle biopsy of primary bone tumours. *J Bone Joint Surg Br.* 2000;**82**:50–54.

Stoker DJ, Cobb JP, Pringle JAS. Needle biopsy of musculoskeletal lesions. A review of 208 procedures. *J Bone Joint Surg Br.* 1991;**37**:498–500.

Open biopsy of bone
Preoperative planning
Indications
- Patients who are not suitable for a needle biopsy.
- Patients in whom tissue from a needle biopsy was insufficient to make the diagnosis.

Open biopsy can be incisional where a sample of the lesion is taken or it can be excisional where the whole lesion is removed. Excisional biopsy is generally reserved for lesions which, on radiology, have diagnostic features of a benign lesion.

Contraindications

Lesions where a satisfactory needle biopsy can be performed.

Consent and risks

- Neurovascular injury
- Infection
- Seeding of the tumour
- Unexpected histological result with need for further surgery

Templating

The incision should be planned with the surgeon and be made in the line of the surgical approach that will be used to remove the tumour.

Thought should be given as to how to localise the tumour, e.g. with image intensifier intraoperatively if necessary.

Anaesthesia and positioning

Regional/general anaesthesia and patient positioned to enable good access.

Surgical technique

Landmarks and incision

The incision should be made in line with an extensile approach that can be utilised at the time of definitive surgery to excise the biopsy tract together with the specimen.

Dissection

Dependent on the location.

Technical aspects of procedure

It is important to minimise potential complications of biopsy such as infection and haematoma as a poorly performed biopsy *carries significant morbidity*. When a tourniquet is used, the limb should be elevated rather than exsanguinated and the tourniquet deflated prior to closure to ensure adequate haemostasis. If a drain is used, the exit point should be in the line of any further incision.

Only one compartment of the limb should be violated during the approach. Muscles should be split and meticulous haemostasis applied to minimise haematoma formation and spread of fluid through tissue planes. The area to be biopsied should be carefully exposed, taking care not to disrupt the capsule or expose more of the tumour than is necessary. If a capsule is opened then it should be closed carefully.

A *representative sample* of tissue should be taken to include the transition from normal to abnormal tissue if possible. If there is any doubt then frozen section should be undertaken to ensure a diagnostic specimen.

Closure
Routine.

Postoperative instructions
Neurovascular observations.

Recommended references
Ashford RU, McCarthy SW, Scolyer RA et al. Surgical biopsy with intra-operative frozen section. An accurate and cost-effective method for diagnosis of musculoskeletal sarcomas. *J Bone Joint Surg Br.* 2006;**88**:1207–1211.

Mankin HJ, Lange TA, Sapnnier SS. The hazards of biopsy in patients with malignant primary bone and soft tissue tumours. *J Bone Joint Surg Am.* 1982;**64**:1121.

Pollock RC, Stalley PD. Biopsy of musculoskeletal tumours – Beware. *A NZ J Surg.* 2004;**74**:516–519.

Excision of benign bone tumour
Preoperative planning
Common indications
- Impending fracture, e.g. aneurysmal bone cyst
- To prevent further bony destruction and/or functional loss in aggressive lesions – e.g. giant cell tumour
- Mechanical symptoms – osteochondroma
- Pain – osteoid osteoma
- Risk of malignant transformation

Contraindications
No definitive characterisation of the lesion on either imaging or pathology.

Consent and risks
Depend on anatomical location and pathology of the lesion.

Templating
The approach depends on access required to perform resection while also taking into consideration any future potential reconstructive procedures.

Anaesthesia and positioning
Usually general anaesthesia and routine positioning.

Surgical technique
Landmarks and incision
As per preoperative plan.

Dissection
The exposure is dependent on the anatomical location and whether the plan is to perform curettage of the lesion (intralesional excision) or to excise it (marginal excision) and reconstruct it. It is *unwise to* attempt tumour excision and reconstruction through 'minimally invasive' approaches.

Technical aspects of procedure
Again, these depend on procedure and location. If *en bloc* resection is planned then reconstruction options need to be available, including any autograft or allograft necessary, in conjunction with any hardware for fixation. If curettage is planned, graft or adjuvant treatments, such as cement, liquid nitrogen or phenol, may be required to fill/treat the resulting cavity.

Necessary imaging modalities need to be available, such as computed tomography for localisation of an osteoid osteoma or image intensifier to localise a larger lesion.

Closure
Routine – procedure dependent.

Postoperative care and instructions
- Routine
- Weightbearing and physiotherapy regimen – depend on procedure

Recommended reference
Malawer MM, Dunham W. Cryosurgery and acrylic cementation as surgical adjuncts in the treatment of aggressive (benign) bone tumours. *Clin Orthop Relat Res.* 1991;262:42.

Bone cyst curettage with or without bone graft
Preoperative planning
Indications
- Risk of fracture or repeated fracture.
- Failure of other methods of treatment, such as a steroid injection into the cyst.

Contraindications

If radiology is not classical of a bone cyst, then histopathological diagnosis should be sought.

Consent and risks

- General risks and that of recurrence
- Depend on the location

Operative planning

Planning of the approach to allow good access to the whole cyst while not threatening the physis or nearby neurovascular structures.

Anaesthesia and positioning

General anaesthesia; positioning depends on the access required.

Surgical technique

Landmarks and incision

Utilisation of a recognised surgical approach in most cases.

Dissection

Dissection to bone, following described approaches and avoiding neurovascular structures, exposing the periosteum over the length of the cyst. The image intensifier is often necessary to locate the lesion or to confirm the position and extent of the cavity.

Technical aspects of procedure

Once the cyst has been located, a 2.5 mm drill bit is used to drill (at 5–10 mm intervals) the outline of a cortical window through which curettage is going to take place. By drilling, it confirms the presence of the cyst and avoids stress risers in the bone or the propagation of a fracture. The holes are joined up with a small osteotome or saw blade (**Figure 2.3**).

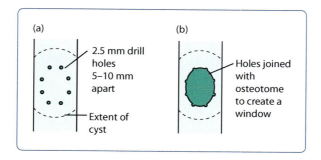

Figure 2.3 (a,b) Technique for making a cortical window for curettage of a bony lesion.

Once the cyst is entered, thorough curettage can take place, attempting to remove tissue from all bone surfaces. A communication is made from the cyst to the medulla of the bone to allow the cyst to fill with blood (which reduces recurrence rate). Screening with an image intensifier (**Figure 2.4**) confirms that the whole cavity has been treated.

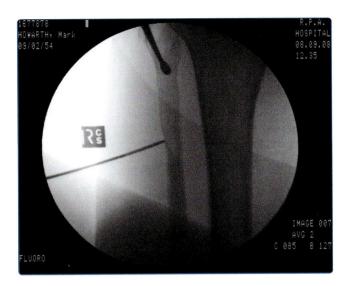

Figure 2.4 Screening the extent of the cavity to be curetted.

If the cyst is close to the growth plate, the cortical window is made distant to the physis; curettage of the growth plate is avoided as this may lead to a growth disturbance. The cyst can be grafted with a cancellous or corticocancellous autograft from the ileum, tibia or fibula. An allograft or synthetic graft may also be used to fill the defect.

The cortical window, if large enough, may be replaced and held with a screw or periosteal sutures.

Closure
Routine.

Postoperative instructions
Restoration of the range of motion of neighbouring joints is undertaken as soon as possible. Weightbearing status is dependent on the anatomical location and the size of the defect.

Recommended reference
Aboulafia AJ, Temple HT, Scully SP. Surgical treatment of benign bone tumors. *Instr Course Lect.* 2002;51:441–450.

Malignant tumour principles

Preoperative planning

Common indications
- Excision of an isolated primary tumour
- Excision of a primary tumour with metastatic disease depending on life expectancy
- Excision of isolated metastases
- Excision of a fungating tumour for local control
- Excision of tumour recurrence

Contraindications
- Poor life expectancy
- Co-morbidities
- Malignancies treatable by chemotherapy alone such as lymphoma

> ### Consent and risks
> Depend on the anatomical location and magnitude of the procedure.

Operative planning

The tumour, the surrounding compartments and the whole bone must be satisfactorily imaged to allow adequate planning of the procedure and reconstructive method. This will usually involve plain films, computed tomography and magnetic resonance imaging.

Planning of the surgical approach needs to enable sufficient access to remove the tumour and any structures to be sacrificed to *ensure tumour clearance with wide margins*, which means removal of a layer of the normal tissue surrounding the whole tumour (**Figure 2.5**).

Structures at risk and the method of reconstruction have to be considered. Surgical approaches that are not routinely used may have to be employed and plastic surgical techniques may be necessary to provide soft tissue coverage after resection. In cases of highly vascular tumours or particularly renal and thyroid metastases, preoperative embolisation should be considered to reduce the intraoperative blood loss.

Anaesthesia and positioning

General or regional anaesthesia as appropriate and positioning to allow sufficient access.

Surgical technique

Landmarks and incision

Depend on anatomical location of the tumour.

Malignant tumour principles

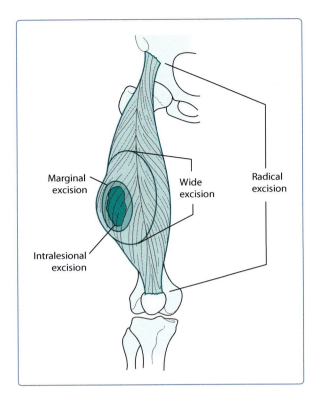

Figure 2.5 Intralesional, marginal, wide and radical margins for the excision of bone and soft tissue tumours. (Note the diagram shows a soft tissue lesion.)

Dissection

Dissection must enable *removal of the tumour* en bloc *with a layer of normal tissues surrounding it* to provide a wide margin. In some cases neurovascular structures may be preserved and therefore a marginal excision around these structures is performed. Postoperatively, an opinion regarding adjuvant therapy is obtained. However, if cure is sought, and the neurovascular structures are involved then they must be sacrificed. This may mean an amputation or reconstruction of the vessels. In certain soft tissue sarcomas, a course of preoperative radiotherapy may be advocated, and repeat imaging is acquired prior to surgical excision. Wound complication rates are higher in this group of patients.

Technical aspects of procedure

Margins and structures to be sacrificed can usually be anticipated from good-quality imaging. However, during the procedure the surgeon needs to decide, based on experience and the feel of the tissues, what has to be sacrificed, in conjunction with the imaging.

The parts of the procedure that have the easiest anatomical access are undertaken first. Samples from remaining surrounding tissues are sent for histology if the resection margin is questionable. Intraoperative frozen section can be used to ensure an adequate resection margin if there is any doubt.

The wound should be thoroughly washed with water (as water is highly hypotonic, it may aid in lysis of any spilled tumour cells) after removal of the tumour. If any spillage of the tumour or invasion of the capsule of the tumour has taken place intraoperatively then after washing, new instruments, gloves and gowns should be used for reconstruction and/or closure.

If it is found postoperatively on histological examination that an inadequate margin has been taken then a repeat wide local excision should be considered.

Closure
- Routine closure
- Drains to be placed in line of incision to facilitate tract excision if re-excision is necessary

Postoperative care and instructions
- Routine
- Weightbearing and physiotherapy – depend on procedure

Recommended reference
Enneking WF, Maale GE. The effect of inadvertent tumour contamination of wounds during the surgical resection of musculoskeletal neoplasms. *Cancer.* 1988;**62**:1251.

Recommended references (for whole chapter)
General information relating to all of the topics in this chapter can be found in the following:

Enneking WF. *Musculoskeletal Tumour Surgery.* New York, NY: Churchill Livingstone, 1983.
Malawer MM, Sugarbaker PH. *Musculoskeletal Cancer Surgery Treatment of Sarcomas and Allied Diseases.* Dordrecht: Kluwer Academic, 2001.
O'Sullivan B. Preoperative versus postoperative radiotherapy in soft tissue sarcoma of the limbs: A randomised trial. *Lancet.* 2002;**359**(**9325**):2235–2241.
Sim FH, Frassica FJ, Frassica DA. Soft tissue tumours: Diagnosis, evaluation and management. *J Am Acad Orthop Surg.* 1994;**2**:202–211.

Viva questions
1. What do you understand about the principles of biopsy of a tumour?
2. How would you perform a biopsy of a bony lesion?
3. How would you perform a biopsy of a soft tissue lesion?
4. How would you choose between a needle biopsy and an open biopsy?
5. What must be avoided during biopsy?
6. How would you make a cortical window in bone?
7. How would you treat a benign bone cyst?
8. What are the indications for excision of a benign bone tumour?

Malignant tumour principles

9. What considerations have to be taken into account when excising a benign bone tumour?
10. What are the indications for excision of a malignant bone tumour?
11. How would you plan the excision of a malignant bone tumour?
12. What are the principles involved in the excision of a malignant bone tumour?
13. What is the difference between an open biopsy and an excision biopsy?
14. What does a marginal resection mean?
15. What is the difference between a wide and a radical resection?
16. How would you ensure that you have an adequate biopsy?
17. What do you understand by the term *limb salvage*?
18. Why might it not be possible to salvage a limb?
19. Where and by whom should a biopsy be carried out?

3 Surgery of the Cervical Spine

Julian Leong and Kia Rezajooi

Anterior approach to the cervical spine (C3-T1) — 25	Posterior approach to the upper cervical spine (C1-C2) — 35
Posterior approach to the cervical spine (C2-C7) — 31	Halo vest fixation of the cervical spine — 36
	Viva questions — 41

Cervical spine	Clinical range of motion	Radiological upper spine (C1-C2) range of motion	Radiological lower spine (C3-C7) range of motion
Flexion	45°	15°	40°
Extension	55°	15°	25°
Lateral bending	40°	0°	50°
Axial rotation	70°	40°	45°

Position of arthrodesis

- Maintain the sagittal contour (lordosis) and avoid local kyphosis.
- During anterior interbody fusion surgery, the graft or artificial cage selected is wedge shaped with greater anterior vertebral height.
- The rods are contoured into lordotic shape during posterior fusion/stabilisation procedures.

Anterior approach to the cervical spine (C3-T1)
Preoperative planning
Indications
- Anterior decompression for spinal canal or foraminal stenosis
  - Presenting symptoms – myelopathy, radiculopathy, neurological deficit
  - Herniated disc from degenerative or traumatic causes

- Osteophytes
- Bony element (traumatic causes)
- Subluxation of the vertebra due to degenerative process
- Tumour
- Infection
- Congenitally narrow canal
- Ossification of posterior longitudinal ligament
- Anterior intervertebral fusion
  - Degenerative pathology
  - After anterior decompression for indications listed previously
- Anterior stabilisation
  - Trauma
  - Degenerative subluxation
  - After decompression/fusion
- Cervical disc replacement
  - Degenerative disc disorders
- Biopsy/excision/drainage of collection
  - Tumour
  - Infection

Consent and risks

- *Dysphagia*: 50% in short term; 10% long term (more common in multilevel surgery, longer retraction time, older patients). This complication can be reduced by keeping retraction time to a minimum, using smooth contour retractors, lower profile plate, good tissue handling and haemostasis.
- *Recurrent laryngeal nerve injury*: 0.2%; it produces paralysis of one side of the vocal cord, and leads to hoarseness of the voice, airway problems and aspiration. This is more common in the right-sided approach. The reason for its vulnerability on the right side is because of its course, as it crosses from lateral towards the trachea in the midline, in the lower part of the neck. Some consider it to occur due to the dual compression of the nerve from the self-retaining deep retractor on the lateral aspect and medially by the cuff of the endotracheal tube within the trachea. This can be avoided by relaxing the retractor often and deflating and reinflating the cuff after application of the retractor.
- *Other neurological injuries*: Superior laryngeal nerve, hypoglossal nerve, sympathetic nerve and stellate ganglion causing Horner's syndrome.
- Spinal cord injury.
- *Vascular injury*: Inferior thyroid artery, common carotid artery, vertebral artery, internal jugular vein.
- Haematoma.
- *Visceral injury*: Oesophagus, trachea.
- *Infection*: 0.5%.
- *Cerebrospinal fluid (CSF) leak and fistula*: 0.1%.
- *Death*: 0.1%.

Risks for fusion/stabilisation
- Bone graft donor site morbidity
- *Non-union/pseudarthrosis*: 4%–20% in single-level fusion, 25%–50% in multilevel fusion
- Implant pull out/failure
- Anterior graft migration

Operative planning

An image intensifier should be available from the start of the procedure. If an operative microscope is to be used it should be pre-booked. Some prefer to use magnification loupes, along with headlights for improved illumination of the operative field.

All radiological investigations should be available. Check/pre-order the specific implants and instrumentation.

If iliac bone crest graft is required, then the side and draping need to be pre-planned; a tri-cortical graft is best. In high-risk cases, the spinal cord integrity is monitored intraoperatively using evoked potentials (somatosensory or motor), and this needs to be organized.

Anaesthesia and positioning

The operation is performed under general anaesthesia. The head end of the patient is positioned opposite to the anaesthetist; therefore, long tubing is needed which must be safely placed and well secured. The outer end of the endotracheal tube is positioned and fixed away from the side of the incision. Prophylactic antibiotics are given as per protocol.

Place the patient in a supine position on the operating table with or without Mayfield skull clamp attachment. Head ring and adhesive tape are used to position the head securely if the Mayfield clamp is not used. The Mayfield skull clamp attachment provides a three-point rigid cranial fixation and allows greater flexibility in positioning of the cervical spine and better visualisation during imaging. It is particularly useful in surgery for cervical spine fracture. It enables better control of cervical spine position and allows change in position and manipulation during the surgical procedure.

A rolled-up pad or saline bag or sandbag is placed between the scapulae to enable slight extension of the cervical spine as desired. The head end of the table is tilted up to minimise venous bleeding. The foot end of the bed may need levelling to prevent migration of the patient down the bed. To enable adequate visualisation of the lower cervical spine image intensifier and for improved access, broad strips (10 or 15 cm [4 or 6 inches]) of adhesive are used to pull the shoulders down and anchor them to the operation table.

The accessibility of the image intensifier and the ability to visualise the required field must be checked. The positioning of the image intensifier and the microscope during the procedure needs to be planned.

Surgical technique

Choosing the side for the approach

For the upper and middle cervical spine, the right- or left-sided approach can be used. The right-sided approach is usually preferred by the right-hand dominant surgeon and vice versa. The site of the pathology (e.g. in tumour) can sometimes influence the choice.

For the lower cervical spine (C6 and below), some prefer the left-sided approach, because of the increased risk of injury to the recurrent laryngeal nerve injury with the right-sided approach.

If previous surgery has been carried out on one side of the neck, the vocal cord function must be checked before considering operating on the opposite side.

Choosing the incision

Depending on the number of vertebral levels to be exposed, the incision can be transverse, oblique or longitudinal. The transverse approach is most commonly used and can give access to up to three vertebral body levels, although for more extensive oncological approaches an expansile longitudinal approach along the anterior border of sternocleidomastoid may be used.

The cosmetic appearance is better with transverse and mild oblique incision along the neck's skin creases/cleavage lines.

Landmarks

Few palpable structures in the anterior aspect of the neck give an approximate estimation of the vertebral level and incision (**Figure 3.1**). It is common practice to use an image intensifier to identify the level of the incision, and the incision site is marked.

The following guidelines can be applied for the transverse incision for the approaches to the following vertebral levels:

- C3 and C4 level – level of the hyoid bone or two finger breaths below the mandible
- C4 and C5 level – level of the thyroid cartilage
- C5 and C6 level – level of the cricoid cartilage
- C6 and below – two finger breadths above the clavicle

The anterior border of the sternocleidomastoid muscle and the midline are identified and marked.

Incision

The skin incision extends from the anterior border of the sternocleidomastoid muscle to the midline, extending further if necessary.

Anterior approach to the cervical spine (C3–T1)

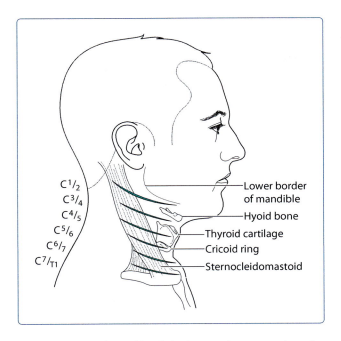

Figure 3.1 Anatomical landmarks and levels in the anterior approach to the cervical spine.

Superficial dissection

Structures at risk

- Longitudinal and traversing veins in deep cervical fascia
- Inferior thyroid artery
- Carotid sheath (enveloping the common carotid artery, internal jugular vein and vagus nerve)
- Trachea and oesophagus
- Recurrent laryngeal nerve and superior laryngeal nerve

The platysma muscle is cut in the same direction as the skin incision or split longitudinally along its fibres. The platysma is supplied by the cervical branch of the facial nerve, and it receives its branches in the mandibular region, superior to the incision site. However, dividing the platysma does not cause any significant morbidity.

The anterior border of the sternocleidomastoid is identified, and the deep cervical fascia is incised medially. The longitudinal and traversing vein may need retraction or ligation. The sternocleidomastoid muscle is gently retracted laterally, and the strap muscles and thyroid gland are retracted medially. The superior belly of the omohyoid muscle can be divided if it traverses the operating field or if an extensive approach is required.

This dissection exposes the carotid sheath and the pretracheal fascia (**Figure 3.2**). The carotid pulse is palpated and the pretracheal fascia incised medial to the carotid sheath using blunt dissection (peanut surgical swab). *The carotid sheath enveloping the common carotid artery, internal jugular vein and vagus nerve are retracted laterally and the trachea and the oesophagus are retracted medially.* The prevertebral fascia and the longus colli muscle are visualised.

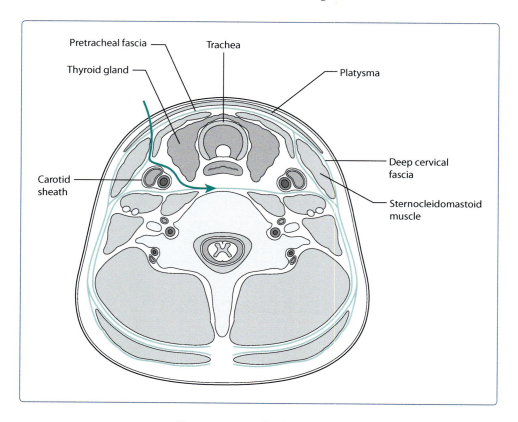

Figure 3.2 Superficial dissection.

Deep dissection

Structures at risk
- Vertebral artery
- Sympathetic nerve and stellate ganglion
- Spinal cord injury

The prevertebral fascia is incised with blunt dissection to expose the anterior surface of the cervical spine with the two longus colli muscles. The right and left longus colli muscles are stripped subperiosteally from the anterior vertebral bodies, using cautery good haemostasis (**Figure 3.3**). The smooth-ended retractor blades are placed underneath the

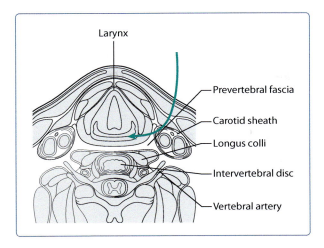

Figure 3.3 Deep dissection.

two longus colli muscles to improve the exposure; this helps to protect the oesophagus, recurrent laryngeal nerve, trachea and carotid sheath from injury by the retractors.

The appropriate level is identified using a bent needle as a marker (bent at about 1 cm to act as a stop) seen on a lateral radiograph using an image intensifier. After the level is identified, the further procedure of decompression, fusion or stabilisation is carried out.

Closure

After removal of the retractors, special attention is paid to haemostasis of all the layers, as a retractor could have acted as a temporary tamponade. Also, check for any injury to the visceral structures.

A deep drain is placed with care and kept for 24 hours. The platysma is approximated well by interrupted suture. The subcutaneous layer is closed by 2-0 Vicryl. Skin is closed by subcuticular stitches or skin clips. Check for bleeding at the Mayfield clamp pin site and apply Opsite spray or dressing as required.

Postoperative care and instructions

Prescription of neck collars varies according to the pathology, type of surgery/stabilisation and surgeon's choice.

Posterior approach to the cervical spine (C2-C7)
Preoperative planning
Indications
- Posterior stabilisation/fusion
  - Trauma, degenerative subluxation, after decompression/fusion

- Posterior decompression of the spinal canal or foraminae stenosis
  - Presenting symptoms – myelopathy, radiculopathy, neurological deficits
  - Degenerative pathology – facet joint arthritis, osteophytes, ligamentum hypertrophy, instability
  - Trauma – instability, bony and disc encroachment
  - Others – congenital stenosis, ossification of posterior longitudinal ligament, tumour, etc.
  - Posterior decompression is preferred to anterior decompression in multilevel (more than two levels) degenerative stenosis if suitable
- Biopsy/excision/drainage of collection
  - Tumour
  - Infection

Consent and risks

- *Haemorrhage*: Usually caused by straying away from subperiosteal plane and entering intermuscular plane. Extension of the exposure lateral to facet risks bleeding from the segmental vessels and venous plexus. Cervical canal also has a rich epidural venous plexus which can bleed profusely.
- Dural tear.
- *Cord or nerve root damage (rare)*: It is important to use bipolar cauterisation while controlling bleeding near the cord and nerve roots. Cord handling needs to be kept to a minimum and care taken not to plunge instruments into the interlaminar space. The laminae can be surprisingly thin and fragile.
- *Vertebral artery injury (rare)*: Vertebral artery is at risk when the exposure extends over the transverse process and in surgery involving C1 and C2. Injury bilaterally endangers the blood supply to the hindbrain.
- General morbidity and mortality are shown to be increased in patients of older age and those with myelopathy.

Operative planning

An image intensifier should be available at the start of the procedure, for example to check for spine alignment during positioning in patients who have instability of the cervical spine. The image intensifier is also used perioperatively to identify level, check spinal alignment, and check implant, screw and graft position. For other considerations at this stage, see 'Anterior approach to the cervical spine (C3-T1)' earlier in this chapter.

Anaesthesia and positioning

The operation is performed under general anaesthesia. The patient is placed in the prone position on the operating table. The head end of the patient is positioned at the opposite side to the anaesthetist. The long anaesthetic tubing is secured safely.

The head is positioned in a special head ring or brace, or held by a Mayfield skull clamp attachment, which provides three-point rigid cranial fixation, allows greater flexibility in positioning and better visualisation during imaging. The eyes should be protected appropriately during prone positioning. During exposure, the neck is positioned in slight flexion, to allow easier dissection and avoid skin creasing.

The spinal stability needs to be taken into account and the spinal alignment checked with imaging if necessary. As with the anterior approach, broad strips (10 or 15 cm [4 or 6 inches]) of adhesive tape are used to pull the shoulders down, and the positions of the image intensifier and microscope are checked. The head end of the table is tilted upwards to minimise venous bleeding.

Surgical technique

Landmarks

Identification of the level is important to avoid unnecessary dissection of the wrong levels. The external occipital protuberance and the longer spinous processes of C2, C7 and T1 vertebrae are easily palpable landmarks to guide the location of the incision. An image intensifier may be used to verify the level as needed.

Incision

A midline straight incision centring over the exposure is required. The skin in this area is vascular and thick and adrenaline can be injected to reduce bleeding.

Superficial dissection

> **Structures at risk**
>
> Segmental vessels and venous plexi. (Bleeding is much worse if dissection strays from the midline or into muscle. Lateral extension of the dissection beyond the facet joint risks bleeding from the segmental vessels.)

The fascia is incised at the midline. Retractors and palpation are used to keep dissection in the midline. The nuchal ligament is split in the midline, and the spinous process is reached. The spinous processes of C3, C4, C5 and C6 are normally bifid.

Using Cobb elevators and diathermy, further dissection is carried out in the subperiosteal plane reflecting the paracervical muscles off the spinous process and the lamina, either bilaterally or unilaterally as required. The extent of lateral extension depends on the procedure planned, e.g. need to expose the facet joint or transverse process.

Deep dissection

> **Structures at risk**
> - Dura
> - Cord and nerve root
> - Vertebral artery
> - Epidural venous plexus

Care should be taken to avoid plunging instruments into the interlaminar space. If required, the ligamentum flavum is detached from the inferior lamina using a spatula, Kerrison punch or triple zero curette. Further laminotomy, laminectomy or laminoplasty are carried out as needed (**Figure 3.4**).

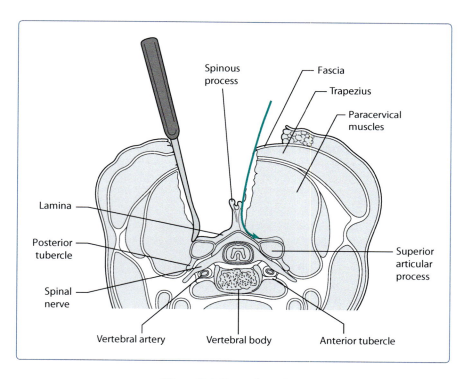

Figure 3.4 Deep dissection.

Closure
- Approximation of fascia with musculature and the nuchal ligament.
- Approximation of the subcutaneous tissue and the skin. The posterior neck skin is thick, and owing to skin creases, it is better to keep the neck in slight flexion if possible to attain better approximation, typically with subcutaneous sutures.

Postoperative care and instructions

Prescription of neck collars varies according to the pathology, type of surgery/stabilisation and surgeon's choice.

Posterior approach to the upper cervical spine (C1-C2)

The approach is very similar to that of the lower cervical spine, and it is recommended that this section is read in conjunction with the previous one.

Preoperative planning

Indications

- Posterior stabilisation and fusion (C1-C2, occipitocervical):
  - Trauma
  - Degenerative subluxation
  - Following decompression from other causes
- Posterior decompression:
  - Spinal canal stenosis from various aetiologies, e.g. rheumatoid arthritis, trauma, degeneration, tumour

---

Consent and risks

- Similar to posterior approach of C2–C7.
- *Haemorrhage*: The venous plexi are rich around the C2 nerve root and posterior to C1-C2 facet, and they tend to bleed profusely.
- *Vertebral artery injury*: Vulnerable at C1 level, passing through the foramen transversarium of the C1 it turns medially and runs in the groove of C1 to pierce the posterior atlanto-occipital membrane and enter the foramen magnum.
- *Nerve injury*: The greater occipital nerve (branch of posterior rami of C2), third occipital nerve (branch of posterior rami of C3) and suboccipital nerve are prone to injury if you stray away from the subperiosteal plane, while dissecting laterally.

Operative planning

This is similar to the posterior approach of C2-C7. Three-dimensional computed tomography (CT) reconstruction is needed to plan the appropriate angle for C1-C2 transarticular screw fixation.

Anaesthesia and positioning

See 'Posterior approach to the cervical spine (C2-C7)' earlier in this chapter.

Surgical technique
Landmarks
- External occipital protuberance in the posterior aspect of the skull in the midline (midpoint of the superior nuchal line)
- The spinous process of C2 vertebra (the longest in the upper cervical spine)

An image intensifier can also be used to verify the level as needed.

Superficial dissection

> ### Structures at risk
> - Suboccipital venous plexus
> - Vertebral artery

See 'Posterior approach to the cervical spine (C2-C7)' earlier in this chapter. The Cobb elevator and diathermy are used to separate the musculature from the occiput (superior nuchal line to superior margin of foramen magnum). Subperiosteal dissection is carried out separating the muscles from the C1 and C2 spinous processes and lamina, taking care of the interlaminar spaces, venous plexus and vertebral artery.

Deep dissection
If required, the ligamentum flavum is detached between C1 and C2 and the posterior atlanto-occipital membrane between occiput and C1, using a triple zero curette, spatula or Kerrison punch.

Postoperative care and instructions
Prescription of neck collars varies according to the pathology, type of surgery/stabilisation and surgeon's choice.

Halo vest fixation of the cervical spine
Preoperative planning
Indications
- Cervical spine trauma (temporary or definite stabilisation), e.g. odontoid and upper cervical spine fracture, fracture of the occipital condyles
- External stabilisation following surgery as a primary stabiliser or as an adjuvant, e.g. after osteotomy for ankylosing spondylitis
- Instability due to infection or tumour
- Paediatric patients: Trauma, after fusion, scoliosis and other pathologies
- Halo traction (halo-gravity traction, halo-wheelchair traction, halo-pelvic traction): Trauma, scoliosis, after surgery, etc.

Contraindications

- Active infection at the pin site area or in the area of the skin covered by the vest
- Patients with conditions where pin purchase in the skull bone is unlikely to provide adequate support for the required duration, e.g. rheumatoid arthritis
- Doubt about patient compliance, understanding and ability to cope, e.g. dementia
- Patients experiencing recurrent, significant falls

Consent and risks

- *Pin loosening*: 36%–60% (The pin should be retightened regularly using 8 inch-pounds torque [2–5 inch-pounds torque for children].) It is retightened 48 hours after initial application and thereafter every week. If the resistance is not met after a few full turns, then a fresh pin is applied in a new adjacent location as appropriate. This complication can be minimised by selecting an appropriate pin insertion site on the skull, adopting a perpendicular pin insertion angle and using the correct pin insertion torque
- *Pin site infection*: 20%
- Pin migration and dural puncture
- *Loss of reduction*: More common in anterior column insufficiency/poor reduction/poorly fitted vest mainly in obese or very thin individuals
- Pressure sores and skin problems underlying the vest area
- Restricted ventilation and pneumonia
- Restricted arm elevation
- Scar
- *Dysphagia*: 2%. Can be prevented by avoiding immobilisation at extreme range of neck extension
- Palsy of the sixth cranial nerve with traction

Operative planning

Templating

The patient's head circumference and chest circumference are measured to determine the crown and vest size, respectively. The manufacturer of the halo vest provides a rough guidance with regard to selection of the sizes (paediatric, small, medium and large). The halo ring can be trialled to check that it provides a *clearance all round the head circumference of 1–2 cm*. Availability of the correct size of the crown and vest, and other equipment and materials, is confirmed.

Three or more people are usually needed for the application of the vest and for logrolling the patient, if required. The nature and type of the neck instability should be taken into account by the surgeon. An image intensifier can be used, if needed, to assess cervical position. A crash trolley should be available for emergency resuscitation.

Anaesthesia and positioning

The operation is performed under local anaesthesia, enabling recognition of any changes in the neurological status during the procedure and manipulation. General anaesthesia is occasionally required if concomitant surgical procedures are carried out.

A hard cervical spine collar is applied for provisional additional support, to improve stability and prevent neurological deterioration. The patient is positioned supine, with the head close to the edge or beyond the edge of the bed, so that the posterior portion of the ring can be positioned appropriately. Most modern systems have either the posterior position of the ring open or curved superiorly to enable easy positioning. If slight extension of the cervical spine is desired to improve alignment, then a saline bag is placed between the scapulae.

The positioning of the image intensifier during the procedure needs to be planned. The accessibility of the image intensifier and the ability to visualise the required field must be checked.

Surgical technique

Selection of pin insertion sites

Anterior pin sites

Anterolateral aspect of the skull, about 1 cm superior to the supraorbital rim, above the lateral two-thirds of the eyebrows (**Figure 3.5**). This site is optimal (relatively safe zone) for the following reasons:

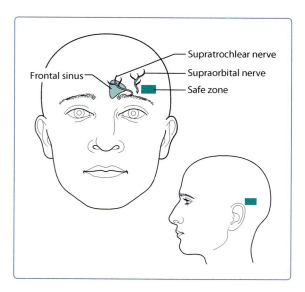

Figure 3.5 Safe zones for anterior and posterior pin placement.

- It is lateral to the frontal sinus, supratrochlear nerve and supraorbital nerve (structures at risk).
- It is medial to the temporalis muscle (pin penetration can lead to pain during mastication and speaking), temporalis fossa (thin bone) and zygomaticotemporal nerve.

- There is adequate skull thickness.
- It is below the equator (largest circumference) of the skull (prevent cephalad migration).

Posterior pin sites

Posterolateral aspect of the skull at the 4 o'clock and 8 o'clock positions, roughly diagonal to the contralateral anterior pins (**Figure 3.5**). These sites are

- Below the equator of the skull, but still 1 cm above the upper tip of the ear
- Where the skull is more uniformly thick
- Away from at-risk neurological and muscular structures

Halo application

Appropriate sterile precautions are undertaken during halo ring application using sterile pins and ring. Care is taken to avoid injury to the eye during the procedure.

The halo ring is positioned about 1 cm above the superior ear tip and eyebrows, but below the equator of the skull. It is temporarily stabilised using three positioning baseplates (**Figure 3.6**) at the 12 o'clock, 5 o'clock and 7 o'clock positions. The appropriate locations for the pin sites and the corresponding holes in the ring are identified. Hair is shaved or trimmed over the posterior pin sites, if required. The skin over the chosen pin site area is prepared with antiseptic solution and is infiltrated with local anaesthetic solution.

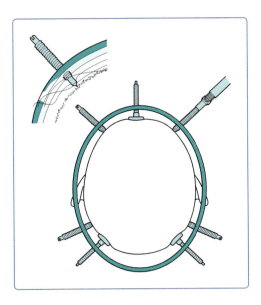

Figure 3.6 Pin sites and temporary positioning baseplates.

The pins are positioned in the corresponding holes and advanced through the skin as perpendicular as possible to the skull surface. (A perpendicular bone-pin interface enables increased contact area of the pin tip and so better purchase.) The patient should gently close the eyes and relax the forehead when the anterior pins are fixed. This avoids skin tethering and problems with eyelid closure. Direct insertion of pins into the skin without a prior skin incision is preferred. A single-use torque-limiting device, which breaks off when a torque of 8 inch-pounds is reached, is available in some halo systems. These are used to advance the pins if available; if not a torque-limiting screwdriver is used.

The pins are tightened in diagonal fashion, by working on the contralateral pins concurrently (see **Figure 3.6**). Each pin is secured using a locknut to prevent loosening. The locknuts are tightened gently, as over-tightening can result in backing out of the pin. After the locknut comes in contact with the ring, it is tightened further by one-eighth turn with the spanner supplied. If skin tenting is noted around the pin, a skin release can be performed with a scalpel. Now the secured halo ring can be used to control and position the cervical spine for further procedures.

Vest application

The posterior and anterior halves of the vest are separated, but left connected to their respective two upright posts. The bolts, nuts and connectors are loosened but dismantling of various parts of the vest is best kept to a minimum, to avoid confusion and save time. After the neck is stabilised to the trunk manually, the trunk is lifted or logrolled for the placement of the posterior vest and the two upright posts.

The anterior vest is applied next. Both halves of the vest are connected and tightened to a level that will allow two fingers to slide between the vest and chest. The patient should be able to breathe comfortably. Both the shoulder straps are also fixed and tightened. The two right posts are connected loosely to the right connector and similarly the left two posts are connected to the left connector. Both the connectors are then slackly fixed to the halo ring. The head and neck are positioned and all the bolts and nuts are tightened after placing the posts and connectors in the appropriate position. Attach the spanner to the front of the anterior vest for quicker access, to deal with any emergency that requires vest removal.

An image intensifier may be used to check the cervical spine position and to enable correction under image guidance. All of the fixations are retightened when a satisfactory position is achieved.

Halo application in children

Multiple pins and low torque techniques are used. For older children, the torque used for pin application is 2–5 inch-pounds. Six pins or more can be used. For children under 3 years, 10–12 pins can be used. A CT scan of the skull helps to plan pin placements, by avoiding thin bone and suture lines. The pins are hand tightened only. Custom-made halo vest components may be required or a plaster jacket can be applied instead.

Postoperative care and instructions

If an image intensifier was not used, a radiograph is used to check the alignment.

Forty-eight hours after application the locking nuts are unlocked and all of the pins retightened to 8 inch-pounds. The locking nuts are retightened. The pins and other fixations must be rechecked regularly – at least every 2 weeks thereafter. Regular care is required for the pin sites and the skin under the vest. Regularly check imaging as appropriate, as loss of reduction is common. One spanner should always be attached to the anterior vest and the rest of the application tools and spares to be kept by the patient.

Recommended references

Bauer R, Kerschbaumer F, Poisel S. *Atlas of Spinal Operations*. New York, NY: Thieme Medical, 1993.

Clark CR. *The Cervical Spine*, 3rd ed. Philadelphia, PA: Lippincott Raven, 1998.

Fountas KN, Kapsalaki EZ, Nikolakakos LG et al. Anterior cervical discectomy and fusion associated complications. *Spine (Phila Pa 1976)*. 2007;**32(21)**:2310–2317.

Gokaslan ZL, Bydon M, De la Garza-Ramos R et al. Recurrent laryngeal nerve palsy after cervical spine surgery: A multicenter AO Spine Clinical Research Network Study. *Global Spine J*. 2017;**7(1 Suppl)**:53S–57S.

Nordin M, Frankel VH. *Basic Biomechanics of the Musculoskeletal System*, 3rd ed. Philadelphia, PA: Lippincott Williams & Wilkins, 2001.

Viva questions

1. How do you position a patient for anterior cervical spine surgery?
2. Describe the steps of the anterior cervical approach and the reasons behind them.
3. What are the structures at risk in anterior cervical surgery and how are they avoided?
4. Describe the radiological signs indicating cervical spine instability.
5. Describe how you will position a patient for the posterior approach to the cervical spine.
6. What are the structures at risk during a posterior approach to the lower cervical spine and how can they be avoided?
7. What are the structures at risk during a posterior approach to the upper cervical spine and how are they avoided?
8. How do you apply a halo to stabilise the cervical spine?
9. What complications occur in halo stabilisation of the cervical spine?
10. How is a halo vest looked after following application?

4 Surgery of the Thoracolumbar Spine

Daniel P Ahern, Joseph S Butler, Matthew Shaw and Sean Molloy

| Thoracic spine | 43 | Viva questions | 60 |
| Lumbar spine | 53 | | |

Thoracic spine
Posterior thoracic surgery
Scoliosis correction
Choice of approach
- There is an increasing trend towards posterior-only surgery. However, much depends on the characteristics of the curve and on the surgeon's training and preference.
- Thorough discectomy is only possible with an anterior approach; thus very stiff curves may benefit from anterior release prior to posterior surgery.
- Thoracolumbar/lumbar curves are often treated with anterior instrumentation, especially if there is no thoracic curve.
- Posterior instrumentation allows fixation to the pelvis – an advantage in long fusions in the elderly and in non-walking patients with neuromuscular-type curves.

Indications
- Severe deformity
- Curve progression
- Radicular pain or neurological deficit (degenerative cases)
- Back pain failing conservative measurement (rare)

Risks
- Mortality 0.03%
- Respiratory dysfunction
- Neurological deficit: complete 0.03%; incomplete 1.5%
- Revision surgery 5%
- Failure to achieve complete curve correction
- Damage to sympathetic chain, major vessels
- Infection 1%–2%
- Blood loss

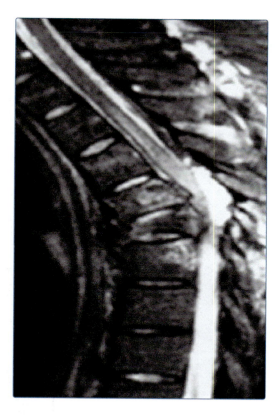

Figure 4.1 A thoracic flexion compression fracture with kyphosis.

- Scar
- Imbalance, shoulder height discrepancy
- Back pain
- Blindness 0.028%–0.2%

Operative planning
- Full history and examination
- Full spine radiographs including bending films:
  - Bending films to assess flexibility of spine
  - Identifying the correct level in the thoracic spine is more of a challenge as the reference points of the sacrum or C2 are not available. Therefore, it is important to check the number of ribs a patient has on plain X-ray, as these can be used to mark the skin using fluoroscopy prior to incision
- Whole spine MRI
- Multidisciplinary team involvement
- Anaesthetic and medical workup
- Lung function tests, chest radiograph, electrocardiogram (ECG)
- Cord monitoring arrangement
- Intensive care unit (ICU) bed arranged

Thoracic spine 45

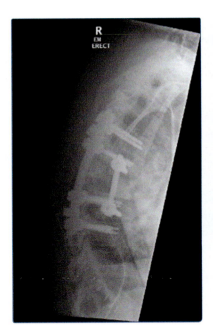 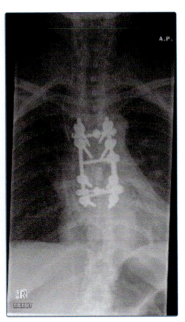

Figure 4.2 Thoracic vertebrectomy with posterior stabilisation for a solitary metastasis.

Surgical procedure
- General anaesthesia
- Prone positioning:
  - Montreal mattress, Jackson table, four-post frame or similar
  - Arms can be placed by the patient's side or out in front (depending on the level of surgery and the need to use X-ray)
- Protect pressure areas, eyes:
  - It is important that the shoulders are not hyperflexed or abducted and there is no pressure on the axilla, which could cause a nerve palsy
  - Padding is used under the patient's elbows to avoid an ulnar nerve palsy
  - No pressure on the eyes
  - Table should be slightly head up to decrease central venous pressure
- Mechanical deep vein thrombosis prophylaxis
- X-rays on display
- Incision:
  - Skin:
    - Note the pedicle entry point will be above the spinous process of the vertebra counted and therefore the skin incision should allow for this
- Dissection:
  - Subcutaneous fat and fascia
  - Spinous process identified and subperiosteal dissection:
    - Ensure haemostasis – diathermy, gauze packing
  - Dissection to identify transverse processes, medial and lateral borders of the facet joints, and the pars

- Pedicle screw insertion:
  - In general, at the junction of the medial two-thirds and lateral one-third of the facet joint
- Decortication of facets and lamina
- Reduction
- Rod insertion
- +/− Cross-links
- Closure in layers
- +/− Drain insertion

Postoperative care
- Neurovascular observations and analgesia
- Postoperative haemoglobin and renal function
- No spinal precautions – mobilise as pain allows
- Postoperative full spine X-rays

Posterior thoracic decompression and fusion

Indications
- Unstable thoracic fracture
- Posterior cord compression from a tumour or degenerative process
- Palliative procedure from an anterior compressive pathology
  - Where patient condition does not allow for anterior approach
- Disc pathology as part of costotransversectomy
- Coronal or sagittal deformity correction

Risks
- Mortality
- Infection: 2%

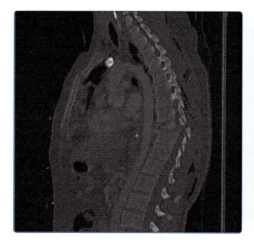
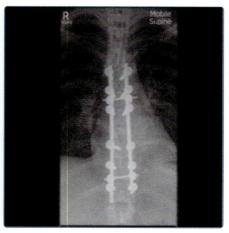

Figure 4.3 A fracture dislocation of the thoracic spine stabilised with posterior thoracic rods and screws.

- Neurological injury
  - Higher rate in the thoracic spine as canal dimensions smaller
- Wrong level surgery
  - Higher rate in thoracic spine – reference points of C2 and sacrum not available
- Blindness 0.02%–0.2%
- Thromboembolism
- Respiratory infection
- Failure/fracture of fixation

Operative planning
- Full history and examination
- Radiographs/computed tomography (CT)/magnetic resonance imaging (MRI)
- Anaesthetic and medical workup/optimisation as appropriate

Surgical procedure
- General anaesthesia
- Prone positioning
  - Montreal mattress, Jackson table, four-post frame or similar
- Arm positioning
  - May be placed on patient's side or out in front
    - Dependent on level of surgery and use of intraoperative imaging
  - Beware not to hyperflex or abduct when position arms overhead (less than 45° abducted and less than 90° hyperflexed)
- Pressure area padding
- Midline incision
- Dissection
  - Skin, fat and fascia with haemostasis control
- Paraspinal musculature stripped from spine
- Dissection for landmark identification
  - Transverse processes, medial and lateral borders of the facet joints and the pars

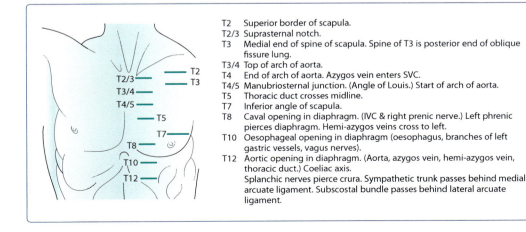

T2 — Superior border of scapula.
T2/3 — Suprasternal notch.
T3 — Medial end of spine of scapula. Spine of T3 is posterior end of oblique fissure lung.
T3/4 — Top of arch of aorta.
T4 — End of arch of aorta. Azygos vein enters SVC.
T4/5 — Manubriosternal junction. (Angle of Louis.) Start of arch of aorta.
T5 — Thoracic duct crosses midline.
T7 — Inferior angle of scapula.
T8 — Caval opening in diaphragm. (IVC & right prenic nerve.) Left phrenic pierces diaphragm. Hemi-azygos veins cross to left.
T10 — Oesophageal opening in diaphragm (oesophagus, branches of left gastric vessels, vagus nerves).
T12 — Aortic opening in diaphragm. (Aorta, azygos vein, hemi-azygos vein, thoracic duct.) Coeliac axis. Splanchnic nerves pierce crura. Sympathetic trunk passes behind medial arcuate ligament. Subcostal bundle passes behind lateral arcuate ligament.

Figure 4.4 Thoracic structures corresponding to various vertebral levels.

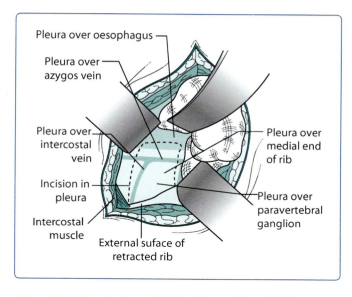

Figure 4.5 The selection of rib level in anterior scoliosis surgery.

- Pedicle screw insertion
  - Medial and lateral borders of the facet joints give the medial and lateral starting points for the pedicle screws
  - In craniocaudal direction, pedicle screw direction is approximately 90° to the translamina line
- Decompression
  - After instrumentation gives more protection to the neural elements than during instrumentation
- +/− Drain insertion
- Closure in layers

Postoperative care
- Adequate analgesia
- Neurological observations including formal postoperative neurological examination
- No spinal precautions – patient allowed to sit to any angle and mobilise as pain allows
- Postoperative radiographs

Anterior thoracic surgery

Scoliosis (anterior release)

Indications
- Same as posterior procedure
  - Severe deformity
  - Curve progression
  - Radicular pain or neurological deficit (degenerative cases)
  - Back pain failing conservative measurement (rare)

Risks
- Mortality 0.03%
- Respiratory dysfunction
- Neurological deficit: complete 0.03%; incomplete 1.5%
- Revision surgery 5%
- Failure to achieve complete curve correction
- Damage to sympathetic chain, major vessels, thoracic duct
- Infection 1%–2%
- Blood loss
- Scar
- Imbalance, shoulder height discrepancy
- Back pain

Operative planning
- Full history and examination
- Full spine radiographs including bending films
  - Bending films to assess flexibility of spine
- Whole spine MRI
- Multidisciplinary team involvement
- Anaesthetic and medical workup
- Lung function tests, chest radiograph, ECG
- Cord monitoring arrangement
- ICU bed booked

Surgical procedure
- General anaesthetic
- Lateral position
  - Convexity of the curve facing upwards
- Pressure areas padded
- Incision
  - In line with proposed rib
  - Note that rib level to be entered should be two levels above the superior vertebra being instrumented due to downward slope of ribs
- Dissection
  - Skin, fat and muscle are incised in line with the rib
  - Maintain haemostasis
- Periosteum stripped off the rib as far posteriorly as possible
- Anteriorly, rib is exposed to costochondral junction, then cut and removed
- Expose and carefully incise pleura and expose lung
- Retract lung superiorly using wet packs
- Posterior pleura is then incised
- Beware underlying segmental vessels
- If procedure is to cross the thoracolumbar junction, the diaphragm will need to be taken down
  - Before or after entering pleural cavity, costal cartilage is incised
  - Abdominal musculature is divided inferomedially
    - Beware risk of damage to peritoneum

- Retroperitoneal fat entered deep to the costal cartilage
- Peritoneum is reflected anteriorly using blunt finger dissection/gauze swabs
- Dissection is carried down to the spine, anterior to the psoas muscle
- Diaphragm is divided (with electrocautery)
  - A 2 cm peripheral cuff is left for repair
- Great vessels and viscera are carefully reflected anteriorly and protected with blunt retractors throughout procedure
- Once exposure is complete, individual segmental vessels can be tied, cauterised or preserved
- Disc material is removed piecemeal until posterior longitudinal ligament is visualised
- Cartilaginous end plates are removed using a Cobb, osteotome or curette
  - Ideally, bony end plates should not be breached as this markedly increases blood loss
- Instrumentation
  - Important to appreciate rotation of the curve and relationship of vertebral body to spinal canal
  - Achieving a 'cadence' of screw insertion with the apical screw being most posterior will assist in de-rotation of the spine
  - Bicortical fixation aids stability
- Following screw insertion, a rod is applied
- Reduction
- Screw and rods are applied to the convexity of the curve; therefore, compression between individual screws aids reduction
- Closure
  - Posterior pleura may be left open or closed – surgeon preference
  - Diaphragmatic repair
  - Chest wall closed in layers
  - Chest drain inserted
  - Superficial closure

Postoperative care
- Neurovascular observations and analgesia
- Postoperative haemoglobin and renal function
- No spinal precautions – mobilise as pain allows
- Postoperative full spine X-rays

Thoracic discectomy +/− corpectomy

Indications
- Disc prolapse
- Other compressive pathologies
  - Fracture
  - Tumour

Risks
- Mortality less than 1%
- Respiratory infection

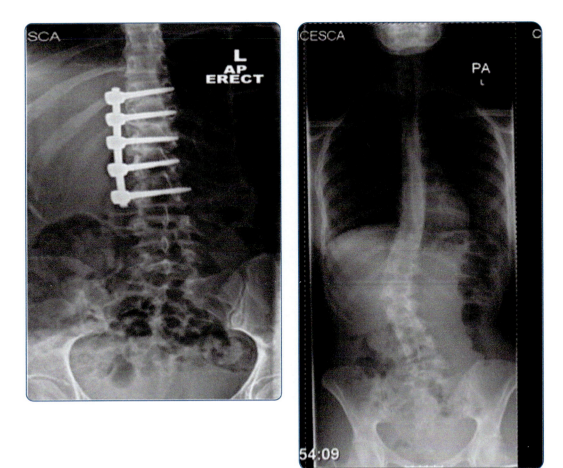

Figure 4.6 Anterior scoliosis correction.

- Anterior chest wall pain
- Major vessel damage 2%–15%
- Neurological compromise
- Cosmesis of scar
- Thromboembolism less than 1%
- Back pain
- Wrong level surgery

Operative planning
- Full history and physical examination
- Imaging – radiographs, CT, MRI
- Anaesthetic and medical workup/optimisation
- Appropriate cardiothoracic/vascular backup available

4 Surgery of the Thoracolumbar Spine

Surgical procedure
- General anaesthesia
- Lateral position
  - Sand or bean bag commonly placed underneath operative site to aid exposure and open disc spaces
  - Pressure areas padded
- Incision
  - In line with proposed rib
  - Note that rib level to be entered should be two levels above the superior vertebra being instrumented due to downward slope of ribs
- Dissection
  - Skin, fat and muscle are incised in line with the rib
  - Maintain haemostasis
- Periosteum is dissected off the rib and rib freed circumferentially from underlying soft tissue
- Rib cutters are used to remove the rib
- Underlying pleura carefully incised and lung protected with a chest pack
- Rib spreader is positioned to optimise exposure
- Posterior pleura incised and plane developed between segmental blood supply

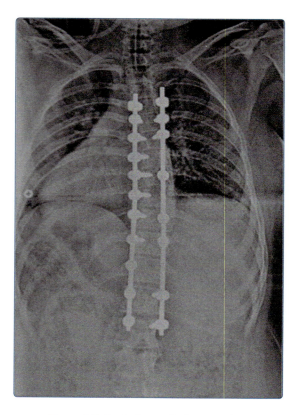

Figure 4.7 Posterior scoliosis correction.

- Segmental blood vessels may be tied, cauterised or preserved
- Discs are incised and removed piecemeal
- Cartilaginous end plates are removed (aiding fusion)
- Thoracic corpectomy
  - Discs above and below the vertebra in question are removed
  - Vertebral body is cut and removed piecemeal
  - Implant positioning
- Closure
  - Chest drain insertion
  - Chest wall closed in layers
  - Superficial closure

Postoperative care
- Neurovascular observations and analgesia
- Postoperative haemoglobin and renal function
- No spinal precautions – mobilise as pain allows
- Postoperative chest and spine X-rays

Lumbar spine
Posterior lumbar surgery
Microdiscectomy
Indications
- Acute disc prolapse symptomatic following 6 weeks non-operative measures
- Earlier surgery if
  - Features of cauda equina syndrome
  - Neurological deficit
  - Intractable pain

Risks
- Nerve root injury: 1%
- Epidural haematoma
- Dural tear: 5%
- Infection: 1%–2%
- Wrong level surgery: Less than 1%
- Cauda equina: 0.01%
- Dural tear
- Ongoing pain
- Post-discectomy instability leading to lower back pain
- Blindness

Operative planning
- Full history and physical examination
- MRI lumbar spine
- Plain X-ray lumbar spine
  - Useful for assessing transition levels in lumbar sacral spine

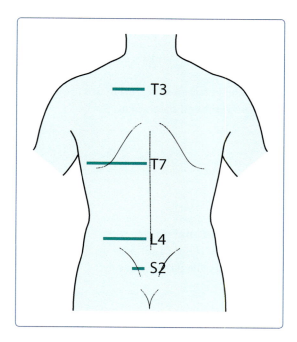

Figure 4.8 Anatomical levels in the lumbar spine.

Surgical procedure
- General anaesthesia
- Positioning
  - Prone on Montreal mattress, Wilson frame, or Jackson table
  - 'Knees-to-chest' prone position
- Skin prep
- Level check
  - Needle into estimated level
  - Cross-table lateral radiograph
  - Needle adjusted until inserted onto spinous process of correct level
- Midline incision
- Dissection
  - Fat, fascia
  - Diathermy used to dissect the musculature off the posterior elements of the spine
  - Soft tissue swept laterally using a Cobb elevator
- Identification of landmarks
  - Lamina of vertebra above
  - Inferior edge delineated
- Ligamentum flavum identified and incised
- Level check recommended
- Development of interlaminar window
  - Important not to remove more than one-third of facet so as not to develop instability
- Careful exposure of dura

- Identification and protection of nerve root
  - Using nerve root retractors
- Incision of posterior longitudinal ligament
  - If intact; with large disc prolapses, disc will have 'broken through' this layer
- Incision of disc and piecemeal removal
- Washout with saline
- Closure in layers
- Skin closure

Postoperative care
- Adequate analgesia
- No spinal precautions
- Postoperative neurological examination

Posterior lumbar decompression +/− fusion
Indications
- Lumbar spine trauma
- Spondylolisthesis
- Spinal stenosis
- Degenerative deformities

Risks
- Nerve injury: 1%
- Cauda equina injury: 0.1%
- Infection 1%–2%
- Venous thromboembolism: 1%
- Persistence/worsening of symptoms: 5%–10%
- Non-union: 5%
- Dural tear

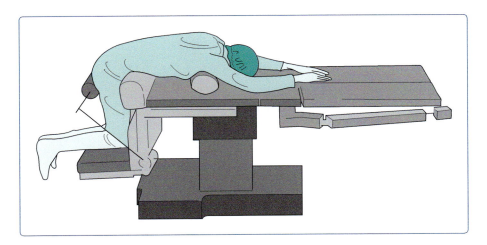

Figure 4.9 The knees-to-chest position for lumbar discectomy.

Operative planning
- Full history and physical examination
- Plain X-rays
  - Deformity evaluation
  - Baseline for levels intraoperatively
- MRI lumbar spine
- Single-photon emission computed tomography lumbar spine
- Anaesthetic and medical optimisation

Surgical procedure
- General anaesthesia
- Prone position
  - Montreal mattress or Jackson frame
  - Pressure area padding
- Skin prep
- Level check
  - Needle into estimated level
  - Cross-table lateral radiograph
  - Needle adjusted until inserted onto spinous process of correct level
- Midline incision
- Dissection
  - Fat, fascia
  - Diathermy used to dissect the musculature off the posterior elements of the spine
  - Soft tissue swept laterally using a Cobb elevator
- Identification of landmarks for instrumentation/pedicle entry points
  - Pars
  - Junction of the transverse process and facet
  - Continue soft tissue dissection until transverse process clearly seen
- Level check
- Pedicle screw insertion
  - At the confluence of the pars, transverse process and facet
- Rod application
- Decompression
  - Laminectomy
  - Burr and osteotome
  - Nerve roots identified and explored
  - Undercutting facetectomy
    - Ensure nerves are decompressed both in lateral recesses and foramen
- If dural leak occurs (5%)
  - Repair using 5.0 Prolene
  - Blood, fascia or fat patches
  - Dural 'glues'
  - Maintain supine for 48 hours postoperatively
- Closure in layers

Postoperative care
- Adequate analgesia
- Neurological observations and formal neurological assessment
- No spinal precautions

Transforaminal lumbar interbody fusion and posterior lumbar interbody fusion

Indications
- Isthmic and degenerative spondylolisthesis
- Discogenic back pain
- Post-discectomy pain syndromes failing conservative management

Risks
- Nerve injury
- Infection
- Pseudarthrosis
- Persistence of symptoms following non-operative management

Operative planning
- Full history and physical examination
- X-ray
- MRI

Surgical procedure
- General anaesthesia
- Prone position
- Montreal mattress, Jackson table, four-poster frame
- Midline incision
- Dissection
  - Fat, fascia
  - Diathermy used to dissect the musculature off the posterior elements of the spine
  - Soft tissue swept laterally using a Cobb elevator
    - Unilaterally – transforaminal lumbar interbody fusion (TLIF)
    - Bilaterally – posterior lumbar interbody fusion (PLIF)
- Identification of landmarks
  - Transverse processes
- Pedicle screw insertion
- Resection of superior and inferior articular processes of identified facet joint (TLIF) or laminotomy (PLIF)
- Exposure of disc
  - Ensure haemostasis of epidural veins running superior to the pedicle in the neuroforamen
- Piecemeal disc removal

- Cartilaginous endplate removal
- Cage insertion +/- bone graft
- Rod application (under slight compression)
- Closure in layers

Postoperative care
- Adequate analgesia
- Neurological observations and formal neurological assessment
- Postoperative X-rays
- No spinal precautions

Minimally invasive spinal surgery

New, less invasive techniques have and are continually developed in relation to the above procedures due to technological advances in access instrumentation and visualisation, as well as a desire to reduce approach-related comorbidities.

Indications
- Degenerative disc diseases
- Spinal stenosis
- Trauma
- Curvatures
- Pseudoarthrosis
- Tumour

Risks
- Increased operative length

Operative planning
- Full history and physical examination
- Spinal imaging
  - Plain X-rays
  - CT spine
  - MRI spine

Surgical procedure
- General anaesthetic
- Prone position
- Sterile prep and drape with fluoroscopy/navigation system
- Approach consists of multiple
  - Stab incision at desired angle from midline
  - Guidewire to posterior elements of spine
  - Sequential dilators or pedicle screw guide
    - Guidewire removed after first dilator to prevent advancement
  - Dilated retractor allows adequate visualisation of bony elements for decompression, discectomy, etc.

Anterior lumbar surgery

Anterior lumbar interbody fusion

Indications
- Degenerative disk disease
- Discogenic disk disease
- Revision of failed posterior fusion

Risks
- Approach-related complications
  - Retrograde ejaculation
  - Vascular injury
  - Visceral injury
- Infection
- Persistent pain

Operative planning
- Full history and examination
- Comprehensive surgical history (previous abdominal surgery)
- Plain X-rays
- MRI

Surgical procedure
- General anaesthetic
- Supine position
- Incision
  - Pfannenstiel
  - Paramedian
  - Lower midline

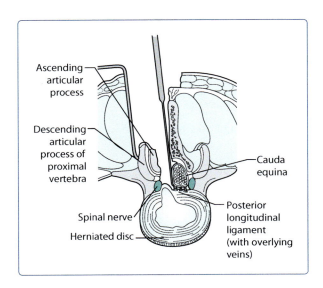

Figure 4.10 The operative view in lumbar discectomy.

- Retroperitoneal dissection
- Identification of
  - Iliac arteries and veins
  - Aortic bifurcation
  - Vena cava
- Mobilisation of great vessels
  - Allows greater exposure of disc space
- Ligation of midline tributaries
  - L4-L5 – iliolumbar and segmental vessels
  - L5-S1 – midline sacral vessels
- Débridement of anterior longitudinal ligament at desired level and exposure of disc space
- Incision into disc with subsequent discectomy
- Exposure to ventral dura
- Interbody cage insertion +/− bone graft
- Closure in layers

Postoperative care
- Adequate analgesia
- Neurological observations
- Postoperative X-rays
- No spinal precautions – sit to any angle and mobilise as tolerated

Viva questions

1. Describe the relevant surgical landmarks when planning an anterior approach to the T10 vertebral body.
2. What are the indications for performing an anterior approach to the spine?
3. Describe where the segmental blood supply of the vertebral body lies in relation to the disc.
4. At what level of the thoracic spine does the inferior border of the scapula lie when the arms are by the sides? Where, in relation to the spinous process, does the corresponding pedicle of the same vertebra lie?
5. Describe what steps you would take to minimise wrong level surgery in the thoracic spine.
6. What role do chest drains have in thoracic spinal surgery?
7. What factors are involved in selecting patients for scoliosis surgery?
8. Give a brief account of the preoperative management of a patient due to undergo scoliosis surgery.
9. Describe the positioning and the peripheral nerves at risk from prone positioning of a patient.
10. Which nerve runs in the lateral recess at the L5-S1 level?

11. Describe your intraoperative and postoperative management of a dural tear.
12. What might be the presentation and management of an acute epidural haematoma?
13. Describe the approach for a lumbar discectomy.
14. What nerve root would be compressed by an L4-L5 far lateral disc?
15. An L4-L5 left-sided paracentral disc protrusion will impinge on which nerve root?
16. What is the incidence of nerve root injury with a discectomy?
17. Describe the orientation of the facet joints at different levels of the spine.
18. Following temporary success of facet blocks, which other radiological procedure can be performed with potential for longer-lasting benefit?
19. Which nerve root leaves the spinal canal via the L4-L5 foramen?

5 Surgery of the Peripheral Nerve

Ravikiran Shenoy, Gorav Datta, Max Horowitz and Mike Fox

Carpal tunnel decompression	63	Principles of surgery on peripheral nerves	76
Ulnar nerve decompression at the wrist	68	Principles of brachial plexus surgery	80
Ulnar nerve decompression at the elbow	72	Viva questions	84

Carpal tunnel decompression

Preoperative planning

Indications
- Median nerve compression neuropathy at the wrist
- As part of a fasciotomy for compartment syndrome/decompression after distal radial fracture
- Drainage of sepsis

Contraindications
- Active overlying skin infection
- Uncertainty over diagnosis – may warrant further investigation before proceeding

Consent and risks
- *Nerve injury*: Median nerve injury less than 1%; palmar cutaneous nerve injury less than 1%
- *Radial artery injury*: Less than 1%
- *Failure to relieve symptoms*: 1%–10%; the incidence is highest in heavy/repetitive manual workers
- *Pillar pain*: Quoted at up to 10%; this is tenderness around the site of ligament release
- *Scar tenderness*: The incidence is reduced by massage in the postoperative period
- Complex regional pain syndrome (rare)
- Infection

Operative planning

History and clinical examination remain the mainstay of diagnosis. It is essential to examine the entire limb as well as the cervical spine to exclude a 'double-crush' lesion. Nerve conduction studies are useful and should be available on the day of surgery. They are considered essential in cases of recurrent carpal tunnel syndrome and complex upper limb lesions. Prolonged sensory latency is the earliest and most reliable nerve conduction abnormality. Magnetic resonance imaging (MRI) is rarely indicated, unless there is clinical evidence of a space-occupying lesion causing the symptoms. Conventional radiography is not generally indicated. Consideration should be given to extraneous causes such as diabetes mellitus, rheumatoid and other arthritides, amyloidosis and thyroid dysfunction; where appropriate these may also require investigation prior to operation.

Anaesthesia and positioning

The procedure may be carried out under local, regional or general anaesthesia. Most primary decompressions are performed under local anaesthesia. A local anaesthetic consisting of 1% lidocaine and 0.5% bupivacaine in a 1:1 mixture is infiltrated into the wound prior to surgical draping. General anaesthesia is usually reserved for revision procedures.

The patient is positioned supine on an operating table and the arm is positioned on an arm table in supination, with a padded lead hand used to maintain finger extension. A tourniquet is inflated to 250 mm Hg. In obese patients, a forearm tourniquet is recommended.

Surgical technique

Landmarks

The tendon of palmaris longus (absent in about 10%) is easily seen and palpated by opposing the thumb and little finger and then flexing the wrist to around 30°. The distal end of the tendon bisects the anterior surface of the carpal tunnel. Other useful landmarks include the thenar skin crease (running at the base of the thenar eminence) and the transverse skin crease of the wrist joint (running parallel to the joint line). The transverse wrist crease marks the proximal border of the flexor retinaculum. If the thumb is outstretched to 90°, a parallel line drawn across the palm in line with its distal border represents the surface marking of the superficial palmar arch: this is known as Kaplan's cardinal line (**Figure 5.1**).

Incision

The incision runs a few millimetres to the ulnar side of the thenar skin crease, in the line of the long axis of the ring finger. This ensures that any scarring is well away from the median nerve and ensures that proximal extension avoids the palmar cutaneous branch of the median nerve. The extent is from the distal volar wrist up to a few millimetres proximal to the superficial palmar arch. In revision surgery, the proximal extent is increased: this is curved to run along the ulnar side of the palmaris longus tendon (**Figure 5.2**). This avoids crossing the wrist joint crease at a right angle and, once again, minimises any damage to the palmar cutaneous branch of the median nerve.

Carpal tunnel decompression

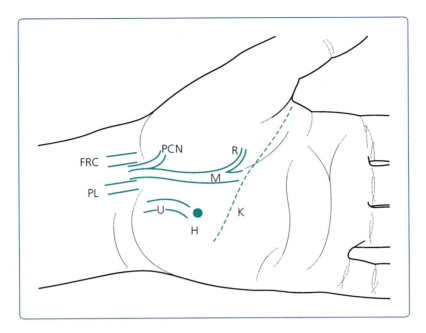

Figure 5.1 Surface anatomy of the wrist and hand. (FCR, flexor carpi radialis tendon; H, hook of hamate; K, Kaplan's cardinal line; M, median nerve; PCN, palmar cutaneous nerve; PL, palmaris longus tendon; R, recurrent motor branch; U, ulnar nerve.)

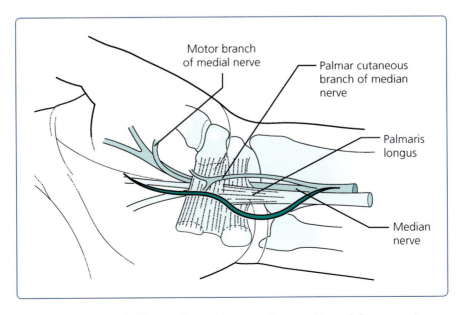

Figure 5.2 Extended incision for revision/complex carpal tunnel decompression.

Dissection

Structures at risk

- Palmar cutaneous branch of the median nerve is at risk if the skin incision is angled to the radial side of the forearm
- Deep motor branch of the median nerve (due to variation in its course) – staying on the ulnar side of the median nerve minimises the risk of damaging the structure
- Superficial palmar arch
- Median nerve

The exposure continues in line with the skin incision until the superficial palmar fascia is exposed deep to subcutaneous fat. Occasionally, the belly of flexor pollicis brevis (FPB) is superficial to the fascia and is divided. The fibres of the superficial palmar fascia are incised in the same line.

Retraction of the skin flaps will reveal the insertion of palmaris longus into the flexor retinaculum. If it is in the way, it can be retracted to the radial side: this exposes the median nerve. Careful dissection through the flexor retinaculum is recommended until the nerve is visualised. A McDonald tissue dissector is passed between the plane of the flexor retinaculum and the median nerve. The dissector must be used with caution and should elevate the retinaculum and not press down on the nerve. The flexor retinaculum is incised with a scalpel, cutting down onto the McDonald tissue dissector, which lies over the nerve and protects it (**Figure 5.3**).

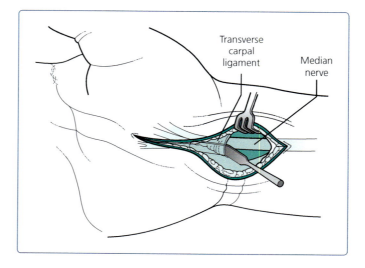

Figure 5.3 Release of the flexor retinaculum.

The nerve is released from proximal to distal. In revision surgery, the nerve should be dissected out proximal to the wrist crease. The perivascular fat pad is the distal border of the flexor retinaculum. This must be retracted to visualise the distal end of the ligament to ensure complete decompression. The proximal end of the wound should also be retracted to ensure complete release under direct vision with either tenotomy scissors or a blade.

The deep motor branch of the median nerve can have a variable course. Usually, it arises on the radial side of the median nerve as the nerve exits the carpal tunnel. The nerve continues radially, entering the thenar muscles between abductor pollicis brevis and FPB. However, variations may include a motor branch arising from the median nerve within the carpal tunnel, running distally to pierce the retinaculum supplying the thenar muscles. Bearing this in mind during the dissection, it is prudent to stay on the ulnar side of the median nerve to prevent damage to the motor branch.

External neurolysis need only be performed if the nerve is adherent to adjacent structures. Internal neurolysis is not performed.

The tourniquet should be released prior to wound closure. It is important to check for reperfusion of the nerve and to ensure adequate haemostasis before skin closure.

Extensile measures

These are generally not necessary for standard carpal tunnel surgery and are reserved for specific indications.

Proximal
The approach may be extended proximally to expose the median nerve in the forearm. This may be required in cases of fracture fixation with concomitant carpal tunnel decompression. Extension is gained between the tendons of flexor carpi radialis and palmaris longus. The nerve lies on the deep surface of flexor digitorum superficialis in the forearm. The median nerve is retracted to the ulnar side and pronator quadratus incised to access the distal radius.

Distal
The incision may be extended distally with a zigzag incision (Brunner incision) to access any digit, providing a complete palmar exposure. This is useful in procedures requiring the drainage of sepsis.

Closure
Skin closure is performed with 4-0 interrupted nylon sutures. An occlusive dressing is applied, followed by a compressive hand dressing. The compression dressing should allow immediate mobilisation of the fingers and wrist and should not be excessively bulky.

Endoscopic decompression

Endoscopic decompression may be performed through the Brown two-portal or the Agee single-portal technique. The main proven benefits of the endoscopic procedure are restoration of normal grip and absence of a painful scar in the early postoperative period. The procedure, however, has a steep learning curve with complications ranging from nerve injury and an inability to see anatomical variations to incomplete release.

Postoperative care and instructions

The bandage is removed 3–7 days following surgery. The sutures are removed and advice on scar massage given 10–14 days postoperatively. It is imperative that patients are encouraged to mobilise their fingers from day 3 onwards. They should also be counselled that it takes 6 weeks to regain their pinch grip and 3 months to achieve a power grip.

Recommended references

Cobb T, Dalley B, Posteraro R et al. Anatomy of the flexor retinaculum. *J Hand Surg Am*. 1993;**18**:91–99.

Graham B. The value added by electrodiagnostic testing in the diagnosis of carpal tunnel syndrome. *J Bone Joint Surg Am*. 2008;**90**:2587–2593.

Green DP. *Green's Operative Hand Surgery*, 7th ed. Philadelphia, PA: Elsevier, 2017.

Hankins CL, Brown MG, Lopez RA et al. A 12-year experience using the brown two-portal endoscopic procedure of transverse carpal ligament release in 14,722 patients: Defining a new paradigm in the treatment of carpal tunnel syndrome. *Plast Reconstr Surg*. 2007;**120**:1911–1921.

Mintalucci DJ, Leinberry CF. Open versus endoscopic carpal tunnel release. *Orthop Clin North Am*. 2012;**43(4)**:431–437.

Rotman MB, Donovan JP. Practical anatomy of the carpal tunnel. *Hand Clin*. 2002;**18**:219–230.

Smit A, Hooper G. Elective hand surgery in patients taking warfarin. *J Hand Surg Br*. 2004;**29**:206–207.

Steinberg DR. Surgical release of the carpal tunnel. *Hand Clin*. 2002;**18**:291–298.

Upton AR, McComas AJ. The double crush in nerve entrapment syndromes. *Lancet*. 1973;**2(7825)**:359–362.

Ulnar nerve decompression at the wrist

Preoperative planning

Decompression of the ulnar nerve at the wrist is a relatively uncommon procedure. Nerve compression may be associated with space-occupying lesions, anomalous muscles or trauma. It is imperative that the patient is examined from the cervical spine downwards, and clinical findings should be correlated with neurophysiology.

Indications

- Decompression of the canal of Guyon
- Ulnar nerve repair at the wrist (e.g. laceration)

Contraindication

Active overlying skin infection.

Consent and risks

- Nerve injury
- Vascular injury
- Infection
- Failure to relieve symptoms
- Stiffness
- Scar tenderness and hypersensitivity

Anaesthesia and positioning

The procedure may be carried out under local, regional or general anaesthesia. A local anaesthetic consisting of 1% lidocaine and 0.5% bupivacaine in a 1:1 mixture is infiltrated into the wound prior to surgical draping. There should be a low threshold for general anaesthesia if more than a simple exploration is being considered.

The patient is positioned supine on an operating table and the arm is positioned on an arm table in supination, with a padded lead hand used to maintain finger extension. A tourniquet is inflated to 250 mm Hg.

Surgical technique

Landmarks

The hypothenar eminence and transverse wrist skin crease are important surface landmarks. The bony landmarks of Guyon's canal (*Table 5.1*) are palpated and marked; the hook of hamate lies 1 cm radial and distal to the pisiform, which is easily palpated at the base of the hypothenar eminence.

Table 5.1 Boundaries of Guyon's canal

Floor	Pisohamate and pisometacarpal ligaments, flexor retinaculum and opponens digiti minimi
Roof	Volar carpal ligament and palmaris brevis
Medial wall	Pisiform, flexor carpi ulnaris and abductor digiti minimi
Lateral wall	Flexor digiti minimi, hook of hamate and flexor retinaculum
Proximal extent	Flexor retinaculum
Distal extent	Fibrous arch of the hypothenar muscles

Incision

The incision lies in between the two landmarks (hook of hamate and pisiform) and runs distally for approximately 4 cm and proximally for 3 cm (**Figure 5.5**). It is curved to the ulnar side, on crossing the wrist flexor crease, to overlie the tendon of flexor carpi ulnaris (FCU).

Superficial dissection

Structure at risk

A crossing cutaneous nerve between the ulnar nerve and the skin exists in 15% of cases and must be protected.

The subcutaneous fat is incised to the deep fascia of the forearm. The tendon of FCU is identified, and the fascia is incised on its radial border. The FCU tendon is retracted to the ulnar side revealing the ulnar nerve and artery (the artery lies radial to the nerve). If necessary, the incision is followed proximally to release the distal aspect of the antebrachial fascia.

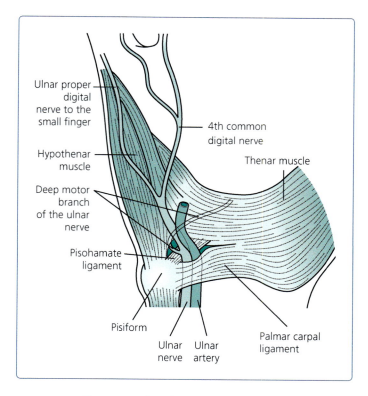

Figure 5.4 The relations of Guyon's canal.

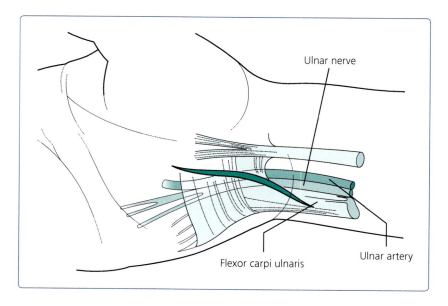

Figure 5.5 The incision for ulnar nerve decompression at the wrist.

Deep dissection

Once the nerve and artery are identified proximally, they are traced distally where they enter Guyon's canal. The volar carpal ligament is incised taking care not to damage the nerve or artery (**Figure 5.6**). The hook of hamate is then identified. Incising the edge of the hypothenar muscles reveals the deep motor branch as it continues around the hook of hamate.

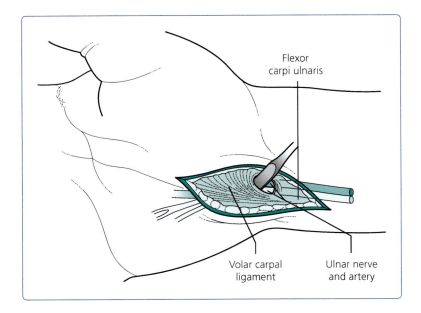

Figure 5.6 Incision of the volar carpal ligament.

Incising the volar carpal ligament, the palmaris brevis muscle and the hypothenar fibrous tissue will decompress the ulnar nerve within Guyon's canal. The nerve need not be completely circumferentially dissected out as this may devascularize it. Distally, the interval between the pisohamate and pisometacarpal ligaments is explored for any masses, fibrous bands or fracture fragments. The superficial branch passes superficial to the fibrous arch of the hypothenar muscles. The ulnar artery must be examined at this point to ensure that it is free of aneurysm or thrombus – it should be smooth and not tortuous.

Despite the ability to accurately diagnose the site of compression, surgical decompression should involve exposure of the nerve from the distal forearm to the hand distal to the bifurcation. The most common causes of compression are ganglia, other space-occupying lesions, fracture fragments and a thrombosed ulnar artery. The tourniquet should be deflated to ensure that there is no iatropathic injury of the ulnar artery and to achieve haemostasis.

Extensile measures

The incision may be extended proximally to the forearm. The deep fascia is incised on the radial border of FCU. A plane is developed between the FCU and the flexor digitorum superficialis (FDS), retracting the FCU to the ulnar side, revealing the ulnar nerve.

Closure
Skin closure is performed with 4-0 interrupted nylon sutures and a bulky, compressive hand dressing is applied.

Postoperative care and instructions
The bandage is removed 3-7 days following surgery, and active finger motion is encouraged at all times. Sutures are removed at 10-14 days postoperatively.

Recommended references
Chen SH, Tsai TM. Ulnar tunnel syndrome. *J Hand Sur.* 2014;**39(3)**:571–579.
Green DP. *Green's Operative Hand Surgery*, 7th ed. Philadelphia, PA: Elsevier, 2017.
Polatsch DB, Melone CP, Beldner S et al. Ulnar nerve anatomy. *Hand Clin.* 2007;**23**:283–289.

Ulnar nerve decompression at the elbow
Preoperative planning
Indications
- Ulnar nerve compression with or without recurrent subluxation of the nerve
- Exploration of the ulnar nerve in trauma

Contraindication
Active overlying skin infection.

Consent and risks
- Nerve injury to the ulna, median or medial antebrachial nerve (the most common at 4%)
- Medial elbow tenderness: 10%
- Failure to relieve symptoms and recurrence: 10%
- Elbow stiffness: 5%–10%
- Elbow instability associated with medial epicondylectomy: 1%–5%

Operative planning
A full neurological examination of the upper limb must take place. This should include an examination of the cervical spine as well as eliciting Tinel's sign at the elbow and wrist. Unlike in carpal tunnel disease, neurophysiological examination should be performed in almost all cases.

It is the authors' preferred choice to manage the majority of cases with simple decompression. Other options include partial medial epicondylectomy or nerve transposition procedures (which can be subcutaneous or submuscular). Partial medial epicondylectomy can be useful where there is significant extrinsic pressure on the nerve (e.g. an osteophyte). Transposition remains controversial because of an increased incidence of haematoma and infection without convincing improvements in results.

Anaesthesia and positioning

The procedure may be carried out under regional or general anaesthesia.

The authors prefer a medial approach as this avoids incision directly over the nerve. It also allows early visualisation of the medial antebrachial cutaneous nerve of the forearm. The patient is positioned supine on an operating table and the arm is positioned on a padded arm table, in supination, with the shoulder externally rotated. If a posterior approach is used, the patient is positioned in the lateral decubitus position with the arm placed in front of the chest, resting on a padded arm gutter. If a tourniquet is used it is inflated to 250 mm Hg. The authors do not routinely use a tourniquet, as pre-infiltration with local anaesthetic mixed with adrenaline provides excellent postoperative analgesia as well as a clear field for surgical dissection.

Surgical technique

Landmarks

The olecranon can easily be palpated posteriorly as it is a subcutaneous structure. Similarly the medial epicondyle is easily palpated. The nerve runs between these two structures and is at its most superficial at this point. **Figure 5.7** shows the relations of the ulnar nerve at the elbow.

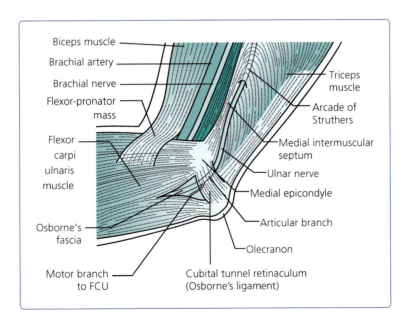

Figure 5.7 The relations of the ulnar nerve.

Medial approach

The medial incision starts 5 cm proximal to the medial epicondyle and extends distally to lie medial to the ulna distal to the elbow joint. It is advisable to place the skin incision anterior to the medial epicondyle so that the nerve does not lie directly under the skin wound. This prevents scarring directly over the nerve, and the medial cutaneous nerve of the forearm branch can be visualised. It is also less likely that a painful medial pressure area will occur. Subcutaneous tissues are reflected proximally and distally exposing the cubital tunnel retinaculum.

Posterior approach

This is recommended for the identification of the nerve in complex elbow trauma.

A longitudinal incision is made in the midline approximately 5 cm above the olecranon. The incision is curved laterally around the lateral side of the olecranon process and then curved medially so that the incision lies over the middle of the ulna distally. Curving the incision laterally moves the suture line away from the midline and avoids any potential pressure area over the olecranon process. The subcutaneous tissues are then dissected medially to expose the medial epicondyle. The advantage of the posterior approach is that frequently patients may have other elbow disorders requiring surgery (e.g. rheumatoid arthritis) and further incisions may be performed through the same scar. The disadvantage is that considerable dissection is necessary to expose the medial side adequately.

Deep dissection

The ulnar nerve is identified proximal to the cubital tunnel by blunt dissection. It is first released at the arcade of Struthers (the hiatus in the medial intermuscular septum through which the ulnar nerve enters the posterior compartment). The roof of the cubital tunnel is Osborne's ligament (the cubital tunnel retinaculum) proximally and Osborne's fascia (the deep component of the aponeurosis of the two heads of FCU) distally. The nerve is followed distally and Osborne's ligament is incised from proximal to distal. The veins lying on the dorsal surface of the medial intramuscular septum should be identified and coagulated. The nerve is traced into the two heads of the FCU to ensure release distally. At this stage it is important to identify and protect the motor branch to the FCU.

The nerve should not be dissected from its groove as this may lead to subluxation and devascularisation. After release, the elbow is moved through its full range; the nerve should be lax in full extension and should remain in the groove in full flexion. Residual adherent structures should be released and if subluxation is a problem then medial epicondylectomy or subcutaneous transposition should be considered.

Medial epicondylectomy

This procedure is useful in patients with a medial epicondyle fracture non-union or space-occupying lesions within the cubital tunnel (e.g. medial osteophyte, exostosis or ganglion). Routine decompression is performed, after which the common flexor origin is elevated off the medial epicondyle in a subperiosteal manner. A sleeve is left around the bone to ensure smooth closure and haemostasis. A partial medial epicondylectomy is performed with a narrow osteotome; bone wax can be placed on the exposed cancellous bone. The periosteal sleeve is closed over the epicondyle stump with a heavy Vicryl suture; this should be done in full extension so that an extension lag is avoided.

The anteroinferior medial collateral ligaments must be avoided and no more than 20% of the depth of the epicondyle should be excised to prevent elbow instability.

Subcutaneous transposition

The theory behind transposing the nerve is to reduce tensile stress on the nerve. This occurs during traction on the nerve in flexion and leads to an increased intraneural pressure and flattening of the nerve around the medial epicondyle. This increased pressure may cause temporary ischaemia.

The medial intramuscular septum must be divided to ensure tension-free transposition. It is essential that the longitudinal vascular supply of branches are protected and allowed to move with the main body of the nerve.

Once the nerve is decompressed and easily transposable anterior to the medial epicondyle, a subcutaneous fascial flap is elevated with a scalpel. The nerve is placed anterior to the deep surface of the flap and the distal flap edges are sutured to deep dermal tissue with an absorbable 3-0 Vicryl suture. The wound is then closed as normal.

Closure

The wound is closed with interrupted 2-0 Vicryl sutures for the subcutaneous layer and a running subcuticular monofilament suture for skin. If a tourniquet has been used it should be released and followed by meticulous haemostasis. A sterile dressing should be applied and then a compressive dressing over it.

Postoperative care and instructions

Dressings are removed at 3-4 days. Range-of-motion exercises within the limits of comfort should be started at the same stage. Active hand and wrist motion is encouraged at all times.

The wound should be checked at 2 weeks and the patient advised on appropriate care of the scar. Heavy lifting should be avoided for 1 month. It is important to counsel the patient that not all symptoms may be relieved by the surgery and that recovery may take up to 6 months.

Recommended references

Catalano LW, Barron OA. Anterior subcutaneous transposition of the ulnar nerve. *Hand Clin.* 2007;**23**:339–344.

Macadam SA, Gandhi R, Bezuhly M, Lefaivre KA. Simple decompression versus anterior subcutaneous and submuscular transposition of the ulnar nerve for cubital tunnel syndrome: A meta-analysis. *J Hand Surg Am.* 2008;**33(8)**:1314.e1–1314.e12.

Mowlavi A, Andrews K, Lille S et al. The management of cubital tunnel syndrome: A meta-analysis of clinical studies. *Plast Reconstr Surg.* 2000;**106**:327–334.

O'Driscoll SW, Jaloszynski R, Morrey BF et al. Origin of the medial ulnar collateral ligament. *J Hand Surg Am.* 1992;**17**:164–168.

Osterman AL, Spiess AM. Medial epicondylectomy. *Hand Clin.* 2007;**23**:329–337.

Staples JR, Calfee R. Cubital tunnel syndrome. *J Am Acad Orthop Surg.* 2017;**25(10)**:e215–e224.

Waugh RP, Zlotolow DA. *In situ* decompression of the ulnar nerve at the cubital tunnel. *Hand Clin.* 2007;**23**:319–327.

Principles of surgery on peripheral nerves

Preoperative planning

The aims of surgery are

- To confirm a diagnosis and establish prognosis
- To restore function
- To relieve pain

Indications

- Closed traction injury of the brachial plexus leading to severe paralysis
- Associated nerve and vascular injury
- Nerve injury with an associated fracture requiring early internal fixation
- Increasing progression of a neurological injury or an entrapment neuropathy
- Failure of recovery of a lesion within an expected time frame
- Failure of recovery in conduction block within 6 weeks of injury
- Persistent pain following injury
- Severe paralysis of a nerve following blunt trauma

Contraindications

- Active infection
- Function unaffected by nerve injury

Consent and risks

- Infection
- Nerve damage/failure of repair
- Vascular injury
- Specific to the site of operation, e.g. local structures at risk

Operative planning

Earlier surgery following nerve injury permits easier identification of tissues (due to less scar tissue) and therefore any repair is easier as it is possible to visualise and match the arrangement of the cut ends of the nerve fascicles. The results of prompt repair are also markedly better due to the favourable biological environment for nerve healing. A nerve stimulator should be available. Magnification of at least three times with loupes is helpful. If nerve grafting is likely to be performed, a suitable donor graft should be identified preoperatively and the patient made aware of the need.

Anaesthesia and positioning

Surgical procedures involving the exploration or repair of peripheral nerves should be performed under general anaesthesia, with antibiotic cover to minimise the chance of any postoperative infection. Where possible, a tourniquet is used to achieve a completely bloodless field, facilitating ease of identification of structures. Remember that after approximately 15 minutes of ischaemia, nerve conduction becomes abnormal so any tourniquet should be released when stimulating a nerve.

Surgical technique

Incision

The course of cutaneous nerves should always be remembered when planning a skin incision. A painful neuroma may result from a transected cutaneous nerve and lead to considerable morbidity to the patient.

Nerve assessment

When nerves have been damaged and surgery has been delayed, a neuroma will have formed. The consistency of a neuroma is important when assessing nerve injury, as a hard neuroma may represent an abundance of connective tissue and little in the way of nerve tissue. Making an incision through the damaged epineurium permits visualisation of any nerve bundles present, and stimulation of the nerve proximally. This may give some indication as to likely recovery. Stimulating the nerve proximally and recording from the nerve distally give the best guide for recovery. An absence of recording distally is a relative indication to resect and repair the nerve, depending on the macroscopic fascicular structure seen. Care should be taken not to undertake excessive mobilisation, as this may lead to devascularisation of a nerve.

Bipolar diathermy should be used at all times when coagulating blood vessels around nerves.

Methods of repair

Primary repair

The ends of an injured nerve are cut back progressively until the cut surfaces show bulging healthy nerve bundles. An end-to-end anastomosis is performed, which is possible if the resection gap has been small, little mobilisation of the nerve has been necessary, and the nerve is not under tension. Flexing a nearby joint reduces tension on a nerve, and extra length can be gained by transposition (e.g. anterior transposition of the ulnar nerve) of a nerve. The two principal types of primary repair are *epineural* repair and *fascicular* repair. Epineural repair is technically less demanding and faster to complete. Fascicular repair (**Figure 5.8**) is performed if there has been a clean transection of a nerve trunk (e.g. in the brachial plexus). In each method of repair, the true epineurium is exposed. In a fascicular repair, the matched bundles are opposed and sutured with perineurial 11-0 nylon sutures, and then 10-0 nylon sutures are passed through the perineurium and epineurium. This is done circumferentially to complete the repair. In an epineurial repair (**Figure 5.9**), the fascicular groups in the nerve ends are matched as closely as possible and the ends are then sutured with 10-0 nylon sutures through the epineurium. An initial suture is placed at each of the lateral ends of the nerve, with interrupted sutures subsequently placed on the anterior and posterior aspect of the nerve to complete the repair.

5 Surgery of the Peripheral Nerve

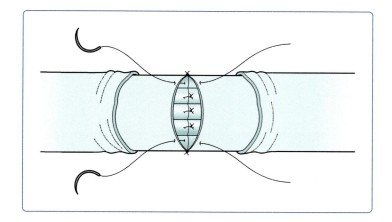

Figure 5.8 Fascicular nerve repair.

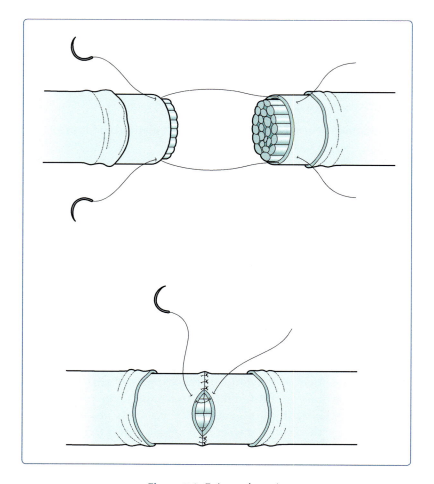

Figure 5.9 Epineural repair.

Nerve grafting

Cable grafts (**Figure 5.10**) are the gold standard for bridging gaps between two cut ends of a nerve where primary repair is not possible. Nerve bundles are matched to bundles; this is achieved by viewing and matching the nerve ends either using loupes or a microscope, using magnification to get the best possible match. Cable grafts consist of multiple cutaneous nerve strands from a donor nerve. The most common donor nerves used are the medial cutaneous nerve of the forearm and the sural nerve in the lower limb. As many grafts as required are used to give good coverage of the cut face of the nerve. The length of the graft should be approximately 15% longer than the gap to be bridged. The grafts can either be fixed with a tissue glue or sutured in place. If a gap to be bridged is greater than 10 cm, grafting is unlikely to be of great benefit.

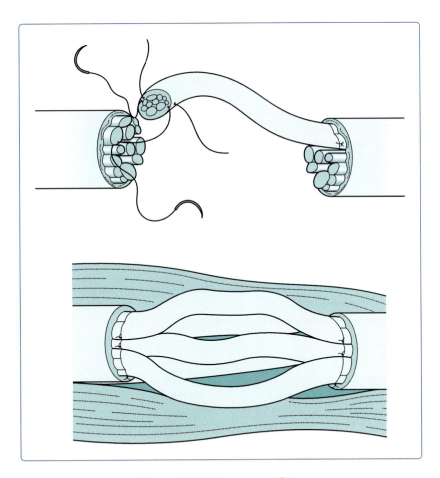

Figure 5.10 Cable nerve grafting.

If a nerve has been severely damaged to the extent that repair and grafting are not possible, nerve transfer (neurotisation) is performed: a distal nerve is reinnervated using an intact donor proximal nerve.

Nerve transfer

Nerve transfers where a nerve, serving a less important function or where the structure innervated by a nerve is damaged beyond repair, is used as a donor to restore a more useful function are an alternative to nerve repair and grafting. These are particularly useful where nerves are injured proximally and need a lengthy period of regeneration following proximal repair or where proximal repair is not possible in cases of brachial plexus avulsions. By anastomosing the donor to the recipient stump closer to the innervation point, the time to regeneration is shortened and also need for a graft is avoided. The technique of anastomosis is similar to that of primary repair. Surgical loupes, meticulous dissection, knowledge of fascicular anatomy of the nerve, and the use of intraoperative nerve stimulators are essential to isolate motor nerve fascicles from the main nerve. Unlike tendon transfers, motor nerve transfers, when successful, restore a more natural function, but they need to be performed before degeneration of the end target taking into account the time taken for the nerve to regrow across the anastomosis to the end target.

Common nerve transfers include spinal accessory nerve transfer to the suprascapular nerve in cases of C5 avulsion/injury to restore posterosuperior shoulder cuff function, Somsak procedure where a branch of the radial to one of the heads of triceps is anastomosed to the anterior motor branch of the axillary nerve to restore deltoid function, and modified Oberlin procedure where the ulnar nerve and/or the median nerve fascicle innervating a wrist flexor is divided at the level of mid arm and anastomosed to the motor fascicle of the musculocutaneous nerve innervating biceps and/or brachialis. Anterior interosseous nerve transfer to the ulnar nerve motor fascicle at the wrist helps restore function of hand intrinsics in cases of high ulnar nerve lesions or injury to the lower trunk of the brachial plexus. Nerve transfers have also been shown to improve function in spinal cord injury and by targeted muscle innervation increase the range of movements in amputation prosthesis.

Postoperative care and instructions

After nerve decompression, patients are told to leave their bulky dressings in place until they have a wound inspection 2 weeks postoperatively. Instruction to begin early hand and finger mobilisation is encouraged in upper limb surgery.

After nerve repair and grafting, the limb is generally protected in a plaster with a sling (or crutches in the lower limb) for a period of between 3 and 6 weeks. Either outpatient or inpatient therapy (as in the case of a brachial plexus repair) is required to overcome any residual stiffness and deformity. This may include appropriate splintage and is often multidisciplinary, with occupational therapy, physiotherapy and pain team input.

Principles of brachial plexus surgery

Preoperative planning

The principles of brachial plexus surgery are similar to those of other peripheral nerve operations (see previous section).

The five roots of the brachial plexus lie in the posterior triangle of the neck between scalenus anterior and scalenus medius muscles. Injuries between the posterior root ganglion and the spinal cord are termed *preganglionic*. The three trunks of the brachial plexus lie in front of one another and in the posterior triangle of the neck. The divisions of the plexus lie posterior to the clavicle. The medial, lateral and posterior cords of the plexus are related to the second part of the axillary artery deep to pectoralis minor.

Indications
- Section/rupture/avulsion of the plexus
- Associated vascular and nerve injuries
- Open wounds
- Compressive neuropathy

Anaesthesia and positioning
The procedure is performed under general anaesthesia, with the patient supine and the head elevated to approximately 30°.

Supraclavicular approach to the brachial plexus
- Cervical and brachial plexus (root/trunk) surgery
- Spinal accessory nerve surgery
- Suprascapular nerve surgery
- Sympathetic chain surgery

Landmarks
The landmarks for the supraclavicular approach are those of the posterior triangle of the neck. The base is formed by the clavicle, the medial border is formed by the medial border of the sternocleidomastoid muscle and the lateral border is formed by the edge of the trapezius muscle.

Incision

> ### Structure at risk
> - Supraclavicular nerves

The skin incision is made approximately one finger's breadth above the clavicle in line with the bone. Care must be taken not to damage the supraclavicular nerves, as a painful neuroma may develop.

Dissection
Skin flaps are raised exposing the apex of the posterior triangle superiorly and the clavicle inferiorly. Next the plane between the external jugular vein and the sternocleidomastoid is developed, with the omohyoid muscle displayed inferiorly in the wound. The muscle is divided and reflected. Deep to the fat pad, the transverse cervical artery is present and is at risk; it is ligated. The phrenic nerve is visualised running across the scalenus anterior. The

nerve is followed proximally, revealing C5. The deep cervical fascia is incised, and C5 and C6 are seen emerging from the lateral aspect of scalenus anterior; C7 is visualised between the scalenus anterior and the upper trunk. The lower trunk is seen following division of the scalenus anterior. By following the plane between the subclavian artery and the lower trunk, C8 and T1 are visualised.

Infraclavicular approach to the brachial plexus
Indications
- Complete exposure of brachial plexus (when combined with supraclavicular approach)
- Infraclavicular brachial plexus repair

Dissection
Essentially this is analogous to the deltopectoral approach to the upper humerus. The difference lies in mobilising the cephalic vein medially and detaching and reflecting the pectoralis minor muscle from the coracoid process. In a full exposure, the pectoralis major insertion on the humerus may also be detached.

Fiolle Delmas approach
Indications
The Fiolle Delmas approach combines the supraclavicular and infraclavicular approaches and is useful in an extensive injury to the plexus.

Incision
The platysma, with skin flaps, is elevated and the mid-portion of the clavicle is exposed superiorly and inferiorly. An extension is made of the collar incision to expose the supraclavicular portion (**Figure 5.11**). This extension starts at around the mid-portion of the supraclavicular incision and extends distally over the mid-portion of the clavicle running over the delto-pectoral groove to the axilla. It is a true extensile approach and can be continued distally, if necessary, as the anterior approach to the humerus. When the infraclavicular is combined with the supraclavicular approach, full exposure is given from the second part of the subclavian artery to the terminal portion of the axillary artery, with exposure of the brachial plexus from the spinal nerves to the terminal branches of the plexus.

Dissection
A clavicular osteotomy may be required to facilitate access, especially if there is a vascular injury. In this case a plate should be precontoured and holes predrilled for easy fixation at the end of the procedure, remembering that the bone will be shortened by the thickness of the saw blade. Distally the pectoralis major muscle is detached from the humerus in its upper portion or, if required, its entirety. The muscle is then reflected medially exposing the clavicle, pectoralis minor muscle and clavipectoral fascia (**Figure 5.12**). The pectoralis minor muscle is divided at its tendon taking care not to damage the musculocutaneous nerve. The subclavius muscle is divided with the suprascapular vessels (once ligated). This exposes the entire plexus and vasculature from the first rib to the axilla.

Principles of brachial plexus surgery

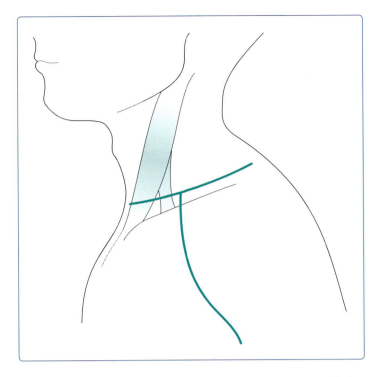

Figure 5.11 Incision for the Fiolle Delmas approach to the brachial plexus.

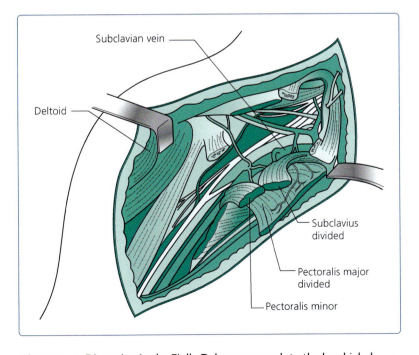

Figure 5.12 Dissection in the Fiolle Delmas approach to the brachial plexus.

Postoperative care and instructions

Following nerve repair/transfer, the limb may require immobilisation in a cast for 3 weeks after which the patient can start motion progressively. In the case of brachial plexus surgery, a sling is applied with a body strapping for 3 weeks, followed by readmission for a week at 6 weeks after index operation to start the rehabilitation process.

Recommended references

Birch R. *Surgical Disorders of the Peripheral Nerves*. London, UK: Springer London, 2011.
Henry HK. *Extensile Exposure*, 2nd ed. Edinburgh, Scotland: Churchill Livingstone, 1957.
Isaacs J, Cochran AR. Nerve transfers for peripheral nerve injury in the upper limb. *Bone Joint J*. 2019;**101–B(2)**:124–131.
Ray WZ, Chang J, Hawasli A, Wilson TJ, Yang L. Motor nerve transfers: A comprehensive review. *Neurosurgery*. 2016;**78(1)**:1–26.
Tupper JW, Crick JC, Mattich LR. Fascicular nerve repairs. *Orthop Clin North Am*. 1988;**19**:57–69.

Viva questions

1. Describe the landmarks and incision for a carpal tunnel decompression.
2. Describe the main structures at risk in a carpal tunnel decompression.
3. What are the sites of compression of the ulnar nerve at the elbow?
4. What are the surface landmarks for Guyon's canal?
5. Which structures commonly cause ulnar tunnel compression neuropathy at the elbow?
6. Describe the techniques used in primary nerve repair.
7. What options are available if primary repair is not possible?
8. What are the principal considerations for successful nerve transfer surgery?
9. What are the priorities in gaining function after brachial plexus injury?

6 Surgery of the Shoulder

Nick Aresti, Omar Haddo and Mark Falworth

Diagnostic shoulder arthroscopy	85	Shoulder arthroplasty	108
Arthroscopic procedures	90	Viva questions	112
Open shoulder procedures	98		

Since the publication of the first edition of this book, arthroscopic shoulder surgery has seen a significant expansion and consequentially open procedures have become increasingly less common. Thankfully, the principles behind the various procedures have stayed the same. Similarly, several large and well-published randomised controlled trials have questioned the efficacy of commonly used procedures and the practice of many surgeons is changing as a result.

We describe the process of a diagnostic shoulder arthroscopy and then expand on how therapeutic procedures are performed, describing open alternatives. We also discuss the treatment of degenerative joint disease with arthroplasty.

Diagnostic shoulder arthroscopy

Diagnostic shoulder arthroscopy can be used as part of arthroscopic treatment of various pathologies, but also purely for diagnostic purposes given the relatively low complication rates.

Contraindications are few and only really include

- Infection of overlying skin
- Lack of proper arthroscopic instrumentation

Complication rates are as mentioned very low, but informed consent of all the possible risks should be discussed with patients. These include

- *Nerve injury*: The musculocutaneous nerve (anterior portal) and the axillary nerve (lateral portal) are most at risk. The suprascapular nerve can be damaged by the inexperienced arthroscopist.
- *Chondral or labral injuries*: Relatively uncommon.

- Fluid imbalance due to fluid extravasation.
- *Infection*: Very rare.
- *Vascular injury*: Very rare.

Operative planning

Recent radiographs and when relevant, ultrasound, computed tomography (CT) and magnetic resonance (MR) images (with or without arthrograms), should be available. Although only basic equipment is necessary for a diagnostic procedure, standard equipment should be available so that therapeutic treatment can be undertaken if necessary. This includes

- Camera with imaging and recording equipment
- Xenon light source
- Fluid management system (pump set at 30–70 mm Hg)
- 5 mm 30° (±70°) scopes with high-flow sleeve
- Shaver
- Burr
- Vaporiser
- Arthroscopic instruments
- Cannulas
- Arthroscopic implants

Anaesthesia and positioning

General anaesthesia is preferred with the use of an interscalene block if certain procedures are planned. The use of a block alone is possible; however, the posterior portal is often not covered as the upper thoracic nerve roots innervate the corresponding area. A 'top up' of local anaesthetic to the surrounding tissues may be required.

Two options for patient positioning exist: lateral and beach chair. The choice is very much surgeon dependent.

- If the lateral position is used, the patient should be as far back towards the edge of the table as possible, with 15° of posterior tilt (horizontal glenoid). Front and back supports are required to secure the patient. The patient's head is placed in a gel ring. Four kilograms of longitudinal skin traction is applied with the arm in 30°–50° abduction and 20°–30° forward flexion (**Figure 6.1**). The brachial plexus should be palpated to ensure that it remains soft and that excessive traction is not being applied.
- If the beach chair position is used, the appropriate operating table (with removable lateral corner) is required. Prior to raising the table into the beach chair position, the table should be tilted into a Trendelenburg position to prevent the patient sliding down the table. A pillow should also be used under the knees. Traction can be added based on surgeon preference. This approach is helpful if progressing to an open procedure.

The surgical field is prepared with a germicidal solution, and waterproof drapes are used with adhesive edges to provide a seal to the skin.

Diagnostic shoulder arthroscopy

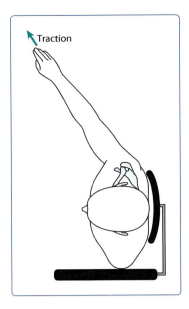

Figure 6.1 Positioning and traction for shoulder arthroscopy.

Landmarks

It is very important to identify and draw on the landmarks of the shoulder, particularly given the difficulty in identifying them once it has swollen with fluid. These landmarks should include

- Spine of the scapula.
- Acromion – the posterolateral corner, lateral acromion, and anterolateral corners.
- Supraclavicular fossa.
- Distal clavicle and acromioclavicular joint (ACJ).
- Tip of the coracoid.
- A line from the anterolateral corner of the acromion heading towards the upper arm signifies the position of the long head of the biceps tendon.
- Lateral orientation line, which aids in the placement of a lateral portal.

Portals

The accurate placement of arthroscopic portals is essential in shoulder arthroscopy. A variety of portals can be used.

Posterior portal

This is the most common viewing portal. A stab incision to the skin is placed 2 cm medial and 2 cm inferior to the posterolateral corner of the acromion. This correlates to a palpable soft spot, which denotes the plane between the infraspinatus and teres minor.

To access the glenohumeral joint, a trocar is aimed inferomedially towards the tip of the coracoid. The glenoid rim and the humeral head can be palpated and the trocar can be pushed between them. Balottement of the humeral head posteriorly or first infiltrating the glenohumeral joint with saline could aid in the placement of the trocar. A popping sensation is usually felt as the joint is entered. The introducer of the trocar is removed and the camera inserted. Normal saline is then attached and the joint irrigated.

To enter the subacromial space, the same posterior portal skin incision is used; however, the scope is aimed superolaterally towards the anterolateral corner of the acromion. The scope must enter the bursa and show the acromion and the bursal aspect of the cuff clearly. If cobweb-like tissue is seen, then the scope is outside the bursa and should be repositioned. This is important as the bursa helps to contain the irrigation fluid, thus limiting soft tissue swelling around the shoulder.

Anterior portal

Once the posterior portal is established, all other portals are made using an outside-in technique in which a spinal needle is used to determine the exact location and angle of entry into the joint. A standard low anterior portal is placed above the lateral half of the subscapularis but medial to the medial biceps pulley. Once the needle has been placed in the appropriate position the portal is made using a size 11 scalpel, which is inserted in the same direction as the needle taking care to avoid the long head of the biceps (LHB), conjoint tendon and rotator cuff.

Superolateral portal

This portal provides access to both the biceps tendon and the labrum anteriorly. It is placed around 1 cm lateral to the anterolateral edge of the acromion and is used for suture management and anchor placement during subscapularis and anterior labral repairs.

Lateral portal

The lateral portal is 5 cm (three fingers breadth) distal to the acromion and 1 cm anterior to the mid-lateral line (in line with the posterior line of the ACJ). This portal is used for instrumentation of the subacromial space (**Figure 6.2**) during subacromial decompressions and rotator cuff repairs.

Accessory portals

Other portals can be made on demand. These include the anterosuperolateral, accessory anterior, accessory lateral, accessory posterior, port of Wilmington and Neviaser (superior) portals. A cannula may be used if proceeding to a therapeutic procedure. Clear cannulas are recommended as they allow visualisation and aid in suture management.

Procedure

A systematic approach to evaluation of the shoulder is imperative so that pathologies are not missed. With the scope in the posterior portal, the glenohumeral joint is assessed first. By using the LHB tendon as a reference, the camera is adjusted so that the image is shown in the correct superoinferior plane. The authors recommend the following systematic way of assessing the shoulder:

Diagnostic shoulder arthroscopy

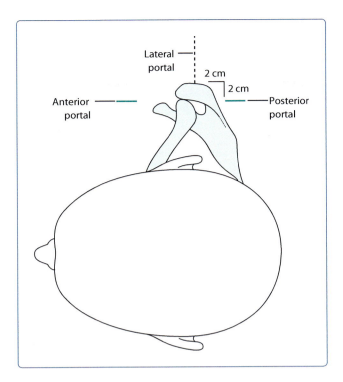

Figure 6.2 Common arthroscopic portals.

- The LHB should first be assessed at its insertion at the superior glenoid tubercle. By raising the arm in 90° abduction and 90° external rotation, the presence of a SLAP (superior labrum from anterior to posterior) tear can be assessed as the labrum rolls off the glenoid rim (peel-back sign). The scope can then be turned laterally and the intra-articular portion of the LHB, and that portion of the biceps tendon that lies within the inter-tubercular grove, can be assessed.
- The stability of the LHB can then be visualised by internally and externally rotating the shoulder. The medial sling/pulley can then be inspected before examining the subscapularis tendon, superior glenohumeral ligament and rotator interval in more detail. The subscapularis tendon insertion can be best visualised with the arm in internal rotation.
- By gently withdrawing the scope and looking laterally, the posterior pulley of the LHB can be viewed and then the supraspinatus and infraspinatus tendons can be examined. The bare area and any Hill-Sachs lesions can now be identified.
- As the arthroscope is taken further inferiorly it enters the inferior recess. The reflection of the inferior capsule and the posterior band of the inferior glenohumeral ligament (hammock effect) can be seen. By then rotating the scope, the posterior inferior labrum can be visualised and then the entire posterior and superior labrum examined before assessing the chondral surfaces of both the humeral head and glenoid.
- The anterior stabilising structures can now be examined. Superiorly the sublabral foramen, labrum and middle glenohumeral and anterior band of the inferior glenohumeral ligaments can all be visualised.

- An anterior portal can be made through the rotator interval for the introduction of a probe for further assessment of any soft tissue pathology or if any glenoid bone loss needs to be further assessed.
- The subacromial space should then be examined by repositioning the trocar above the rotator cuff. Superiorly the acromion is seen, anteriorly the coracoacromial ligament and inferiorly the bursal side of the rotator cuff. The presence of bursal side rotator cuff tears, impingement lesions and acromial and ACJ pathology can all be assessed.

This is just one example of a systematic assessment of arthroscopic shoulder anatomy. Each surgeon can develop their own system; however, it is essential that all surgeons are familiar with arthroscopic anatomy and normal variations.

Closure and postoperative care

Wounds can be closed with suture or Steri-Strips or left open. A pressure dressing assists with a swollen joint. If the procedure was purely diagnostic, a sling is only necessary for comfort and to assist with weakness while a block wears off.

Arthroscopic procedures

Subacromial decompression

Over the last decade, arthroscopic subacromial decompressions (ASDs) have superseded open acromioplasty, and their use has increased exponentially. Recent notable publications have questioned this overuse. Symptoms of impingement are often associated with an underlying diagnosis, be it instability, rotator cuff pathology, biceps tendonitis, etc. We must ensure ASDs are performed in the correct patient groups.

Recommended reference

Beard DJ, Rees JL, Cook JA et al.; CSAW Study Group. Arthroscopic subacromial decompression for subacromial shoulder pain (CSAW): A multicentre, pragmatic, parallel group, placebo-controlled, three-group, randomised surgical trial. *Lancet*. 2018;**391(10118)**:329–338.

Risks

In addition to those described in the diagnostic arthroscopy section, patients should be warned of acromial fracture, as well as ongoing and recurrence of symptoms.

Procedure

Imaging should be interrogated for underlying pathology. In particular, radiographs should be assessed to ensure an os acromiale is not present. The arthroscopic pump is set between 30 and 70 mm Hg. The arthroscope is introduced through the posterior portal and a diagnostic arthroscopy performed. It is then introduced into the subacromial bursa. The bursal surface of the cuff is inspected to confirm the presence of an impingement lesion (inflammation, roughening and fibrillation). Next, the undersurface of the acromion is examined for a corresponding 'kissing' lesion. The acromion can be further assessed using an arthroscopic probe for any acromial hooks or spurs. The coracoacromial ligament is also inspected. The lateral portal is used for instrumentation. A spinal needle is used for the outside-in technique of portal placement. Although this portal is at the level of the axillary nerve, the nerve is not usually threatened as the instruments are aimed proximally towards the acromion. No cannula is required.

A successful decompression has three main components:

1. Resection of the bursa
2. Release of coracoacromial ligament
3. Burring of the acromion

Soft tissue resection and haemostasis can be performed with an electrocautery probe/vaporiser. The soft tissue on the undersurface of the acromion is then resected and the coracoacromial ligament detached. Radial cuts can be made to ensure the ligament does not reform, but care must be taken not to damage the branches of the thoracoacromial artery. The lateral edge of the acromion must be exposed to ensure adequate lateral decompression.

A barrel burr/shaver is used for bone resection. If the acromion has a lateral down-slope then a lateral bevel is performed. The decompression is then performed by excising the anterior acromion, from lateral to medial. The acromial branch of the coracoacromial vessel is at risk at this stage also. Anterior resection is usually approximately 4 mm (the width of the burr) or until the anterior deltoid attachment is reached. Medially, the resection is limited by the ACJ. The undersurface of the acromion is then chamfered, to smooth out any ridges (**Figure 6.3**).

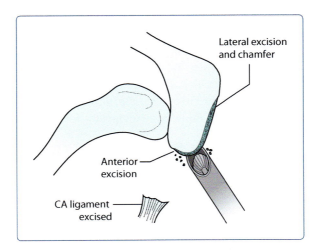

Figure 6.3 Arthroscopic subacromial decompression; CA, coracoacromial.

Further refinement of the acromioplasty can be performed by placing the arthroscope in the lateral portal and the shaver posteriorly. Any residual bone can be resected using the posterior acromion as a 'cutting block', thus creating a flat undersurface to the acromion.

Wounds can be closed as per a diagnostic arthroscopy. No postoperative restrictions are required, and rehabilitation can be commenced immediately.

Acromioclavicular joint excision

ACJ excision can be performed arthroscopically for symptomatic ACJ arthritis which has failed conservative treatment. Stability of the joint is maintained through preservation of the superior ACJ ligaments.

Risks

Risks are much the same as a subacromial decompression with the added possible complication of joint instability. Of all the arthroscopic shoulder procedures, ACJ excision is possibly the most painful postoperatively and patients should be warned accordingly.

Procedure

Essentially, a subacromial decompression is performed; however, the anterior portal should be made in line with the orientation of the ACJ, which occasionally places it slightly more laterally. Accurate placement can be performed via an outside-in technique, ensuring the needle is parallel to the joint line. Identifying the joint is aided through placing a needle through the joint and by palpating the lateral end of the clavicle. A shaver or vaporiser can be used through the lateral portal to expose the ACJ. Scar tissue and the remnants of the meniscus are resected and any inferior osteophytes excised. To ensure adequate visualisation of the ACJ the fibrofatty tissue in the region of the scapular spine and distal clavicle should be resected.

A barrel burr is used to excise the distal clavicle from inferior to superior and from lateral to medial. To ensure that adequate bone is resected, especially posteriorly, the entire circumference of the resected distal clavicle must be visualised. This is often only achieved if both the anterior and posterior acromioclavicular ligaments are excised. However, care must be taken not to excise the superior acromioclavicular ligament or to resect too much bone as this can destabilise the joint. The aim is for approximately 10 mm of bone resection from the medial acromial facet to the distal clavicle, which can be assessed by measuring against the width of the shaver. Occasionally, a Neviaser portal is required to complete the resection.

Wounds can be closed as per a diagnostic arthroscopy. No postoperative restrictions are required, and rehabilitation can be commenced immediately.

Recommended reference

Flatow EL, Duralde XA, Nicholson GP et al. Arthroscopic resection of the distal clavicle with a superior approach. *J Shoulder Elbow Surg.* 1995;4:41–50.

Biceps tenotomy/tenodesis

The LHB is often a cause of pain as it degenerates. If its pulley is damaged it may also sublux in the joint providing difficulty identifying the relevant structures, and possibly 'cheese-wire' through the superior subscapularis. In symptomatic patients, the LHB may be either tenotomised or tenodesed with no clear evidence either way, but a tenodesis being preferred in the younger and active patient. Other indications for interventions include partial thickness tears or SLAP tears. Options for a tenodesis include mini-open approaches, tenodesing the screw in the bicipital groove, and subpectoral tenodesis, some of which can be performed arthroscopically.

Risks

Once again, all the risks of an ASD must be relayed to the patient. In addition, patients who have a tenotomy may develop a 'Popeye sign' or weakness of the biceps. Morbidity is associated with a tenodesis, and this includes 'biceps groove' pain, particularly when a tenodesis screw is used, fracture or re-rupture.

Procedure

During an arthroscopy, an anterior portal is created. A knife or vaporiser may be used to directly divide the LHB under vision. Care must be taken not to damage the superior labrum and the overlying supraspinatus tendon. Some advocate taking a large soft tissue sleeve which gets trapped in the biceps tunnel, creating a 'soft tissue tenodesis'. Alternatively, once a tenotomy has been performed, a mini-open approach may be used to tenodese the remnant biceps tendon to the humerus using an endo-button or an interference screw.

Postoperative management is the same as for a decompression; however, patients who have a tenodesis should avoid resisted biceps activities for up to 6 weeks.

Recommended reference

Moon SC, Cho NS, Rhee YG. Analysis of "hidden lesions" of the extra-articular biceps after subpectoral biceps tenodesis: the subpectoral portion as the optimal tenodesis site. *Am J Sports Med*. 2015 Jan;**43(1)**:63–68.

Rotator cuff repair

Despite large trials showing no difference in outcomes between mini-open and arthroscopic rotator cuff repairs, the latter has become increasingly popular. Techniques and experience have improved such that even massive and retracted cuff tears can be repaired arthroscopically. Indications include

- Shoulder pain, including night pain on a background of a chronic tear
- Loss of function or quality of life
- Traumatic rotator cuff tear
- Failure of conservative management of a chronic rotator cuff tear

Many options exist to treat cuff tears, including anterior deltoid strengthening alone, suprascapular nerve ablation, partial cuff repair, superior capsular reconstruction and even a reverse polarity joint replacement. Patient age, expectations and severity of the tear should all be taken into account when making a decision on how to proceed.

Risks

In addition to the previously mentioned, patients should be warned of damage to nerves (e.g. axillary or suprascapular), stiffness, reduced range of movement, failure of the repair, re-rupture and continued weakness.

Procedure

Posterior, anterior, lateral and accessory lateral portals are often required. The superior Neviaser portal can be useful for passing sutures through the cuff, particularly in massive tears. Glenohumeral arthroscopy is performed and any concurrent pathology assessed and treated as necessary. The cuff is then assessed with respect to its size, shape and mobility. The arthroscope is inserted into the subacromial space and a subacromial decompression (with or without ACJ excision) is performed as necessary. Any releases are then undertaken and the footprint is prepared with the vaporiser and burr, so the exposed bone bleeds, helping the rotator cuff to heal.

Various techniques are described for tendon fixation. The type of anchor and whether a single- or double-row fixation is used remains debatable. However, the principle is to have a large contact area between the tendon and the bone to encourage healing. To achieve this a variety of arthroscopic instruments are required. The suture anchor is inserted percutaneously or through the superolateral portal, such that the correct bone entry angle is achieved. During anchor placement the choice of viewing portal is often determined by the size of the tear with small or partial tears requiring an intra-articular camera position and larger tears requiring visualisation from the subacromial space. The sutures can now be passed using antegrade techniques, using suture passers, or with retrograde techniques where penetrators or suture shuttling instruments are used. When passing sutures, a posterior or lateral viewing portal is used depending on the size and location of the tear.

Sutures are placed approximately 1 cm apart. Suture management is critical in rotator cuff repairs as it is easy to confuse or tangle the sutures. To avoid difficulties only two sutures should be used per portal and if a cannula is not used then sutures must be passed through the same portal together to avoid interposing soft tissue when tying knots. Knot tying is done under direct vision in the subacromial space. Alternatively, knotless techniques may be employed.

For large and massive tears, side-to-side convergence sutures can be used to reduce the size of the tear (**Figure 6.4**). Retracted tears can be mobilised using interval slides. The final construct can be viewed from both the subacromial space and the glenohumeral joint to ensure footprint reconstruction.

Closures of cannula portals are more likely to require sutures. The postoperative regimen depends on the size of the tear, and of course surgeon preference.

- Small and medium tears
  - Sling for 6 weeks
  - Passive/active assisted exercises to 30° external rotation (if no subscapularis tear) and elevation to 90° for first 6 weeks
  - Passive overhead elevation at 6 weeks with further increase in external rotation as able
  - Active exercises once range is normal and strengthening at 12 weeks
- Large/massive tears
  - Immobilise in sling (with or without abduction pillow) sling for 6 weeks
  - Passive/active assisted exercises – elevation to 90° and external rotation to 0° in the presence of a subscapularis repair, otherwise 30° for first 6 weeks

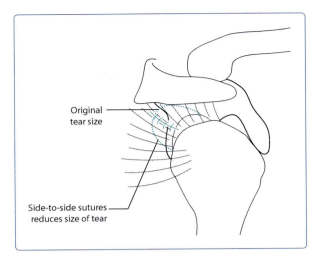

Figure 6.4 Side-to-side sutures used to reduce the size of a rotator cuff tear.

- Passive overhead elevation at 6 weeks with further increase in external rotation as able
- Active exercises at 12 weeks and strengthening at 16 weeks

Arthroscopic soft tissue repair for instability

The glenohumeral joint is the most likely joint to dislocate and recent evidence has moved many units to offering earlier surgical intervention with a view to prevent recurrent dislocations and maintain bone stock. Of all the types of shoulder instability, acute traumatic anterior dislocations fare best with surgical intervention, and multidirectional atraumatic fare the worst. In cases of significant bone loss, bony procedures are generally most suitable.

Risks

Patients should be consented for recurrence, stiffness, early arthritis, neurovascular injury and cuff pathology, particularly in posterior repairs.

Procedure

Prior to commencing the operation, shoulder stability should be assessed with an examination under anaesthesia. The humeral head is translated anteriorly and posteriorly, the direction noted and its excursion graded and documented:

- 1 – Minimal
- 2 – To the edge of the labrum
- 3 – Dislocates

A standard posterior viewing portal is used to assess the labral and capsular pathology. Using an outside-in technique, an anterosuperolateral portal is placed at the junction of the anterior border of the supraspinatus tendon and the upper rotator interval. It should allow a 45° angle of approach to the superior labrum. This will provide both an anterior viewing portal and an accessory portal for SLAP repairs or for suture management.

A further anterior portal is placed just above the subscapularis tendon for anterior repairs and in posterior repairs, a Wilmington portal should be created with a longitudinal split in the infraspinatus tendon. Both are placed such that the angle of approach allows accurate suture anchor placement. This can be best assessed using the anterosuperior viewing portal. A clear cannula is recommended for better visualisation.

The degree of tissue separation and amount of capsular laxity are assessed. The drive-through sign is noted. This reflects the ease with which the scope is passed between the humeral head and the glenoid and is a sign of significant laxity. Whether anterior or posterior, the Bankart lesion (i.e. detached labrum) is released all the way down to the 6 o'clock position on the glenoid with sharp elevators. A sufficient release is confirmed by grabbing the inferior tissue with a manipulator and elevating it superiorly against the glenoid rim. The anterior or posterior glenoid is decorticated with a rasp and burr or shaver (ensure that suction is clamped during this stage).

Anchors are then sequentially placed, starting from an inferior position. Anteriorly the first should be at the 5 o'clock position on the glenoid rim and posteriorly at the 7 o'clock position. A suture is passed through the tissue inferiorly using a penetrator or suture shuttle technique. The amount of tissue included in the suture is critical, as it will dictate the degree of stability following the repair. To help reduce the labral tissue back to the glenoid rim the knot can be tied with the arm in flexion and internal rotation for anterior repairs and abduction and external rotation for posterior repairs. Capsular plication (weaving of sutures through the capsule) can also be performed in cases of marked capsular laxity. Further anchors are placed at 4 and 3 o'clock positions anteriorly or 8 and 9 o'clock positions posteriorly to approximate the labrum and perform a distal to proximal shift of the capsule (**Figure 6.5**). Anterior repairs should aim for a south to north shift to prevent over-tightening of the shoulder.

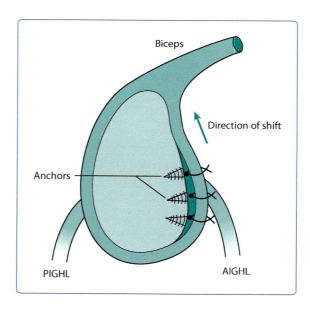

Figure 6.5 Capsulolabral reconstruction with anterior inferior glenohumeral ligament reconstruction (AIGHL). PIGHL, posterior IGHL.

Postoperatively, patients should be placed in a poly sling or brace. These should aim to prevent external rotation in anterior repairs and internal rotation in posterior repairs. Often if the repair is not in too much tension, a body belt or external rotation brace can be avoided. Pendulum exercises can start in the first week, progressing to active rotation after 4 weeks, depending on surgeon and physiotherapy preferences.

Capsular release

Adhesive capsulitis is a common and debilitating pathology. Lots of interest has developed as to the merits of surgical release rather than physiotherapy and hydrodilation alone. While it is generally a self-limiting pathology, the desire to return to function faster with an increased residual range of movement is a relative indication. Care should be taken to rule out the other two main causes of a lack of external glenohumeral rotation: shoulder osteoarthritis and a locked posterior dislocation.

Risks

Capsular releases require a large amount of tissue dissection so the risk of damage to the intra-articular structures and surrounding nerves increases. A manipulation under anaesthesia risks fracturing the proximal humerus.

Procedure

Preoperative range of movement should be assessed by locking the scapula through palpation of the acromion and coracoid process. Standard anterior and posterior viewing portals are created, which can be particularly difficult given the thickened and fibrosed capsule.

Once inside the joint, a shaver, burr and capsular punch can all be used to excise the fibrosed capsule. The majority of work is performed anteriorly by taking down the rotator interval, to the conjoint tendon, coracoid process and anterior deltoid. The LHB may be tethered in scar tissue and if so should be freed. If this does not suffice, the superior, posterior or inferior capsule may be excised. Once finished, the shoulder should be manipulated using a short lever arm to prevent fracture. Once the patient has had their wounds closed and a pressure dressing applied, elevation in a Bradford sling helps to maintain mobility. Demonstrating the increased range of movement to a patient prior to the block wearing off often helps with the rehabilitation.

Postoperative physiotherapy should commence as soon as possible. Patients should be warned that approximately half of the obtained range of movement would remain long term.

Recommended reference

Brealey S, Armstrong AL, Brooksbank A et al. United Kingdom Frozen Shoulder Trial (UK FROST), multi-centre, randomised, 12 month, parallel group, superiority study to compare the clinical and cost-effectiveness of Early Structured Physiotherapy versus manipulation under anaesthesia versus arthroscopic capsular release for patients referred to secondary care with a primary frozen shoulder: Study protocol for a randomised controlled trial. *Trials*. 2017;**18**:614.

Open shoulder procedures

Many of the now performed arthroscopic procedures were for many years successfully performed utilising open techniques. While arthroscopic procedures are less invasive and traumatic, they remain difficult to master. Knowledge of their limitations is important, as are their 'bail-out' options, most of which are open techniques. In this section of the chapter, we describe the principles of open techniques of the aforementioned procedures.

Acromioplasty

The principles are much the same as arthroscopic. In cases of significant cuff tears, acromioplasty should be avoided as loss of the anterior structures may lead to anterosuperior escape of the humeral head.

Risks

Risks include

- Infection
- Neurovascular injury
- Stiffness
- *Fracture of the acromion*: Can occur if the osteotomy is performed in the wrong plane or if excess bone is resected
- Detachment of the deltoid
- *Failure of procedure*: Wrong indications, incomplete decompression, missed cuff tear

Procedure

Anaesthesia is usually general, regional or combined. Where general anaesthesia is used alone, local anaesthetic is recommended for pain relief. The patient is in the beach chair position. A small sandbag is put under the operated shoulder. An arm board can be attached to the side of the table to rest the arm on. The surgical field is prepared and adequately draped.

Landmarks include the

- Acromioclavicular joint
- Anterolateral corner of acromion
- Tip of the coracoid

This procedure is rarely performed as an isolated open procedure as it is most commonly performed arthroscopically or in association with a larger open procedure. As such, the skin incision will be dictated by the other procedure; however, if it is to be performed as an isolated open procedure, a 2–3 cm anterosuperior incision is made over the anterior acromion. The incision is continued through subcutaneous fat and down to the deltoid fascia. The anterior deltoid raphe is split in the line of its fibres. The anterior acromion is located and then an osteoperiosteal flap raised such that a strong deltoid repair can be performed at the end of the procedure.

Deep to the anterolateral tip of the acromion is the coracoacromial ligament. A swab can be used to sweep the soft tissue medially further exposing the ligament and separating its medial border from the clavipectoral fascia. An oscillating saw is used to excise the anteroinferior acromion. The osteotomy is aimed so that it is in continuation with the undersurface of the acromion (**Figure 6.6**). The bony fragment, with its attached coracoacromial ligament, is excised. Traction is applied to the patient's arm and the undersurface of the acromion is smoothed using bone nibblers. The underlying rotator cuff should then be examined for any associated pathology.

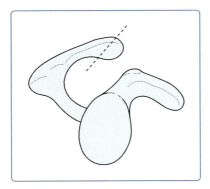

Figure 6.6 The correct orientation for the acromion osteotomy.

A good deltoid reconstruction is essential. If the quality of the osteoperiosteal flaps is poor, a transosseous repair using number 2 Ethibond is performed followed by subcutaneous 2/0 Vicryl and 3/0 Monocryl to skin.

Postoperative care and instructions

Passive-/active-assisted exercises are started from day 1 – 90° forward elevation and 30° external rotation for 3 weeks increasing to full range by 6 weeks. Strengthening exercises can be started at 6 weeks and repetitive overhead exercises at 3 months.

Acromioclavicular joint (ACJ) excision

Open ACJ excisions are indicated as revision procedures or when the orientation of an ACJ precludes arthroscopic resection.

Procedure

If performed in combination with an open acromioplasty, the same approach as previously described is made, although the incision and subsequent dissection will need to be extended medially. If performed in isolation, a 2–3 cm strap incision is made over the distal clavicle and then a transverse incision is made in the deltotrapezoidal fascia to expose the ACJ.

Retractors are placed to expose the distal clavicle and then an oscillating saw is used to resect enough distal clavicle such that there is a 10 mm gap between the medial acromion and the resected distal clavicle (**Figure 6.7**). Care must be taken not to resect too much distal clavicle otherwise distal clavicular instability can occur. Any osteophytes on the undersurface of the acromion are trimmed with bone nibblers and any residual meniscus removed.

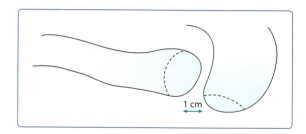

Figure 6.7 Excision of the acromioclavicular joint.

The superior acromioclavicular ligament and deltotrapezoidal fascia are then repaired. If performed in association with an acromioplasty, the deltoid is repaired in the manner already discussed.

Rotator cuff repair

Open cuff repairs are often considered if the tear is large and retracted, or when used in combination with other procedures. It is imperative to understand the principles of open surgery for the cases where arthroscopy is not possible. Preoperative planning and consent are much the same as in open procedures, although there is a greater risk of neurovascular injury.

Procedure

The patient is essentially set up the same as for an arthroscopic procedure. The important landmarks are

- Acromioclavicular joint
- Anterolateral and posterolateral corners of acromion
- Tip of coracoid

The patient is in the beach chair position. A small sandbag is put under the shoulder. An arm board can be attached to the side of the table to rest the arm on. The surgical field is prepared and adequately draped.

> ### Structure at risk
>
> The axillary nerve is approximately 5 cm distal to the lateral acromion and therefore the inferior limit of any incision must not extend beyond this point. This position corresponds to the lower limit of the inferior reflection of the subdeltoid bursa.

An anterosuperior approach is used. An 8 cm incision is made just posterior to the anterior aspect of the ACJ and is directed towards the anterolateral corner of the acromion and down the anterior deltoid raphe. A smaller incision can be performed if an arthroscopic decompression has already been performed such that a mini-open procedure can be undertaken.

The deltoid is bluntly split at the anterior raphe (junction of the anterior and middle thirds). The deltoid is detached off the anterior acromion with an osteoperiosteal sleeve. The bursa is split longitudinally. The inferior reflection of the bursa denotes the position of the axillary nerve, which can be palpated and avoided thereafter (**Figure 6.8**). The coracoacromial ligament is detached from the undersurface of the acromion.

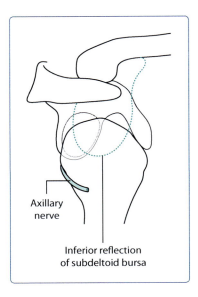

Figure 6.8 The relationship of the subdeltoid bursa to the axillary nerve.

Anterior acromioplasty (with or without ACJ excision) can be carried out as required. The size of the tear is measured and traction sutures are placed through the cuff. The cuff is then mobilised sequentially, initially with blunt dissection; however, a sharp release of the superior capsule and the coracohumeral ligament may be necessary. In massive retracted tears anterior and posterior interval slides may also be necessary. These can also be performed arthroscopically such that only a mini-open approach need be adopted. The configuration and tension of the mobilised cuff tear are then assessed in order to plan the repair. A shallow bony trough/footprint is prepared using an osteotome (or burr in a mini-open) at the level of tendon insertion. This should be made just lateral to the articular surface. The method of the tendon repair is determined by the operating surgeon. Single- and double-row anchor repairs can be undertaken depending on the size of the tear or alternatively a transosseous suture repair can be performed. In the latter method the tendon is repaired with a number 2 Ethibond Mason Allen suture. In each method the aim is to achieve healing of the tendon to the footprint.

A good deltoid reconstruction is essential. If the quality of the osteoperiosteal flaps is poor a transosseous deltoid repair, using number 2 Ethibond, is performed. The deltoid raphe should be closed with 2/0 Vicryl and then 2/0 Vicryl for closure of the subcutaneous tissues and 3/0 Monocryl to skin.

Acromioclavicular joint reconstruction

ACJ disruptions are being increasingly treated non-operatively in line with recent literature, with Rockwood grade III and IV disruptions not necessarily requiring acute surgery. If the disruption becomes symptomatic at a later date, the ACJ can be reconstructed. There are several options for reconstruction, using either allograft, autograft or synthetic materials. These can be used in the modified Weaver-Dunn (described later), a LARS ligament, Tightrope or a Lockdown procedure. Using autografts or allografts should be avoided where the donor tendon has the potential towards hyperlaxity. Describing all procedures is outside the remit of this chapter. Instead we discuss the modified Weaver-Dunn procedure, as it is popular with the authors.

Risks

Infection, neurovascular injury, stiffness and recurrent instability are all possible. Postoperative rehabilitation protocols tend to be demanding so the correct patient should be selected for surgery.

Procedure

Anaesthesia is usually general, regional or combined. Where general anaesthesia is used alone, local anaesthetic is recommended for postoperative pain relief.

The patient is placed in the beach chair position. A small sandbag is put under the shoulder. An arm board can be attached to the side of the table to rest the arm on. The surgical field is prepared and adequately draped. Landmarks include the

- ACJ
- Anterolateral corner of the acromion
- Tip of coracoid

The technique will vary depending on whether an acute or chronic injury is being addressed. Acute injuries do not require a ligament transfer procedure as part of the reconstruction. Chronic injuries are best managed with a biological reconstruction, which is supplemented by another fixation device until healing has occurred approximately 3 months after repair. A strap incision is made, 1 cm medial to the ACJ, and extending down to the coracoid.

The deltotrapezoidal fascia is incised longitudinally along the distal clavicle with an extension across the superior acromioclavicular capsule/ligament and further laterally over the anterior acromion. The deltoid fibres are elevated off the clavicle and, at the acromion, an osteoperiosteal flap is raised to aid later repair. The coracoacromial ligament is defined by sweeping bluntly laterally with a swab. It is then detached from the acromion with a sliver of bone. It is then mobilised down to the coracoid and a whipstitch applied to the ligament with number 2 Ethibond. The distal 1 cm of the clavicle is excised obliquely with an oscillating saw. The bone fragment is retained for later autologous bone graft.

The clavicle is reduced to its anatomical position by reducing the arm back up to the clavicle and by further reducing the clavicle downwards and forwards. This position must be maintained prior to the ligament transfer. This can be achieved by a number of techniques, including a Bosworth screw, three strands of PDS cord (Johnson & Johnson) looped around the coracoid and clavicle or, with a TightRope reconstruction device (Arthrex Inc; Naples, Florida).

Once held in the reduced position two 2 mm drill holes are then made in the superior cortex of the clavicle. The bony fragment of the acromioclavicular ligament is passed into the intramedullary canal and the two sutures are passed through the holes, tensioned and tied (**Figure 6.9**). An autograft from the resected distal clavicle is then used to graft any redundant space around the transferred ligament.

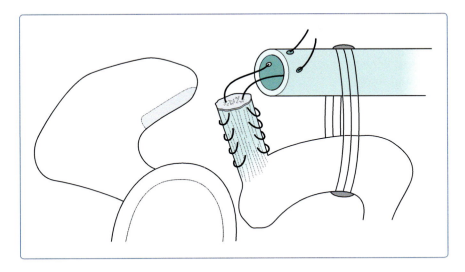

Figure 6.9 Acromioclavicular joint reconstruction.

In acute cases (<3-4 weeks after injury) the coracoclavicular ligaments and superior acromioclavicular capsule/ligament can be repaired and then supplemented with one of the stabilising techniques described earlier. A Weaver-Dunn ligament transfer is not required.

A good deltotrapezoidal reconstruction is essential. If the quality of the anterior acromial osteoperiosteal flap is poor, a transosseous repair using number 2 Ethibond is performed and in cases with significant superior migration of the clavicle any redundant deltotrapezoidal fascia can undergo a 'double-breasted' repair with 1 Vicryl adding further superior support to the reconstruction; 2/0 Vicryl is used for closure of the subcutaneous tissues and 3/0 Monocryl is used for skin.

Postoperative regimens should include

- Six weeks in a sling with passive, and active assisted, forward elevation to 90° and external rotation to 30°
- Progress to active shoulder movement, below shoulder height, from 6 weeks with passive stretching above shoulder height at 10 weeks
- Strengthening at 12 weeks

Soft tissue stabilisation

Arthroscopic stabilisation has largely superseded open procedures, but the outcomes are still comparable, particularly in experienced hands. Indications are similar to those described earlier. Similar to arthroscopic procedures, the shoulder may be stabilised from the front or back depending on the location of the pathology.

Anterior stabilisation

Risks

These are similar to that presented earlier, and include

- Stiffness, particularly loss of external rotation
- Recurrence
- Subscapularis detachment
- Neurovascular injury

Procedure

Anaesthesia is usually general, regional or combined. Where general anaesthesia is used alone, local anaesthetic is recommended postoperatively to aid pain relief. The patient is placed in the beach chair position. A small sandbag is put under the medial scapula of the operated shoulder (this helps to externally rotate the shoulder and 'open' the anterior shoulder joint). An arm board can be attached to the side of the table to rest the arm. The surgical field is prepared and adequately draped and an examination under anaesthesia is performed.

The skin incision runs in the deltopectoral groove, from the coracoid to the axillary fold (with the arm adducted and internally rotated). The subcutaneous tissue is reflected with sharp and electrocautery dissection, exposing the deltopectoral interval which is marked by a fatty streak and the cephalic vein. The fascia overlying the interval is divided and the cephalic vein lateralised with the deltoid muscle. The deltoid and pectoralis major are then defined with sharp and electrocautery dissection.

> ### Structure at risk
>
> - Musculocutaneous nerve – in danger from excessive traction

A retractor can be placed over the coracoid process to enhance the exposure and the clavipectoral fascia is then split vertically starting just lateral to the coracoid. This exposes the conjoint tendon. If required, the lateral third of the conjoint tendon can be divided to allow better exposure (by not detaching the coracoid or the tendon fully, the musculocutaneous nerve is protected from excessive traction). A self-retainer is placed between the coracoid/conjoint tendon medially and the deltoid muscle laterally. The arm is externally rotated to expose the subscapularis muscle. The upper two-thirds of the subscapularis can then be tenotomized approximately 1 cm from its insertion in the lesser tuberosity and dissected free of the underlying capsule. This plane is more easily found inferiorly and becomes easier as the dissection progresses medially. Alternatively, the subscapularis can be split horizontally and retracted, exposing the underlying capsule.

The capsulorrhaphy must now be undertaken. This can be performed either laterally or medially. It is the authors' preference to perform this medially as we feel it gives a more accurate anatomical reconstruction and a more reproducible elimination of the axillary pouch. To achieve a large inferior capsular shift the capsule must be dissected off all of its muscular attachments inferiorly and, indeed, postero-inferiorly in cases of marked laxity. This is best achieved with McIndoe scissors. A bone lever can then be placed inferior to the humeral neck thus protecting the axillary nerve. Depending on the degree of laxity the capsulorrhaphy can involve either a vertical capsular incision or, in cases of greater laxity, a medially based 'T'.

The capsule is split vertically 7–10 mm from the glenoid rim, with a further horizontal incision made midway along the capsule as necessary (**Figure 6.10**). Two stay sutures are placed to mark the superior and inferior apices of the flaps. A Fakuda retractor is used to displace the humeral head posteriorly such that the anterior labrum is exposed. The presence of a Bankart lesion, and the degree of capsule-labral disruption, can now be visualised.

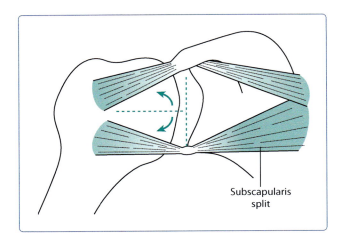

Figure 6.10 The medial 'T'-shaped capsular incision.

The anterior glenoid neck is decorticated using a narrow osteotome or burr, and anchors are used to reattach the anterior labrum to the decorticated area of the glenoid neck. The capsular flaps are overlapped so that the inferior flap is taken superiorly and medially such that it is sutured to the medial capsule. A double-breasted suture technique using 1 Vicryl should be used. The superior flap is then sutured inferiorly taking care not to medialize the flap otherwise external rotation will be restricted. The rotator interval is then closed (**Figure 6.11**).

During the repair, the arm should be held in 30° of external rotation and abduction so that the repair is not over-tightened thus causing postoperative stiffness. Adequate stability and a good passive range of motion should be confirmed before the wounds are closed.

If a large, engaging Hill-Sachs lesion is present a bone block procedure (Bristow-Latarjet or iliac crest bone graft) will be required to increase the depth of the glenoid to prevent recurrent dislocation. A soft tissue procedure alone will not be adequate to restore stability.

If previously tenotomised, the subscapularis should be repaired with number 2 Ethibond. Thereafter, a layered closure using 2/0 Vicryl for the subcutaneous tissues and 3/0 Monocryl to skin is used.

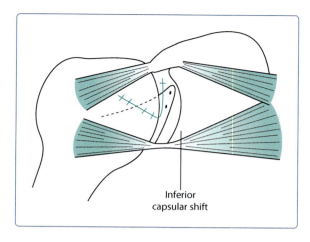

Figure 6.11 Medially based inferior capsular shift.

Posterior stabilisation

Cases of posterior instability will warrant a posterior reconstructive procedure.

Risks

These are much the same as earlier. The posterior circumflex humeral artery and axillary nerve run together in the quadrilateral space, below teres minor. It is therefore safe provided that the correct plane of dissection is used.

Procedure

Anaesthesia is usually general, regional or combined. The patient is positioned in the prone position. A 15 cm posterior vertical incision, which extends over the spine of the scapula in the plane of the ACJ gives good access to posterior structures of the shoulder.

Posteriorly, the deltoid has a tendinous insertion onto the posterior spine of the scapula. This can be incised and reflected inferiorly giving good access to the underlying infraspinatus and teres minor tendons. More laterally an osteoperiosteal flap should be raised off the posterior lateral corner of the acromion with, if necessary, a further extension down the posterior deltoid raphe. The interval between the infraspinatus and teres minor can be developed by blunt dissection exposing the posterior capsule.

The procedure for the repair of a posterior labral injury and/or capsular laxity is similar to that described for an anteriorly based injury. A medial or laterally based capsulorrhaphy can be performed although we favour the former for the reasons described earlier.

The infraspinatus and teres minor do not need formal closure; however, meticulous repair of the deltoid should be undertaken. Thereafter, 2/0 Vicryl to superficial tissues and 3/0 Monocryl to skin are advocated.

A poly sling with body belt is used for the first 4 weeks. At 4 weeks, the body belt is removed and pendular exercises started. At 6 weeks passive stretching exercises are undertaken aiming for full elevation but only half the external rotation of the contralateral side by 3 months. Strengthening exercises are begun at 6 weeks. Contact sports must be avoided for 6–9 months.

Bony stabilisations

In cases of significant bone loss, the threshold of which is around 13% of the glenoid, bony stabilisation procedures are preferred. They fall into two main groups: bone block (Eden-Hybinette – can be anterior or posterior) and anterior coracoid transfers (Latarjet and Bristow). Bone blocks aim to provide stability by increasing the rim of the glenoid, whereas coracoid transfers work in three main ways:

1. Providing a dynamic sling by strengthening the inferior subscapularis muscle through transfer of the conjoint tendon
2. Repair of the capsule and augmentation of the coracoacromial ligament
3. Reconstruction of the glenoid face through transferring the coracoid

While all of these can be done arthroscopically, the benefit over an open procedure is currently questionable. We describe the open Latarjet, which is the most commonly performed.

Risks

General risks described earlier to open soft tissue stabilisations apply here too. There is however also a risk of non-union of the coracoid, early osteoarthritis (particularly if the graft is too lateral) and recurrent instability (particularly if the graft is too medial). The musculocutaneous nerve is particularly at risk as it runs inferomedial to the coracoid, and the axillary nerve is similarly at risk coursing medial to and inferior to the subscapularis.

Procedure

The patient is set up supine with a sandbag between the shoulder blades to bring the glenoid neck into view. A deltopectoral approach is utilised, as already described. The coracoid is identified and the pectoralis minor attaching medially is released, as is the coracoacromio ligament laterally. An osteotomy is then performed to release the coracoid, using an oscillating saw and osteotomes. The conjoint tendon is gently freed from the underlying structures, taking care to protect the musculocutaneous nerve. The coracoid is then turned so that the inferior portion will eventually point to the glenoid. The coracoid is prepared with pre-drilled holes to use later and tucked into the wound.

Attention is turned to the glenoid. Abducting and externally rotating the arm brings the subscapularis muscle into better view. It is split along the border of its superior two-thirds and inferior third. This is extended towards the tendon and held apart using a Gelpi retractor.

An L- or T-shaped capsulotomy is then performed exposing the anterior glenoid. A burr is used to prepare it for the coracoid transfer; bone is removed to a bleeding edge. Ensuring an optimal position of the coracoid is fundamental to the working of the Latarjet: it must be flush with the face of the glenoid. A Fakuda retractor can be used to aid this process.

Once the position of the coracoid is confirmed, two screws should be passed through the coracoid and into the glenoid. These should be tightened sequentially.

The capsule is repaired and the wound closed in a similar manner to the previous descriptions. Bone wax over the coracoid stump may help control bleeding.

Postoperatively the patient should be placed in a sling for 3 weeks, after which stretches and strengthening exercises may begin. After 6 weeks, the patient may progress their range of movement and resistance exercises.

Shoulder arthroplasty

Shoulder arthroplasty can be used to effectively treat advanced degenerative joint disease and unreconstructable trauma cases. The three main types of arthroplasty are humeral hemiarthroplasties, anatomic total shoulder replacements and reverse polarity shoulder replacements. The indication, age of the patient and integrity of the rotator cuff are all important in deciding between the types. Hemiarthroplasties are essentially a humeral replacement of the total anatomical replacement leaving the glenoid intact, and thus are not considered further. Reverse polarity shoulder replacements are indicated in cuff-deficient shoulders. They replace the humeral head with a socket and the glenoid with a glenosphere, with an aim of shifting the centre of rotation of shoulder medially and inferiorly, thus improving the lever arm of the deltoid.

The approach and preparation of the humerus and glenoid are similar for all arthroplasties, so they are considered together and the nuances explained.

Common indications
- Osteoarthritis
- Inflammatory arthritis
- Avascular necrosis
- Trauma – proximal humeral fractures
- Postinfective arthritis
- Instability arthropathy
- Cuff tear arthropathy
- Arthritis secondary to glenoid dysplasia or epiphyseal dysplasia

Contraindications
- Active infection

Risks
Patients should be counselled as to the short-, medium- and long-term risks. These should include

- Infection
- Neurovascular injury
- Stiffness
- Aseptic loosening

- Fracture
- Revision
- Acromial fracture

Procedure

Anaesthesia can be general, regional or combined. Where general anaesthesia is used alone, additional local anaesthetic infiltration or patient-controlled anaesthesia is recommended for pain relief. Antibiotics are given at induction. The patient is placed in the reclining beach chair position and pulled to the side to allow extension and rotation of the arm. A small sandbag is put under the shoulder. The surgical field is prepared and draped.

Landmarks include

- Acromioclavicular joint
- Anterolateral/posterolateral corners of acromion
- Coracoid

Two approaches are possible for shoulder arthroplasty. These are the deltopectoral and the anterosuperior approaches.

Deltopectoral

An incision is made from coracoid toward the axillary fold, extending laterally to the anterior arm. The subcutaneous tissue is reflected with sharp and electrocautery dissection exposing the deltopectoral interval, which is marked by a fatty streak and the cephalic vein. The fascia overlying the interval is divided and the cephalic vein lateralised with the deltoid muscle. In a tight shoulder the pectoralis major tendon can be released at its superior border taking care not to injure the underlying biceps tendon.

> ### *Structures at risk*
>
> The cephalic vein is at risk when entering the deltopectoral interval. The axillary and musculocutaneous nerves are in danger from excessive traction.

To enhance the exposure a retractor can be placed over the coracoid process and then the clavipectoral fascia is split vertically starting just lateral to the coracoid, extending the incision just lateral to the conjoint tendon and its muscle belly.

To improve external rotation the coracohumeral ligament should also be released at its coracoid origin. The deltoid is then mobilised from the tissues of the subacromial space and retracted posterolaterally. Provided that the retractors are placed above the inferior subdeltoid, bursal reflection of the axillary nerve should be safe. If better access is required, as may be the case with a medialized glenoid, the lateral third of the conjoint tendon can be divided to allow better exposure or alternatively a coracoid tip osteotomy can be performed. However, care should be taken not to retract the conjoint tendon excessively as this could put the musculocutaneous nerve at risk. The arm is externally rotated to expose the subscapularis muscle.

The anterior circumflex humeral vessels, which are found at the inferior border of the subscapularis tendon, are then ligated if necessary. The axillary nerve can be exposed so that its position is known and avoided during the remainder of the procedure.

The degree of external rotation that can be achieved should now be assessed. If this is deficient then a subscapularis lengthening procedure may be required. This may involve a layered subscapularis tenotomy or 'Z plasty', and this will need to be planned at this stage. If external rotation is adequate the subscapularis tendon is then tenotomised 1 cm medial to its humeral insertion and raised on stay sutures. This can be taken as one layer with the underlying capsule. In order to lengthen the subscapularis the rotator interval will need to be incised and then the capsule will need to be released from the glenoid neck. Protecting the subscapularis is fundamental to the functioning of both anatomical and reverse prostheses, as the subscapularis-infraspinatus force couple centre the components.

As the capsule is incised an inferior capsular release can be performed, and provided that the axillary nerve has already been identified the nerve should not be at risk. A blunt retractor can be placed inferiorly to protect the nerve and then the humeral head is dislocated anteriorly by applying gentle external rotation to the arm. The LHB tendon should be inspected and tenotomised or tenodesed as necessary. It is often torn in cases of advanced arthritis.

The head is then prepared by removing any osteophytes so that the true anatomical neck of the humerus can be identified. Further preparation will vary depending on the implant; however, the principles are that

1. As much of the tuberosities as possible are retained, important for rotational control of the implant.
2. Enough bone must be resected to allow a suitable implant to function optimally.
3. The arm length should be restored.

For the purpose of this description, a standard stemmed implant will be used. An oscillating saw is used to resect the humeral head at its anatomical neck. If this has been adequately demarcated during preparation, it can be done freehand, otherwise jigs should be used such that the height and version of the resection are appropriate. The resected humeral head is then used as a guide for the size of the subsequent humeral head replacement in the case of an anatomical replacement. With the head resected the remainder of the circumferential glenoid release can be performed and the glenoid inspected. Some implant systems advocate preparation of the humerus at this point, but not definitive implantation, rather a cap can be placed over a prepared humerus to offer protection while glenoid preparation takes place.

Once the capsule is released there should be adequate space to approach the glenoid perpendicular to its face such that preparation can be achieved with the appropriate implant jigs. The labrum and surrounding osteophytes should be excised to aid exposure. Excising the inferior lip of the glenoid may aid implant positioning. The process of this preparation will vary according to the implant. To assess the true version of the glenoid it is useful to place a narrow retractor down the anterior glenoid neck so that the axis of the glenoid is known prior to definitive glenoid preparation. Preoperative planning and templating will aid this step.

If not already done so, the humerus can now be prepared using sequentially sized rasps and when the appropriate size is established a trial prosthesis can be constructed and inserted into the humerus. After reducing the implant the surgeon should check the offset, version and soft tissue tension of the trial prosthesis and if satisfactory the definitive prosthesis can be implanted.

Anterosuperior

An 8 cm incision is started just posterior to the front of the ACJ, directed towards the anterolateral corner of the acromion and down the anterolateral deltoid.

> **Structure at risk**
>
> Axillary nerve – 5 cm below the lateral acromion (below the inferior reflection of the subdeltoid bursa).

The deltoid is bluntly split at the anterior raphe (the junction of anterior and middle third of the deltoid). The deltoid is detached off the anterior acromion with an osteoperiosteal sleeve. This is extended medially to the ACJ. The subdeltoid bursa is split longitudinally palpating the inferior bursal reflection which denotes the position of the axillary nerve.

The coracoacromial ligament is detached from the undersurface of the acromion. Anterior acromioplasty and ACJ excision can be carried out if required.

Blunt soft tissue release is carried out around the cuff. The coracohumeral ligament is released at its coracoid origin. This improves the external rotation. With the arm in external rotation, a bone retractor is inserted on the medial side of the humeral neck, marking the inferior border of the subscapularis muscle. This is detached laterally from its insertion to the lesser tuberosity together with the capsule. Stay sutures are inserted.

If a biceps tenodesis is required, a stay suture is placed and the tendon cut. The humeral head is dislocated anteriorly with external rotation and extension. A Bankart skid is placed between the glenoid and the head. Osteophytes are excised. A bone spike is inserted on the medial side of the humeral neck, under the subscapularis to protect the axillary nerve. Humeral and glenoid preparation is then performed as previously described.

Closure

During closure, the subscapularis tendon is repaired using number 2 Ethibond with the arm held in a position of 30° external rotation. This prevents over-tightening of the tendon repair. A deltoid repair is then performed to the anterior acromion if the anterosuperior approach was used. A 2/0 Vicryl to the subcutaneous tissues and 3/0 Monocryl to skin completes the closure.

Postoperative

A poly sling is used for 6 weeks. Recommended are passive and active assisted exercises to 90° of forward elevation and external rotation to 0° for 6 weeks. Full passive movement to re-establish full range is recommended thereafter followed by active ranging and strengthening exercises as able.

Viva questions

1. What are the treatment options for an irrepairable rotator cuff tear in a 70 year old patient with minimal arthritis?
2. How does a reverse polarity shoulder replacement work?
3. How would you counsel a 16 year old aspiring professional rugby player following a first time traumatic anterior shoulder dislocation?

7 Surgery of the Elbow

Alan Salih, David Butt and Deborah Higgs

Radial head replacement	113	Elbow aspiration/injection	152
Total elbow arthroplasty	123	Elbow arthroscopy	154
Open elbow arthrolysis	137	Viva question	158
Tennis/golfer's elbow release	142		
Lateral collateral ligament reconstruction	148		

	Range of motion	Functional range of motion
Flexion	150°	130°
Extension	0°	30°
Pronation	80°	50°
Supination	80°	50°

Position of arthrodesis
- There is no fixed position of arthrodesis.
- Many authors recommend 90°.
- 110° may be best for activities of daily living, but 60° may suit work activities.

The deep surgical approaches to the elbow may be achieved through a single 'utility' posterior incision or through separate incisions. The approaches described here may be used in their entirety or in part, depending on the anatomy required to be exposed for each procedure. We focus on the approaches that will prove useful for common elbow operations, but this is not an exhaustive collection of all approaches described.

Radial head replacement
Preoperative planning
Indications
- Fractures not amenable to fixation (e.g. >3 fragments) with valgus instability due to medial collateral ligament insufficiency

- Radial head fracture with concurrent distal radioulnar joint injury (Essex-Lopresti injury)
- Instability following radial head resection

Contraindications

- Radial head/neck fractures with no associated injuries can be treated with excision of the radial head.
- Wear or extensive injury to the capitellum chondral surface.
- Inadequate bone and soft tissues around the implant.

> ### Consent and risks
> - Nerve injury
> - Infection
> - Aseptic loosening
> - 'Understuffing' radiocapitellar joint: Recurrent or ongoing instability
> - 'Overstuffing' radiocapitellar joint with increased joint pressure: Pain and stiffness
> - Osteoarthritis

Operative planning

Anteroposterior and lateral radiographs less than 6 months old should be available. Silicone implants are no longer recommended due to high rates of osteolysis and implant fracture.

Other procedures can be utilised for lateral compartment arthrosis or conditions wherein both the capitellum and radial head require addressing, including radiocapitellar replacement, though their indications are distinct from those for radial head replacement.

Types of replacement

The following are implant design characteristics, though there is currently no evidence to suggest that any prosthesis is significantly superior to the others:

Type	Articulation	Stem	Fixation	Material
Monoblock	Fixed bearing	Straight	Cemented	Cobalt-chromium
Modular	Mobile bearing (bipolar)	Curved	Press-fit	Titanium
			Loose-fit or 'floating'	Vitallium
				Pyrocarbon

Bipolar implants provide less stability than fixed-bearing prostheses *in vitro*, but a clinical difference has not been demonstrated. Modular implants allow for easy adjustment of the height of the head and neck, as well as the head size.

Anaesthesia and positioning

Anaesthesia is usually general, augmented by infraclavicular regional nerve blockade if not contraindicated (previous nerve trauma or palsy at the elbow or more proximally). An initial dose of antibiotic is given intravenously. The antibiotic of choice depends on local policy; we use teicoplanin and gentamicin in our practice. Note: If intraoperative biopsies are required to diagnose sepsis, then antibiotics can be withheld until intraoperative samples have been obtained.

The patient is placed in the lateral decubitus position with the operated arm uppermost. Padded lumbar and pelvic supports are used.

A Carter Braine arm support or well-padded drape support is used to cradle the arm, allowing the forearm to move freely in the vertical position, permitting access to the dorsal aspect and both sides of the elbow and to the anterior compartment by external rotation of the shoulder, if required (**Figure 7.1**). Of note in this position: *The ulnar nerve and medial aspect of the elbow are on the side of the elbow facing the feet of the patient.*

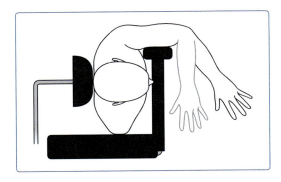

Figure 7.1 Patient position.

A padded narrow tourniquet (inflation to 200 mm Hg is usually sufficient) or an S-MART bandage/tourniquet is used. At least 15 cm of the dorsal aspect of the arm is required for ease of access. The elbow should be sufficiently mobile for appropriate movement intraoperatively. The hand, forearm and arm to the axilla are prepared with a germicidal solution. Waterproof drapes are used with adhesive edges to provide a seal to the skin. An antibacterial adhesive skin drape is applied.

Surgical technique

Any associated injuries will dictate the type of incision required. Posterior, medial and lateral structures can be exposed with the same single posterior incision; if only lateral access is required, a lateral incision can be performed. We delineate the more commonly used Kocher interval, as well as the Kaplan interval.

Posterolateral approach (Kocher)

This is an extensile intermuscular approach to the lateral elbow, between anconeus (supplied by the radial nerve) and extensor carpi ulnaris (supplied by the posterior interosseous nerve, PIN).

Landmarks

Landmarks include the lateral supracondylar ridge, lateral epicondyle, radial head and tip of the olecranon. Palpate the lateral epicondyle and move the fingers distally until a depression is felt. The radial head lies within a palpable depression distal to the lateral epicondyle. It can be felt to move on pronation and supination of the forearm.

Incision

The skin incision extends approximately 5 cm proximal to the lateral epicondyle and continues distally over the epicondyle, along the anterolateral surface of the forearm for approximately 5 cm (**Figure 7.2**).

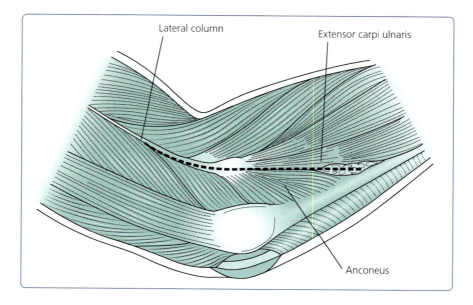

Figure 7.2 The incision for Kocher's approach.

Dissection

> **Structures at risk**
>
> - Radial nerve
> - Lateral antebrachial cutaneous nerve
> - Posterior interosseous nerve

The incision is continued through subcutaneous fat, protecting the lateral antebrachial cutaneous nerve typically lying on the deep fascia, and through the fascia between triceps and origins of the extensor carpi radialis longus (ECRL) and brachioradialis. An interval is developed between the triceps posteriorly and the origins of ECRL and brachioradialis anteriorly (**Figure 7.3**). In the proximal end of the wound, *the radial nerve must be avoided in the interval between the brachialis and brachioradialis muscles.* The common origin of the extensor muscles is elevated from the lateral epicondyle while preserving the origin of the lateral collateral ligament. Campbell's modification of this approach describes taking

Radial head replacement

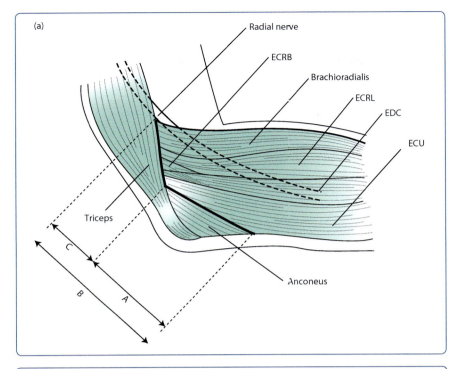

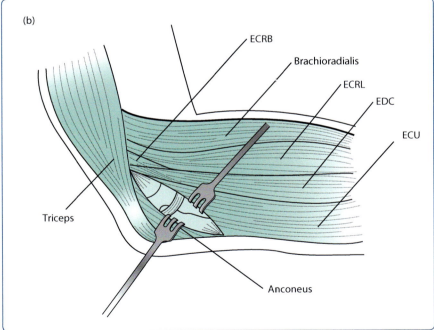

Figure 7.3 (a) Normal lateral anatomy of the elbow, with the Kocher interval highlighted and path of the radial nerve shown. (A) Limited Kocher approach. (B) Extended Kocher approach. (C) Column approach. (b) The limited Kocher approach, between anconeus and extensor carpi ulnaris (ECU). *(Continued)*

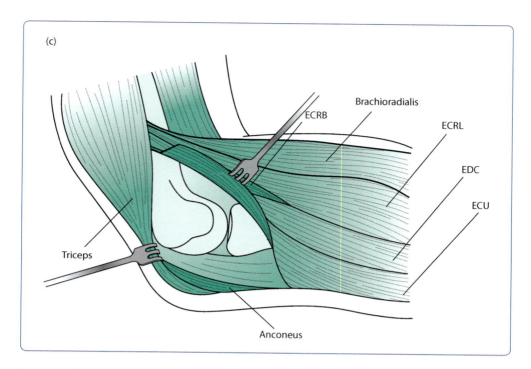

Figure 7.3 (Continued) (c) The extended Kocher approach. The common extensor origin is reflected from the lateral epicondyle.

the common extensor origin together with a thin flake of bone, using a small osteotome. Reflecting the common origin distally exposes the radiocapitellar joint. The PIN is vulnerable as it enters the supinator and must be protected by pronation of the forearm during dissection, careful retractor placement and avoiding dissection into the supinator muscle (**Figure 7.4**).

Lateral approach (Kaplan)

The Kaplan intermuscular approach to the elbow between extensor digitorum communis (EDC, supplied by the PIN) and extensor carpi radialis brevis (ECRB, variable innervation supplied by the PIN, superficial branch of the radial nerve or the undivided radial nerve), which provides excellent radiocapitellar joint visualisation. The radial nerve can translate mediolaterally 1 cm with forearm pronation (**Figure 7.4**), but even so remains in close proximity to the surgical field; therefore, this approach is less commonly undertaken than the Kocher approach for radial head replacement.

Landmarks
Landmarks are the same as those mentioned for the Kocher approach.

Incision
The skin incision extends from the lateral epicondyle approximately 5 cm distally, towards the dorsal radial tubercle. Proximal extension is as described for the Kocher approach.

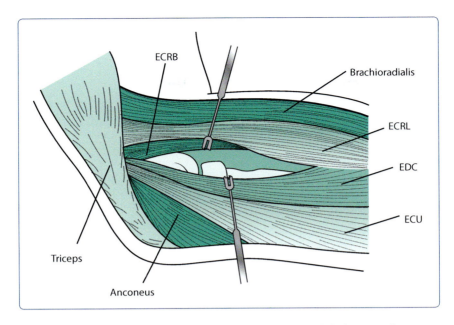

Figure 7.4 The Kaplan approach, between extensor carpi radialis brevis and extensor digitorum communis.

Superficial dissection
Superficial dissection for the Kaplan approach is the same as for the Kocher approach.

Deep dissection
Kaplan's interval lies between EDC posteriorly and ECRL and ECRB anteriorly. The interval can be developed distally to the level of the PIN, until it pierces the supinator at the Arcade of Frohse (**Figure 7.5**). As with the Kocher approach, the common extensor origin can now be elevated from the lateral epicondyle to grant access to the capsule deep to it.

Procedure

The origins of the brachioradialis and ECRL muscles are elevated subperiosteally and the capsule incised to expose the lateral aspect of the elbow joint. By incising the capsule anterior to the lateral ligamentous complex, (overlying the radial head) in line with the radius, the lateral collateral ligament can be avoided. The incision must not stray too far anteriorly as the radial nerve runs over the anterolateral portion of the elbow capsule (**Figure 7.6**).

The annular ligament is incised longitudinally before transecting the radial neck with an oscillating saw using a radial cutting jig (**Figure 7.7**). Exposure distal to the annular ligament risks damaging the PIN and is avoided. The cut surface of the proximal radius should be smooth and even, so that contact between it and the collar of the prosthesis is complete.

The proximal radial medullary canal is prepared with burs or rasps to accept the implant stem. A Hohmann retractor behind the posterior aspect of the radial neck can help to

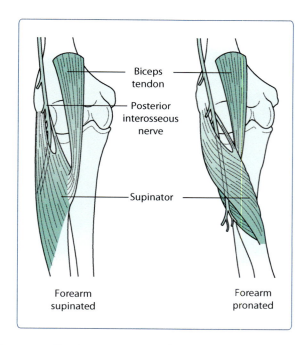

Figure 7.5 The dynamic position of the posterior interosseous nerve.

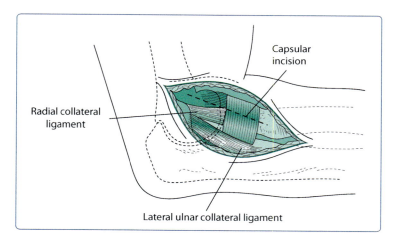

Figure 7.6 Lateral capsule incision, anterior to the lateral ligament complex.

deliver the neck, to facilitate access to the canal. For press-fit stems, the preparation must be tight and accurate; this is less critical for cemented stems. The diameter of the articulating surface of the radial head trial prosthesis should be chosen to match the diameter of the *articulating surface* of the native radial head (**Figure 7.8**). If the radial head diameter is between two available sizes, the smaller of the two should be used. A trial is inserted to

Radial head replacement

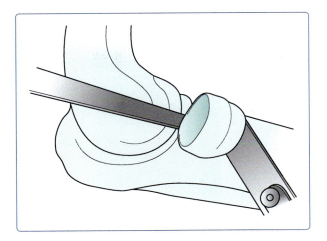

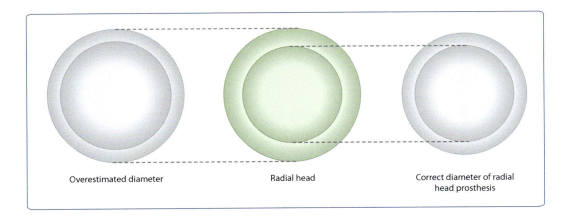

Overestimated diameter　　　Radial head　　　Correct diameter of radial head prosthesis

Figure 7.8 Using the diameter of the radial head (left) may overestimate the size of the prosthesis. The diameter of the articulating surface (right) should be used instead.

Figure 7.7 The radial neck cut.

ensure that contact with the capitellum is satisfactory. To prevent excessive wear of the capitellum from 'overstuffing', the proximal edge of the prosthesis should be level with the lateral edge of the coronoid (**Figure 7.9**). The elbow is taken through a range of flexion and extension in both supination and pronation (**Figure 7.10**). If the elbow tracking is satisfactory in flexion and extension, the final prosthesis is inserted.

Closure of lateral approach

The annular ligament is repaired with an absorbable suture. The common extensor origin is reattached to the lateral epicondyle with transosseous sutures. A suction drain is inserted. The deep dermal layer is approximated with absorbable sutures, then a continuous

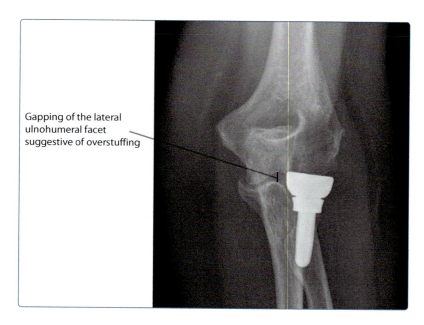

Figure 7.9 Anteroposterior left elbow radiograph demonstrating a radial head replacement with an overstuffed radiocapitellar joint – identified by the separation of the ulnohumeral articulation.

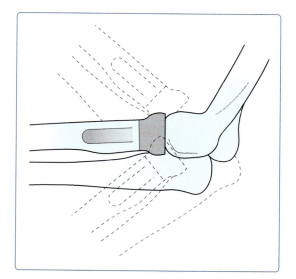

Figure 7.10 Trial reduction to test range of motion.

absorbable subcuticular suture with Steri-Strips to the skin. An occlusive dressing is applied, and the elbow is wrapped with wool and a crepe bandage in extension.

Postoperative care and instructions

The drain, wool and bandage are removed after 24 hours. Gentle active mobilisation of the elbow can begin at this time under supervision. Return to work is allowed after approximately 6 weeks for sedentary jobs, but may be delayed to 3 months or more in active work. The wound should be checked for any signs of abnormal healing or infection at 2 weeks, after which surgical follow-up is recommended at 6 weeks, 6 months and 1 year after surgery. Continuation of follow-up is typically at yearly intervals thereafter. The patient should be advised to return to clinic if there is pain or functional deterioration.

Recommended references

Heijink A, Kodde I, Mulder P et al. Radial head arthroplasty: A systematic review. *JBJS Rev.* 2016;**4(10)**.

Marinelli A, Guerra E, Ritali A et al. Radial head prosthesis: Surgical tips and tricks. *Musculoskelet Surg.* 2017;**101(Suppl 2)**:187–196.

Watkins CEL, Elson DW, Harrison JWK, Pooley J. Long-term results of the lateral resurfacing elbow arthroplasty. *Bone Joint J.* 2018;**100-B(3)**:338–345.

Total elbow arthroplasty

Preoperative planning

With the significant advancements in the medical management of rheumatoid arthritis, the number of patients requiring primary elective total elbow arthroplasty (TEA) is decreasing. Nonetheless, the valuable role of TEA in improving pain and function in the appropriate patient cannot be underestimated. It remains a low-volume procedure, with just over 400 TEAs performed per year in the United Kingdom, compared with over 100,000 hip replacements. Recent guidelines advocate complex primary and revision TEAs being managed in specialist centres, with operations jointly performed by two senior surgeons.

Indications

Indications include painful elbow conditions that have failed non-operative management, including

- Rheumatoid and other inflammatory arthropathies
- Primary and post-traumatic osteoarthritis
- Comminuted distal humeral fractures not amenable to fixation
- Avascular necrosis

Contraindications

- Infection (generalised or of the limb)
- Paralysis or dysfunctional neuropathy of the elbow
- Significant hand dysfunction
- Relative contraindication – patients who will not be able to comply with postoperative restrictions on function

Consent and risks

- Ulnar nerve injury: 3%
- Deep infection: 3%
- Intraoperative fracture: 5%

- Triceps dehiscence or significant weakness: 1%
- Dislocation/symptomatic subluxation: Unlinked, 5%; linked, 1%
- Symptomatic aseptic loosening: Unlinked, 5%; linked, 5%
- Need for revision surgery: 10%–15%

Operative planning

Recent radiographs must be available. The lateral and medial distal humeral columns must be present to provide rotatory stability. In cases with significant bone loss, the surgeon should consider use of a custom implant, modular endoprosthesis (**Figure 7.11**) or structural allograft. Availability of the implants must be checked by the surgeon. Biologic agents for rheumatoid arthritis should be discussed with a specialist to create a perioperative plan for stopping and restarting medication.

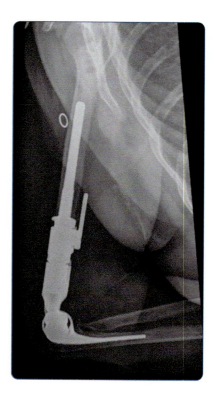

Figure 7.11 Lateral right humeral radiograph of modular distal humeral replacement, used in tumour surgery and revision surgery for humeral loosening and osteolysis.

Types of replacement

There are three types of TEA – linked, unlinked and convertible (which may function as an unlinked or linked arthroplasty and can be converted from one to the other intraoperatively). Fully constrained hinged prostheses are no longer used and instead semi-constrained linked prostheses use varying shapes of polyethylene articulating surface to permit some varus-valgus angulation throughout the arc of motion. Note: Though often used interchangeably in error, constraint is distinct from linkage. Some unlinked prostheses are more constrained than linked prostheses.

Linked	Unlinked	Convertible
Coonrad-Morrey	Capitellocondylar	Acclaim
Discovery	Kudo	Latitude
GSB-III	Sorbie	
Nexel	Souter-Strathclyde	

	Linked	Unlinked
Advantages	• Can be used in cases of ligamentous insufficiency • Allows for more aggressive soft tissue and contracture release • Better postoperative range of motion (further extension)	• Less bony resection required • Lower constraint, possibly lower wear and osteolysis • Can be used as distal humeral hemiarthroplasty (e.g. in trauma)
Disadvantages	• Small risk of linkage dissociation • Increased constraint predisposes to increased bushing wear and osteolysis	• Risk of dislocation • Dependent on soft tissue integrity • Requires accurate component positioning

Issues regarding the radiocapitellar joint and handling the ulnar nerve in a TEA remain contentious. The radial head may be preserved or excised during a TEA. Radial head impingement may occur if preserved, necessitating a secondary procedure to excise the head. The Latitude prosthesis is modular and allows the surgeon to replace the radiocapitellar articulating surface concurrently. The capitellar surface of the humeral component in this design is anatomic so can articulate with a native or replaced radial head, to allow lateral column load sharing, though any benefit has yet to be borne out in clinical studies.

The ulnar nerve may be decompressed or anteriorly transposed during the operation. The approach used in the operation may dictate the handling of the ulnar nerve. Indications for transposing the ulnar nerve in a primary replacement include significant stiffness, preoperative neuropathy or when using a triceps-on approach (see later).

It is the authors' preference to excise the radial head and not to transpose the ulnar nerve routinely.

Anaesthesia and positioning

Anaesthesia and positioning are the same as for radial head replacement.

Surgical technique
For primary total elbow arthroplasty the approach employed is largely at the discretion of the operating surgeon. Each approach offers different degrees of exposure to the bony anatomy and varies with their handling of the extensor mechanism.

Triceps splitting
Many such approaches involve a midline split along the triceps tendon and elevation of each half from the posterior humerus and ulna, as described by Campbell. The Shahane-Stanley modification of this approach splits the triceps towards the medial aspect, with 75% of the muscle bulk laterally and 25% medially in order to avoid the triceps from 'buttonholing', while also providing protection for the ulnar nerve. The triceps is repaired with side-to-side sutures or transosseous sutures through the olecranon.

Triceps reflecting
The Bryan-Morrey approach describes reflection of the triceps from medial to lateral. This provides excellent exposure, but risks postoperative triceps failure if the tendon repair fails. The triceps is reattached to the olecranon with sutures placed through transosseous drill holes. Wolfe and Ranawat described a modification involving osteotomising the triceps attachment on the olecranon with a thin wafer of bone, to aid healing. A lateral to medial reflecting approach can also be used for cases in which lateral-sided pathology requires addressing.

Triceps-on or triceps-preserving approach
The triceps-on approach maintains the triceps in continuity with the olecranon, either with a single incision or more commonly, a dual para-tricipital incision. The Alonso-Llames approach uses medial and lateral incisions either side of the triceps and elevates the muscle from the posterior aspect of the humerus. The distal humerus can then be displaced medially or laterally to expose the proximal forearm. The approach is limited in its exposure by mobility of the bones and is therefore suited to trauma, when the distal humerus is fractured and more readily mobile.

Triceps-turndown approach
Campbell's original description of this approach utilises a V-Y advancement flap in the triceps tendon. This may be required in cases of chronic dislocation or other causes of triceps shortening. This approach has a high rate of triceps disruption and is therefore not commonly used in primary TEA. Instead, it is the authors' preference when performing a turndown to use an approach based on the blood supply to the triceps, as described by Rajeev and Pooley.

Posterior approach to the elbow
Landmarks
- Midline of the humerus
- Lateral epicondyle
- Radial head

- Tip of the olecranon
- Crest of the proximal ulna

Incision

The incision is made in a curvilinear fashion towards the tip of the olecranon starting about 7.5 cm proximal to the olecranon, skirting on its lateral side, leaving between 0.5 and 1 cm between the incision and the lateral border of the olecranon (to avoid placing the incision on the weightbearing skin of the elbow). The incision is continued distally parallel to the crest of the ulna (*not* crossing it or on it) for approximately 6 cm (**Figure 7.12**).

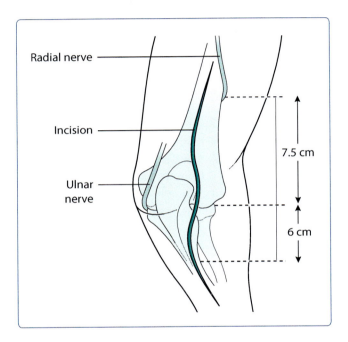

Figure 7.12 Posterior approach to the elbow.

Superficial dissection

Structure at risk

- Ulnar nerve

The triceps tendon is more correctly an aponeurosis. There is a superficial sheet having a median vertical aponeurotic extension, between the lateral and long heads of the triceps, which leads to the deep head. This sheet is the guide to the dissection of the triceps.

The lateral and medial musculotendinous boundaries of the triceps are revealed by epifascial dissection in the proximal part of the wound. Minimal epifascial dissection is used distal to the olecranon over the subcutaneous border of the ulna, sufficient only to see the deep antebrachial fascia over anconeus. Medial dissection is continued, sufficient to reveal the ulnar nerve immediately subjacent to the medial border of the triceps about 6–7 cm proximal to the medial epicondyle.

The ulnar nerve is identified throughout its course, behind the medial condyle, noting the axial vessel and the vena comitans on the deep (articular) surface of the nerve in the cubital sulcus. The fibrous arch between the two bony origins of flexor carpi ulnaris (FCU) is incised, the incision being carried into the muscle for about 2 cm, marking and protecting the nerve branch to FCU, which typically arises proximal to the elbow, and allowing ready displacement of the nerve from the cubital sulcus without tension. A vessel loop can be placed around the nerve to protect and identify it for the remainder of the procedure.

Deep dissection

Triceps-splitting approach

This approach respects the nerve supply to anconeus (an important contributor to elbow stability): this is a distal branch of the radial nerve which crosses the interval between the distal border of the lateral head of triceps and the proximal border of anconeus. Dissection within the lateral head of triceps is to be avoided. The triceps is split between the nerve and blood supply to the long head (a segmental branch can occur very distally) and the nerve to the lateral head, both derived from the radial nerve. The deep head nerve supply is more proximal and is out of the surgical field. The ulnar nerve is protected by keeping dissection lateral and then deep to the long head of the triceps, using the muscular bulk as a protection for the nerve (**Figure 7.13**).

The triceps aponeurosis is incised in the midline and undermined to define the vertical sheet between the two superficial heads of the triceps.

The dissection is then taken down the lateral side of this sheet, i.e. in the intervascular/interneural plane, to the deep head of the triceps. The superficial heads are parted for about 6 cm, uncovering the filmy layer between them and the deep head. The deep head is then incised (the only muscular incision required in this technique) noting the deep transverse epicondylar vessels under the muscle at the proximal margin of the fat pad in the olecranon fossa. The vessels are cauterised. The fat pad is excised and the olecranon fossa exposed. A posterior capsulectomy is performed and any olecranon osteophytes removed.

The antebrachial fascia is incised parallel to and about 1 cm lateral to the crest of the ulna over anconeus. The dissection is taken under the fascia but outside anconeus to the crest and then, on bone, down to the supinator crest, the annular ligament and capsule of the proximal radioulnar joint, lifting anconeus away from the capsule and radial head, but preserving the posterior band of the lateral collateral ligament (to maintain stability in varus strain).

Triceps-reflecting approach

The medial head of the triceps muscle is separated from the medial intermuscular septum and dissected down to the humerus. Note: At this point, the triceps is still 'on' (attached

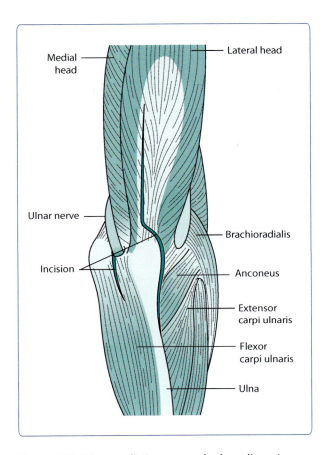

Figure 7.13 Triceps-splitting approach, deep dissection.

to the olecranon) and this is where a triceps-on approach would free the medial border of the triceps from the intermuscular septum. With the triceps-reflecting approach, the medial incision is extended approximately 6 cm distally with subperiosteal dissection of the medial antebrachial fascia to expose the posterior capsule. This fascia is thin over the posterior ulna; therefore, a narrow osteotome can be used to create a series of osteo-periosteo-fascial shingles (small, superficial shards of bone). The periosteo-antebrachial fascia is then sharply dissected from the crest in continuity with the olecranon shingles.

The triceps, fascia and periosteum can then be elevated from the olecranon from medial to lateral as a single flap. This is done at 30° flexion to relieve tension on the flap. The flap is mobilised laterally, elevating the anconeus origin from the distal humerus until it can be reflected over the capitellum (**Figure 7.14**).

Remnants of the triceps and posterior capsule can then be elevated from the posterior humerus.

Triceps-turndown approach
A transverse incision is made through the triceps aponeurosis approximately 4 cm proximal to the triceps insertion on the olecranon. The incision is then extended distally

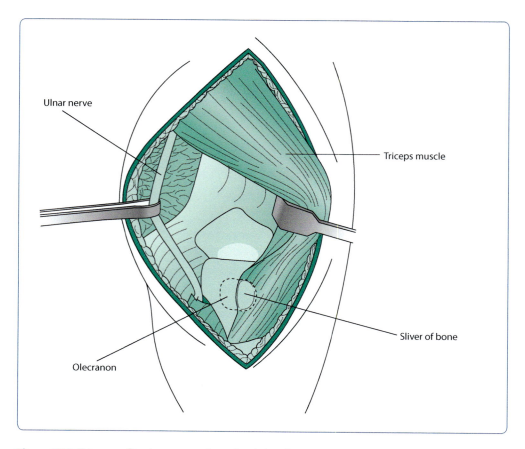

Figure 7.14 Triceps-reflecting approach, maintaining the triceps in continuity while reflecting from medial to lateral.

from its lateral aspect along the deep fascia of the lateral head of triceps and then the deep fascia overlying anconeus midway between the lateral epicondyle and olecranon, until the incision reaches the lateral subcutaneous border of the ulna. The triceps aponeurosis and deep fascia overlying anconeus is then stripped from the muscle bellies, usually requiring sharp dissection proximally and medially. The first transverse incision is extended distally from its medial aspect, to create a fascial flap (**Figure 7.15**).

Anconeus is then elevated subperiosteally from the ulna. The lateral head of triceps is separated from the intramuscular aponeurosis between the lateral and medial heads with sharp dissection. The muscle fibres run parallel to this incision; therefore, the muscle fibres are not transected. The lateral head and anconeus can now be reflected laterally as a single unit (**Figure 7.16**).

Repeat the process of separating the muscle from the intramuscular aponeurosis with the medial head of triceps and retract this medially. The intramuscular aponeurosis can now be divided 2 cm proximal to its insertion on the olecranon, permitting access to the posterior distal humeral and posterior capsule (**Figure 7.17**).

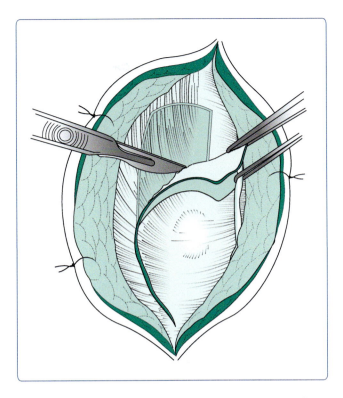

Figure 7.15 Creation of a fascial flap. (From Rajeev A, Pooley J, *Eur J Orthop Surg Traumatol.* 2009;19:467–472.)

Procedure

Preparation of distal humerus and proximal ulna

The forearm is rotated laterally to allow exposure of the distal humerus. The radial head and tip of olecranon, along a line tangent to the posterior-most portion of the olecranon articulation, are excised with an oscillating saw (**Figure 7.18**).

To mark the humeral saw cuts, the olecranon fossa guide is available on the instrument set. To orientate the guide, the shaft of the fossa guide is aligned with the humeral canal. The medial border should lie along the medial trochlea. The guide should also align with the anatomical internal rotation of the trochlea, which approximates the flat surface posterior and just proximal to the olecranon fossa. Using a fossa reamer or burr, a hole is created and an oscillating saw is used to remove the remains of the trochlea, along the lines previously marked, allowing access to the medullary canal of the humerus (**Figure 7.19**).

The canal is identified with a high-speed rotating bur at the proximal aspect of the resection of the olecranon fossa in a proximal direction (**Figure 7.20**). Open the medullary canal to a size sufficient to allow a humeral rasp (about 4 mm).

The humeral rasps are now used to prepare the humeral canal (**Figure 7.21**). Serial rasps increasing in size are used until cortical resistance is met. If a rasp is unable to be advanced fully, use an implant corresponding to the largest size of rasp which was fully introduced.

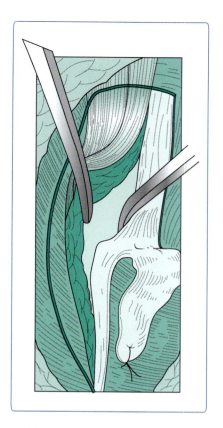

Figure 7.16 Retraction of the lateral head of triceps, together with anconeus. (From Rajeev A, Pooley J, *Eur J Orthop Surg Traumatol.* 2009;19:467–472.)

The medial and lateral portions of the supracondylar columns *must be preserved* during the preparation of the distal humerus. They act as points of reference to ensure satisfactory orientation and alignment. The trial prosthesis is inserted until the margins of the prosthesis are exactly level with the epicondylar articular surface margin on the capitellar and trochlear sides (**Figure 7.22**). Further small pieces of bone are removed with rongeurs or bone nibblers from the distal humerus to aid proper seating of the component.

A high-speed burr is used at an angle of roughly 45° from the vertical in a posterior and distal direction to remove subchondral bone to identify the ulnar medullary canal. Serial rasps are introduced into the medullary canal of the ulnar until cortical resistance is met (**Figure 7.23**). As with the humerus, the size of implant used corresponds with the largest size of rasp fully inserted.

The appropriate rasps are used to shape the proximal ulna, maintaining vigilance to ensure the rasps are aligned down the medullary canal to avoid angular malpositioning.

After the proximal ulna and distal humerus have been prepared, a trial will evaluate the elbow for complete flexion and extension. During trialling, inspect the anterior flange of the humeral component. If there is a space between the anterior humeral cortex and

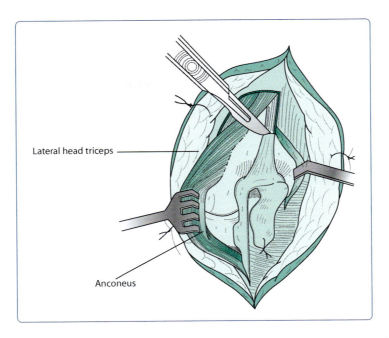

Figure 7.17 Division of tricipital intermuscular septum, 2 cm proximal to its insertion on the olecranon. (From Rajeev A, Pooley J, *Eur J Orthop Surg Traumatol.* 2009;19:467–472.)

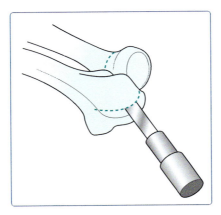

Figure 7.18 Radial head and tip of olecranon excised.

the flange, an allogenic or autologous (from the excised trochlea) bone graft may be used for added rotational stability. The bone graft should measure roughly 1.5 cm × 1 cm, and 2–3 mm in depth and can be placed in the space during cementation to establish contact between the flange and the bone (**Figure 7.24**).

The medullary canals are cleaned with pulsatile lavage and the canals dried. A cement restrictor is inserted into both canals. A cement gun is used for retrograde insertion of low-viscosity cement into the canals. If the components are cemented separately, the ulnar component is inserted first. The centre of the ulnar component is aligned with the centre

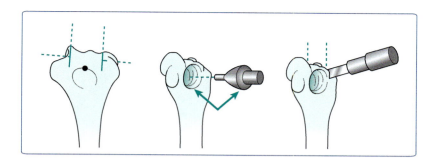

Figure 7.19 Use of guide, fossa reamer and oscillating saw to prepare the humerus.

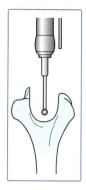

Figure 7.20 A high-speed burr is used to identify the humeral canal.

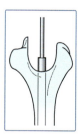

Figure 7.21 Rasping the humeral canal.

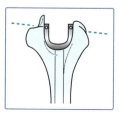

Figure 7.22 Trial of the humeral component.

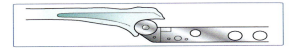

Figure 7.23 Rasping of the ulnar metaphysis.

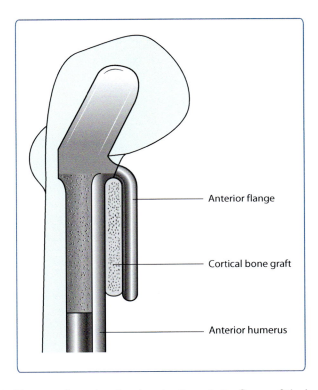

Figure 7.24 A cortical bone graft can be placed under the anterior flange of the humeral component if there is a gap between the prosthesis and bone.

of the sigmoid fossa. The humeral component is impacted down to a point that allows articulation of the device and the placement of the axle and the locking clip or interlocking axis pins (if a linked device is used) (**Figure 7.25**).

The arm is held in extension until the cement has cured, then the humeral device can be linked with the ulnar component.

Closure

The soft tissues that were dissected deeply in each approach are repaired with absorbable sutures (number 2 gauge). The olecranon osteo-periosteo-fascial medallion is repaired by transosseous non-absorbable sutures (number 2 gauge) to the olecranon. A suction drain is placed deep to the triceps muscle. The triceps aponeurosis and antebrachial fascia are closed with the elbow flexed at 90° flexion using absorbable braided number 1 interrupted sutures (continuous suturing reduces the 'give' of the tendon during assisted motion).

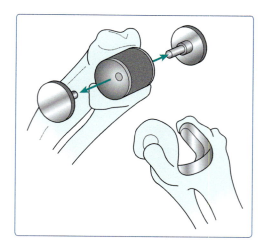

Figure 7.25 Implanted components.

- The skin is closed with a dermal supporting absorbable suture and an absorbable continuous subcuticular suture plus Steri-Strips.
- An occlusive dressing is applied with the elbow in 90° of flexion.
- A bulky wool and crepe bandage dressing is applied in two layers.

Postoperative care and instructions

The drain, wool and bandage are removed after 24 hours. Supervised physiotherapy should allow active- and gravity-assisted extension, as well as active and passive flexion, pronation and supination. It is the authors' practice to apply a removable extension splint, which the patient can wear at night for 6 weeks in order to maintain full extension.

The wound should be checked for any signs of abnormal healing or infection at 2 weeks, after which surgical follow-up is recommended at 6 weeks, at which point the patient can begin strengthening exercises. Thereafter, follow-up should be at 6 months and 1 year after surgery, then at yearly intervals if required. The patient should be advised to return to clinic if there is pain or functional deterioration.

Patients are recommended to avoid lifting with the ipsilateral limb objects weighing more than 1 kilogram on a regular basis or lifting more than 5 kg on a single event.

Recommended references

Rajeev A, Pooley J. A posterior approach to the elbow joint based on the blood supply to the triceps muscle. *Eur J Orthop Surg Traumatol.* 2009;**19**:467–472.

Sanchez-Sotelo J. Total elbow arthroplasty. *Open Orthop J.* 2011;**5**:115–123.

Sanchez-Sotelo J. Primary elbow arthroplasty: Problems and solutions. *Shoulder Elbow.* 2016;**9(1)**:61–70.

Voloshin I, Schippert D, Kakar S et al. Complications of total elbow replacement: A systematic review. *J Shoulder Elbow Surg.* 2011;**20(1)**:158–168.

Open elbow arthrolysis

Preoperative planning

Indications

- Post-traumatic capsular contracture of the ulnohumeral (medial column), radiocapitellar (lateral column), and proximal radioulnar joints (anterior and posterior compartments)
- Degenerative contracture of anterior and posterior compartments
- Intracompartmental adhesiolysis, usually of the radiocapitellar joint
- In association with intra-articular corrective osteotomy of the distal humerus, proximal ulna or radial head
- In association with joint replacement arthroplasty of the elbow, including lateral compartment resurfacing and radial head replacement

Contraindications

- Vascular compromise of the limb
- Infection (generalised or of the limb)
- Compromised skin in the region of the surgical incision
- Inability of the patient to understand the postoperative rehabilitation programme
- Contraindication to regional nerve blockade; previous nerve trauma or palsy (particularly if incomplete nerve lesion) at the elbow or more proximally

Consent and risks

- Ulnar nerve injury: 10% transient ulnar neuritis, 1% tardy ulnar nerve palsy, less than 1% acute permanent lesion
- Infection: Less than 1%
- Heterotopic ossification: 10%
- Recurrence: More common in post-traumatic stiffness syndrome, less common in degenerative or inflammatory contractures
- Failure to achieve desired result (due to surface/topographical articular lesions)
- Need for further surgery, including joint replacement arthroplasty

Operative planning

Anteroposterior and lateral (in flexion and extension) radiographs, less than 6 months old, should be available.

For articular surface lesions a computed tomography (CT) arthrogram is desirable. It should be possible to readily convert from an arthroscopic procedure to an open procedure (see positioning and incision sections).

Anaesthesia and positioning

Anaesthesia and positioning are the same as for radial head replacement and total elbow arthroplasty.

Surgical technique

Arthrolysis can be performed open or arthroscopically.

Open arthrolysis

The choice of approach is governed by which compartment is to be accessed:

- *For the lateral compartment, plus anterior and posterior capsule*: The lateral column (Morrey) approach can be used. This is equivalent to the proximal half of the extended Kocher approach and can be extended proximally into a lateral approach to the humerus and distally into a Kocher approach to the radial head and neck. The anterolateral compartment is readily accessible (see section 'Radial head replacement', p. 113).
- *For the medial side of the anterior compartment*: The direct medial approach anterior to the ulnar nerve (see section 'Tennis/golfer's elbow release', p. 142).
- *For the anterior compartment alone* (e.g. for lengthening of the biceps tendon): The anterior approach. This is a lazy-S incision respecting the flexure crease of the elbow, passing from medial to the tendon of the biceps proximally over the brachial neurovascular bundle, to the medial side of the 'mobile wad' (of Henry) distally (**Figure 7.26**).

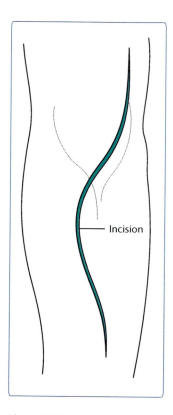

Figure 7.26 Anterior approach.

- *For the dorsal (olecranon fossa) compartment and ulnar nerve*: A dorsal (trans-tricipital) approach may be used, as for elbow arthroplasty. The anterior compartment may then be accessed via a transhumeral approach by making an aperture in the olecranon fossa (the Outerbridge-Kashiwagi or OK procedure).

Column procedure

This procedure provides access to the anterior and posterior capsule, as well as to the coronoid and olecranon, should osteophyte excision be required. The incision can be extended distally to readily access the radiocapitellar joint.

Superficial dissection

The superficial dissection is the same as for Kocher's extended approach, but using only the proximal half of the incision (**Figure 7.27**). If access to the medial side is required (e.g. preoperative ulnar nerve symptoms necessitating release or transposition) or a posterior approach has previously been used, then a dorsal skin incision can be used with subcutaneous dissection to the lateral aspect in order to expose the column.

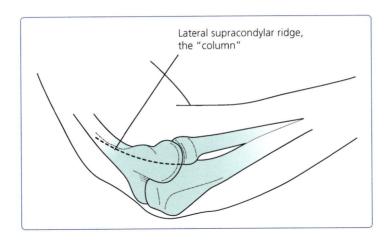

Figure 7.27 The distal lateral humerus that is proximal to the lateral epicondyle is termed 'the column'.

Deep dissection

Release of the origin of ECRL and the distal origin of brachioradialis from the lateral column on the humerus permits access to the superolateral anterior capsule. The brachialis muscle can be swept away from the capsule with a periosteal elevator, which can now be entered at the radiocapitellar joint. Careful retraction will protect the brachialis muscle, median nerve and brachial artery, allowing the anterior capsule to be excised to at least the level of the coronoid. Anterior (coronoid) osteophytes may be excised if required, and the articular surface of the trochlea can be visualised.

If there is still a significant fixed flexion deformity or lateral radiographs identify posterior osteophytes, then the triceps can be elevated from the posterior aspect of the column with

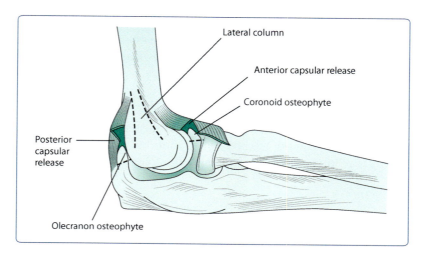

Figure 7.28 The column procedure, with both anterior and posterior releases demonstrated.

epifascial dissection. The posterior capsule may then be released, clearing the olecranon fossa of soft tissue and excising osteophytes from the olecranon, as needed (**Figure 7.28**).

Outerbridge-Kashiwagi procedure

The procedure begins as per the trans-tricipital approach to the distal humerus. An aperture is then made through the distal humerus using a high-speed burr, directing the burr radially and proximally: the medial humeral column is thinner and flatter than the lateral column, so the transhumeral opening should be directed radially immediately medial to the lateral column to avoid iatrogenic medial column fracture. The aperture should exit anteriorly immediately behind the tip of the coronoid process (**Figure 7.29**).

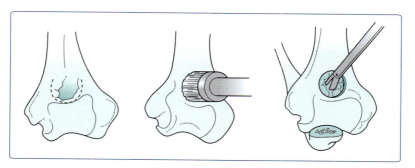

Figure 7.29 The Outerbridge-Kashiwagi procedure.

The diameter of the aperture should be no more than half the transverse diameter of the humerus at this level. The anterior capsule of the radiocapitellar joint, the coronoid tip, and most of the anteromedial capsule can be removed through the aperture, using elbow flexion to bring the capsule into the aperture. It is inadequate for release of the medial capsule, and the anterior band of the ulnar collateral ligament should not be incised, to avoid iatrogenic valgus instability.

Technical aspects

Where total capsulectomy has been required in cases such as post-traumatic contracture, heterotopic ossification and myositis ossificans, the collateral ligaments are often released – the elbow is therefore unstable. Fixed splintage is counterproductive. Dynamic splintage is required: a hinged external fixator is indicated if the ligaments cannot be reattached and should be retained for about 8 weeks, before application of a removable hinged brace for a further 4 weeks. If the ligaments can be restored to their optimal tension an external hinged removable brace can be used. Re-fixation of the ligaments to their footprint origins is facilitated by one of the several varieties of anchors that are available. The elbow must be stable enough to permit full-range assisted sagittal motion with gravity eliminated immediately after the operation.

Closure

A limited lateral release (e.g. anterior column procedure alone) may not require a drain; however, anything more extensive will warrant a suction drain placed deep to triceps. The triceps aponeurosis and antebrachial fascia are closed with the elbow flexed at 90° flexion using absorbable braided number 1 interrupted sutures (continuous suturing reduces the 'give' of the tendon during assisted motion).

- The skin is closed with a dermal supporting absorbable suture and an absorbable continuous subcuticular suture plus Steri-Strips.
- An occlusive dressing is applied with the elbow in 90° of flexion.
- A bulky wool and crepe bandage dressing is applied in two layers.

Arthroscopic arthrolysis

Landmarks

- Lateral epicondyle
- Radial head
- Tip of the olecranon

Approach

The usual portals (as described in the section 'Elbow arthroscopy', p. 154) are used. In principle the arthroscopic portals respect the same incisions, i.e. the portals are placed in the line of the standard skin incisions to permit extension into an open approach as required.

Using the anteromedial and anterolateral portals, fibrous tissue can be resected from the anterior part of the joint, using a combination of a full-radius resector and electrocautery. Any loose bodies are removed. The coronoid fossa is re-created, using the resector and a burr for any bony hypertrophy. The coronoid tip is removed if there is evidence of coronoid impingement. The resector is used to strip the capsule proximally, off the distal humerus, for approximately 2.5 cm proximal to the olecranon fossa until the fibres of brachialis come into view proximally. To complete the release a 1 cm capsulotomy of the anterior capsule from medial to lateral is required.

Using the direct posterior and posterolateral portals, the posterior compartment is debrided similarly. The scope enters through the posterolateral portal and the resector or burr through the direct posterior portal to complete the procedure. Careful release of the contracture, with a full-radius resector, releases the posteromedial and posterolateral gutters. Beware of the ulnar nerve in close proximity medially. Manipulation of the elbow is used to achieve maximum extension.

Closure

- A drain is placed in the direct posterior portal and the portals closed with absorbable sutures.
- Occlusive dressings are applied.
- The elbow is splinted in maximum extension.

Postoperative care and instructions

The arm is rested on pillows at chest height for 48 hours. The bandage is reduced at 24 hours and the drain is removed. A Tubigrip bandage is applied. If there is uncertainty about elbow stability a removable extension splint may be applied, to be worn between exercise periods.

Active assisted sagittal full-range motion exercises are performed for 20 minutes four or five times per day. Fist gripping and forearm pronosupination are undertaken as comfort permits. Supervised physiotherapy for the neck, shoulder and hand is undertaken. If achieving extension is problematic, then a removable elbow splint or brace can be applied at night.

Active unassisted movement is permitted by 6 weeks and axial weightbearing at approximately 12 weeks. Passive motion of the elbow may be indicated for recalcitrant/recurrent arthrofibrosis. However, continuous passive motion equipment is difficult to apply accurately, particularly in the unstable joint. A continuous patient-controlled analgesic infusion, or continuous infraclavicular regional anaesthetic infusion are commonly required.

Recommended references

Mansat P, Morrey BF. The column procedure: A limited lateral approach for extrinsic contracture of the elbow. *J Bone Joint Surg Am.* 1998;**80(11)**:1603–1615.
Morrey BF. The posttraumatic stiff elbow. *Clin Orthop Relat Res.* 2005;**(431)**:26–35.
Nandi S, Maschke S, Evans PJ, Lawton JN. The stiff elbow. *Hand (NY).* 2009;**4(4)**:368–379.

Tennis/golfer's elbow release
Preoperative planning
Indications

Tennis and golfer's elbow release is indicated when conservative management has failed. They are erroneously termed lateral and medial epicondylitis, though do not feature an inflammatory reaction; instead, it is a degenerative process in the tendons involving immature fibroblasts.

Patients with tennis elbow have tenderness at the common extensor origin, with reproduction of symptoms upon resisted wrist extension with the elbow in extension. Non-operative treatment with anti-inflammatories, counterforce bracing and up to three steroid injections to the site of maximal tenderness can achieve success in up to 95% of cases. The ECRB tendon is invariably affected, though the tendon of extensor digitorum communis (EDC) may also be affected in up to 35% of cases and therefore should not be neglected. Tennis elbow occurs at least five times more commonly than golfer's elbow.

In golfer's elbow, pain and tenderness are localised to the common flexor origin. Pain is reproduced by resisted forearm pronation and wrist flexion. Non-operative treatment is similar to that for tennis elbow but usually more difficult to treat.

A number of operative methods have been developed, including open, arthroscopic and percutaneous debridement. Of note, platelet-rich plasma injections have shown promise as a therapeutic intervention and demonstrate greater symptomatic relief than steroid injections alone. Over 90% of patients do not require surgical intervention; of those that do, 85%–95% experience symptomatic relief from any of the above surgical procedures, and there is little evidence to suggest one is conclusively superior to the others. Arthroscopic debridement may be incomplete if much of the pathology is extra-articular, potentially resulting in ongoing pain. Some recent evidence suggests that surgical debridement for tennis elbow may not even have any benefit over sham surgery (i.e. no debridement of the degenerative tendon), though the evidence is not yet conclusive and research is ongoing. Nonetheless, we delineate the operative process for an open debridement of both pathologies.

Consent and risks

- Failure
- Nerve injury: 1%
- Infection
- Heterotopic ossification at surgical site: 10%
- Posterolateral instability: If there is excessive debridement of the collateral ligament origins as well as the origins of the extensor muscles from the lateral epicondyle

Operative planning

Recent anteroposterior and lateral radiographs of the elbow should be available to rule out lateral compartment arthrosis with suspected tennis elbow. Calcification may be visible in the flexor origin in long-standing golfer's elbow.

Anaesthesia and positioning

Anaesthesia is usually general, but may be regional or combined. The supine position is used with the arm placed on an arm board. A pneumatic tourniquet or S-MART bandage/tourniquet is used.

The elbow should be sufficiently mobile for appropriate movement intraoperatively. The surgical field is prepared with a germicidal solution. Waterproof drapes are used with adhesive edges to provide a seal to the skin.

Surgical technique

Extensor origin debridement (tennis elbow)

Landmark

The lateral epicondyle is a landmark.

Incision

A 4–5 cm gently curved skin incision is made centred over the lateral epicondyle (**Figure 7.30**).

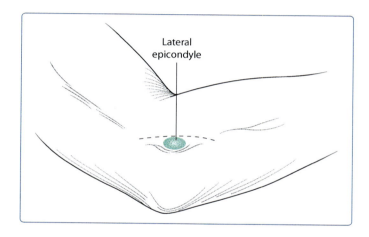

Figure 7.30 Tennis elbow skin incision.

Superficial dissection

The incision is continued through subcutaneous fat and down to fascia. The fascia overlying the posterior edge of ECRL is incised and elevated to expose extensor carpi radialis brevis (ECRB), which lies beneath ECRL. Just posterior to ECRL lies the extensor aponeurosis, the anterior edge of which may be abnormal. ECRL is then dissected sharply off the anterior ridge and displaced anteromedially to expose ECRB. ECRB is inferior to the origin of ECRL and deep to EDC. The border between ECRB and EDC is often poorly defined.

Deep dissection

Degenerate tissue is excised, taking care not to release any normal looking tendon. The procedure is therefore more accurately a debridement than a release. The abnormal tissue may appear fibrillated or discoloured and may contain calcium deposits. The bony site of the ECRB resection (i.e. not the lateral epicondyle) is decorticated with an osteotome, bone nibbler or drill to enhance blood supply and theorised to fill the void with fibrous tissue (**Figure 7.31**).

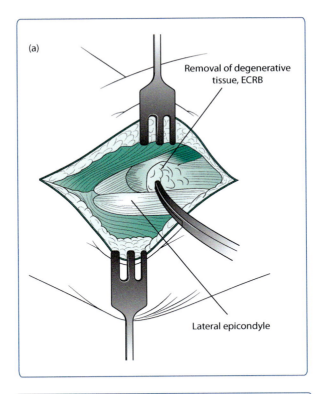

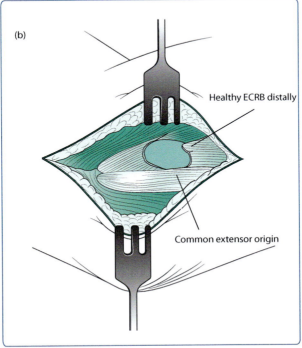

Figure 7.31 Tennis elbow debridement and decortication. (*Continued*)

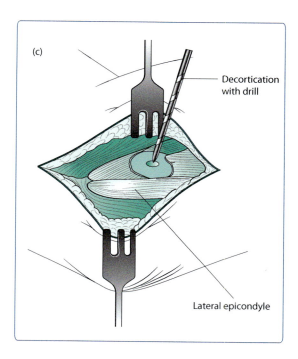

Figure 7.31 (Continued)

Closure of lateral approach

The defect between the posterior edge of ECRL and the extensor aponeurosis is repaired with an absorbable suture to restore the normal anatomical position. Superficial closure utilises absorbable sutures to approximate the subcutaneous fat, then a subcuticular continuous absorbable suture.

An occlusive dressing is applied, followed by a bulky wool and crepe bandage dressing in two layers.

Postoperative care and instructions

Dressings are reduced at 48 hours. Early range-of-motion exercises are begun, followed by strengthening exercises. Strenuous activity is resumed within pain limits at 8–10 weeks, and full power should have returned by 3 months. Follow-up is recommended at 6 weeks, with a wound check by the primary care practitioner at 2 weeks.

Flexor origin debridement (golfer's elbow)

Landmark
The medial epicondyle is the landmark.

Structures at risk

- Medial antebrachial cutaneous nerve

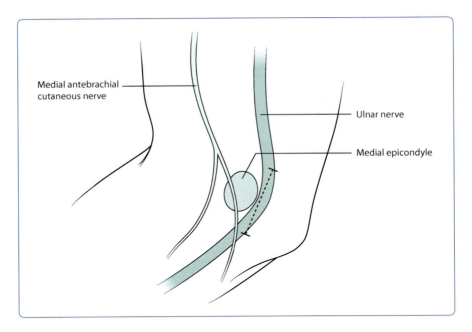

Figure 7.32 Golfer's elbow skin incision.

Incision

A 3–4 cm longitudinal skin incision is made just posterior to the medial epicondyle. This avoids sensory branches of the medial antebrachial cutaneous nerve anterior and distal to the medial epicondyle (**Figure 7.32**).

Dissection

The incision is continued through subcutaneous fat and down to fascia exposing the common flexor origin. Partial debridement of the abnormal tendinosis tissue is usually all that is required, usually involving the flexor carpi radialis and medial side of pronator teres (**Figure 7.33**). Any normal tissue attached to the medial epicondyle is left intact.

Closure of medial approach

The defect in the flexor-pronator origin is closed with absorbable sutures. Superficial closure utilises absorbable sutures to approximate the subcutaneous fat, then a subcuticular continuous absorbable suture.

An occlusive dressing is applied, followed by a bulky wool and crepe bandage dressing in two layers.

Postoperative care and instructions

Dressings are reduced at 48 hours. Early mobilisation of the elbow should be encouraged in all patients.

Follow-up is recommended at 6 weeks, with a wound check by the primary care practitioner at 2 weeks. The patient should be cautioned to return to the clinic if there is pain or functional deterioration.

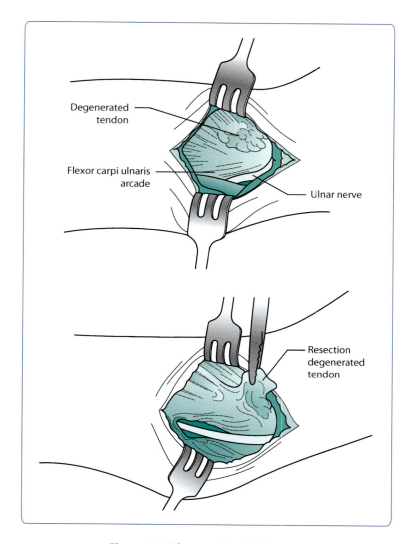

Figure 7.33 Flexor origin debridement.

Recommended references

Amin NH, Kumar NS, Schickendantz MS. Medial epicondylitis: Evaluation and management. *J Am Acad Orthop Surg.* 2015;**23(6)**:348–355.

Kroslak M, Murrell GAC. Surgical treatment of lateral epicondylitis: A prospective, randomized, double-blinded, placebo-controlled clinical trial. *Am J Sports Med.* 2018;**46(5)**:1106–1113.

Pierce TP, Issa K, Gilbert BT et al. A systematic review of tennis elbow surgery: Open versus arthroscopic versus percutaneous release of the common extensor origin. *Arthroscopy.* 2017;**33(6)**:1260–1268.e2.

Lateral collateral ligament reconstruction

The procedure for medial collateral ligament reconstruction was popularised by Jobe and then modified as the 'docking' procedure. Medial collateral ligament insufficiency is common in the United States, as a result of overhead throwing activities, particularly baseball. The lateral ulnar collateral ligament (LUCL) and remaining lateral collateral ligament (LCL) is typically the first structure to be injured during acute elbow dislocation which, despite appropriate initial management can lead to symptomatic posterolateral rotatory instability. The operative procedure for LUCL reconstruction was derived from the procedures on the medial side and therefore shares many similarities. We focus on the lateral side here.

Preoperative planning

Indications

- Symptomatic posterolateral instability in the presence of LCL insufficiency (acute or chronic)

Contraindications

- Infection, generalised or localised around the site of surgery.
- Inadequate bone and soft tissues around the reconstructive graft.
- Open physes in children is considered a relative contraindication, though a modified technique has been described to avoid iatrogenic physeal injury.
- Absence of a radial head has been shown to adversely affect outcomes; therefore, the procedure may still be performed with caution, or can be undertaken with a concurrent radial head replacement.

Consent and risks

- *Inadequate tensioning*: Ongoing instability or stiffness
- *Nerve injury related to tendon donor site*: Median palmar cutaneous nerve, saphenous nerve
- Infection
- Stress fracture
- *Nerve injury in medial collateral ligament reconstruction*: Transient ulnar neuropathy 5%–10%

Operative planning

Rarely in cases of acute injury there may be adequate capsule and ligamentous tissue remaining to permit repair, rather than reconstruction. In the case of reconstruction, choice of autograft or allograft is at the discretion of the operating surgeon. Autografts may be taken from the ipsilateral or contralateral side to the operative site. Described tendon grafts include palmaris, gracilis, plantaris, Achilles tendon (medial sliver) and the toe extensors. The presence of a palmaris tendon should be confirmed if planning to use this as an autograft (absent bilaterally in approximately 16% of patients and unilaterally in 22%).

Diagnosis of posterolateral instability is made with discerning clinical assessment but can be aided with magnetic resonance (MR) imaging, including MR arthrogram. Fluoroscopic assessment can be useful to demonstrate lateral and posterolateral instability on stress tests. Finally, diagnostic arthroscopy may offer a conclusive answer in the face of diagnostic uncertainty.

Surgical techniques include various fixation methods such as the figure-of-eight method, the docking procedure and use of an endo-button prosthesis, though all share the principle of defining a point of isometry on the lateral humerus.

Anaesthesia and positioning

Anaesthesia and positioning is the same as for radial head replacement and TEA, though antibiotics are not routinely required. The entire forearm should be accessible if considering an ipsilateral autologous palmaris graft, otherwise prepare the required limb for the autograft of choice. If the palmaris longus tendon is absent and the surgeon still wishes to use an autograft, the leg should be prepped and draped to allow access to the knee for gracilis tendon harvesting.

Surgical technique

Landmarks/incision/dissection

The limited Kocher approach offers perfect exposure of the lateral ligament complex. The palmaris tendon can be visualised by opposing the thumb and little finger together and should be marked with a skin marker prior to the procedure. The distal flexor crease of the wrist will serve as the landmark for the tendon harvest.

Procedure

On exposure of the deficient capsule/ligament complex, the capsule is incised longitudinally, just anterior to the lateral ligament complex to visualise the radiocapitellar joint. The ulna is drilled at the distal attachment of the lateral ligament complex just anterior to the crest. A second drill hole should be made such that the perpendicular bisector of these two ulnar holes points towards the origin of the LUCL (**Figure 7.34**).

An angled bone curette can then create a bone tunnel between the two holes within the ulna. A suture is placed through the tunnel, held with a haemostat and extended towards the lateral epicondyle while taut. The elbow is taken through flexion and extension until the isometric point of origin on the humerus is found. The suture should remain taut throughout flexion and extension when held at this point. A point *just anterior to the isometric point* is drilled to mark the origin of the ligament. Two tunnels should be drilled from this point, exiting posteriorly on the lateral epicondyle (**Figure 7.35**).

To obtain the palmaris tendon autograft, create a 10 mm transverse incision just proximal to the distal wrist crease over the palmaris longus tendon. Identify the tendon at this level, confirm that it is not the median nerve and harvest the tendon with a tendon stripper. The muscle can be removed from the tendon and the tendon doubled on itself to create a four-ply repair.

The doubled tendon is introduced through the ulnar tunnel and each of the arms can then be taken through one of the humeral tunnels to create a figure-of-eight. The elbow is reduced with a valgus and pronated position and the ends of the tendon can then be measured cut such that approximately 5 mm of the tendon lies within each humeral tunnel (**Figure 7.36**).

Lateral collateral ligament reconstruction | 151

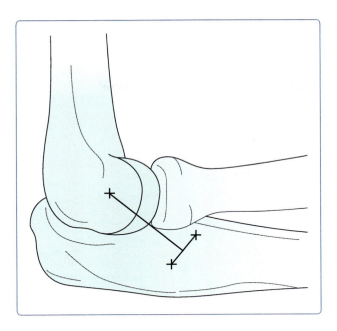

Figure 7.34 Ulnar tunnels in a lateral ulnar collateral ligament reconstruction. The perpendicular bisector of the two ulnar tunnels joins the lateral ulnar collateral ligament origin on the humerus.

A non-absorbable suture is placed in each end of the doubled tendon arm and locked. The capsule is then closed under the tendon graft, and it is imperative that the graft remains extracapsular. The sutures are introduced through the humeral tunnels and the elbow reduced once again in a valgus and pronated position, then the sutures tied together. Further tension is often required at this point, so the two limbs of the graft can be brought together side-to-side along the length of the tendon.

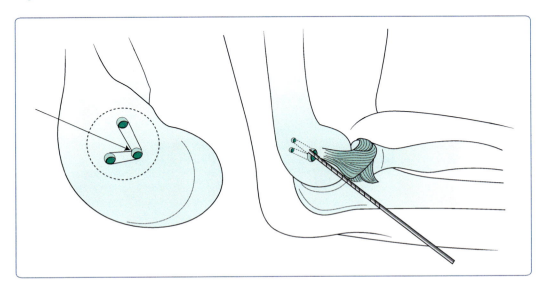

Figure 7.35 Humeral tunnels in a lateral ulnar collateral ligament reconstruction, isometric point arrowed.

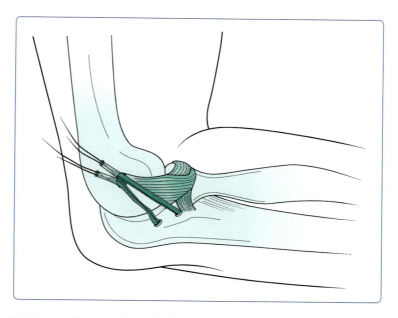

Figure 7.36 Five millimetres of the doubled tendon should lie within each humeral tunnel.

Closure
Closure is routine as for radial head replacement, no drain is required.

Postoperative care and instructions
The elbow should be immobilised in a range-of-motion brace locked at 90° in full pronation for 2 weeks postoperatively. The wound should then be checked and the brace movement range progressively increased with supervised physiotherapy, keeping a 30° extension block until 6 weeks. The patient will be seen in a surgical clinic at 6 weeks and the brace can be removed. Resisted supination should be avoided for 3 months following surgery. Elbow strengthening exercises can begin at 3 months, together with any sport-specific rehabilitation protocol. The patient should be followed up again 6 months postoperatively. Most patients can return to sports at 4–6 months.

Recommended references
Anakwenze OA, Kancherla VK, Iyengar J et al. Posterolateral rotatory instability of the elbow. *Am J Sports Med.* 2014;**42(2)**:485–491.
Jones KJ, Dodson CC, Osbahr DC et al. The docking technique for lateral ulnar collateral ligament reconstruction: Surgical technique and clinical outcomes. *J Shoulder Elbow Surg.* 2012;**21(3)**:389–395.

Elbow aspiration/injection
Indications
- Inflammatory arthritis and other arthropathies
- Suspected infection
- Haemarthrosis

Elbow aspiration/injection

Consent and risks
- Nerve injury: Less than 1%
- Infection: Less than 1%

Landmarks
Landmarks include radial head, lateral epicondyle, and tip of the olecranon (anconeus triangle) (**Figure 7.37**).

Approach
The elbow can be entered either ulnarly or radially, but the radial approach is preferred in order to avoid ulnar nerve injury.

Procedure

Structure at risk
- Radial nerve

The skin is prepared with a germicidal solution. Prior to needle insertion, the elbow is flexed and the forearm pronated to protect the radial nerve. An 18G needle is inserted into the joint, through the soft spot at the centre of the anconeus triangle. With this approach the needle will penetrate only the anconeus and joint capsule. If the needle hits bone, it should be withdrawn slightly and redirected at a slightly different angle. If performing an injection, it is wise to aspirate first to ensure the needle is not in a blood vessel.

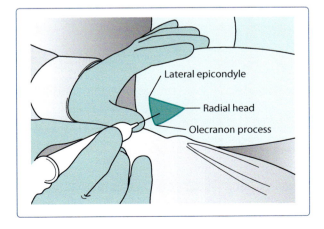

Figure 7.37 Landmarks for elbow aspiration.

Postoperative care and instructions

An occlusive dressing is applied. Mobilisation of the joint depends on the underlying reason for aspiration/injection.

Recommended references

Cardone DA, Tallia AF. Diagnostic and therapeutic injection of the elbow region. *Am Fam Physician.* 2002;**66(11)**:2097–2100.

Foocharoen T, Foocharoen C, Laopaiboon M et al. Aspiration of the elbow joint for treating radial head fractures. *Cochrane Database Syst Rev.* 2014;**(11)**:CD009949.

Elbow arthroscopy

Preoperative planning

Indications

Elbow arthroscopy is indicated in a variety of painful conditions of the elbow. The most frequent are

- Debridement for osteoarthritis
- Osteochondritis dissecans of capitellum
- Arthrolysis
- Removal of loose bodies
- Synovectomy or synovial biopsy
- Septic arthritis
- Radial head resection
- Diagnostic

Contraindications

- Infection of overlying skin
- Bony or severe fibrous ankylosis
- Caution should be taken by the operating surgeon in cases of previous trauma and surgical management as distorted anatomy may predispose nerve injury

Consent and risks

- Nerve injury
- *Infection*: Less than 1%; risk is low, so prophylactic antibiotics are not routinely recommended

Operative planning

Recent radiographs and, where taken, MR images and MR arthrograms, should be available. The correct equipment must be available, and this should be checked by the surgeon. A 30° 4 mm arthroscope should be used. The water flow should be controlled with an inflow pump.

Anaesthesia and positioning

Anaesthesia is general or combined with regional. The lateral decubitus position is used, the position being maintained by side supports. The tourniquet is applied high around the arm, and the arm is placed over a bolster applied to the bed. The elbow should be free to flex to 90° with the hand pointing towards the floor. The TV monitor is placed on the opposite side of the patient. The surgical field is prepared with a germicidal solution. Waterproof drapes are used with adhesive edges to provide a seal to the skin.

Surgical technique

Landmarks

Palpable landmarks are outlined with a marker pen:

- Lateral epicondyle
- Radial head
- Tip of the olecranon
- Medial epicondyle
- Ulnar nerve

Portals

The direct lateral portal is located in the soft spot at the centre of the triangle formed by the lateral epicondyle, radial head and tip of the olecranon, as for an elbow aspiration (**Figure 7.38**, see section 'Elbow aspiration/injection', p. 152). This portal traverses the anconeus muscle. The elbow is initially distended through this portal.

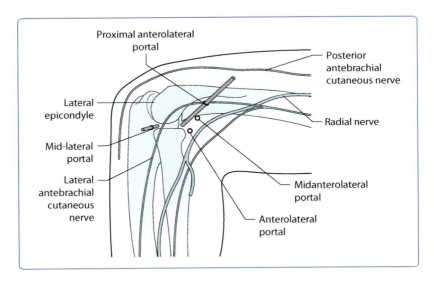

Figure 7.38 Lateral portals for elbow arthroscopy.

Distal anterolateral portal

This portal is usually established first after elbow distension. It is used for instrumentation as well as visualisation of the lateral aspect of the radial head. With the elbow flexed to 90°

the portal is located 3 cm distal and 1–2 cm anterior to the lateral epicondyle. This should bring the portal just anterior and proximal to the radiocapitellar articulation. The skin incision is made with a number 11 blade and a haemostat used to bluntly dissect down to the joint capsule.

This portal traverses the extensor carpi radialis brevis muscle. A blunt trochar is used to enter the joint with the portal driven toward the centre of the trochlea. The elbow joint *must be distended prior to trochar insertion and kept at 90° flexion during insertion* since extension brings the radial nerve closer to the joint (3–7 mm).

Structure at risk
- Radial nerve

Proximal anterolateral portal
This is located 2 cm proximal and 1 cm anterior to the lateral epicondyle. It is further from the radial nerve than other anterolateral portals. It allows for excellent views of the anterior radiohumeral and ulnohumeral joints as well as the anterior capsular margin.

Anteromedial portal

Structure at risk
- Median nerve

Some surgeons prefer to establish this portal first. The elbow should be flexed to 90° as the portal is established. It is situated 2 cm anterior and 2 cm distal to the medial epicondyle. It must be placed *under direct vision*: The median nerve lies 1–2 cm anterior and lateral to this portal.

Proximal anteromedial portal

Structures at risk
- Median nerve
- Ulnar nerve
- Medial brachial cutaneous nerve
- Medial antebrachial cutaneous nerve
- Brachial artery

This portal allows visualisation of the anterior elbow including the anterior joint capsule, medial condyle, coronoid process, trochlea, capitellum and radial head. The joint should already be distended with fluid and the ulnar nerve identified before establishing this portal. The portal is established using a longitudinal skin stab incision and blunt dissection 2 cm proximal to the medial epicondyle and immediately anterior to the intermuscular septum. The trochar is inserted over the anterior surface of the humerus aiming towards the radial head. Contact is maintained with the anterior surface of the humerus *to avoid neurovascular damage*. The ulnar nerve lies 4 mm from the portal. The median nerve lies 7–20 mm from the portal with the elbow in flexion.

Posterolateral portal

Structures at risk

- The posterior antebrachial or lateral brachial nerves can be damaged with deep incisions.

This is 3 cm proximal to the olecranon tip and just lateral to the border of the triceps tendon.

Direct posterior portal

Structures at risk

- The ulnar nerve, if placed too medially

This is 3 cm proximal to the olecranon tip and 2 cm medial to the posterolateral portal. It is *established under direct vision* with the arthroscope in the direct lateral portal (**Figure 7.39**).

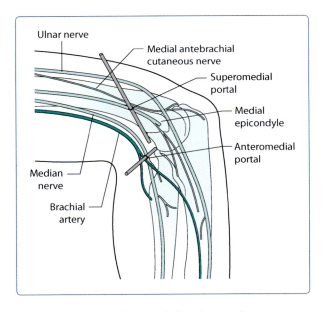

Figure 7.39 Medial portals for elbow arthroscopy.

Procedure

A systematic approach is essential if pathology is not to be missed. To distend the capsule, 15–25 mL of fluid is instilled into the joint through the direct lateral portal using an 18G needle. Backflow of fluid confirms correct placement. The anterolateral portal is established (see earlier) and the arthroscope and cannula inserted. The capsule medial to the articulation is examined first. Medial laxity can be assessed by supinating the forearm and applying valgus stress to the elbow in varying degrees of flexion. Flexing and extending the elbow allows the trochlea to be viewed. The radioulnar articulation is observed as the forearm is rotated and, for coronoid impingement, as the elbow is fully flexed.

The anteromedial portal is established under direct vision and the arthroscope introduced to view the radioulnar and radiocapitellar articulations plus the annular ligament. Extending the elbow reveals more of the capitellum, and forearm rotation exposes more of the radial head. The anterolateral gutter and capsule should also be examined.

Next, the direct lateral portal is established. Via this portal, the radial head (concave) is viewed, articulating with the capitellum (convex). The articulation between the olecranon and the trochlea is also well seen.

Finally, through the posterolateral portal, the olecranon fossa, olecranon tip and posterior trochlea are examined. Loose bodies and osteophytes are sought, particularly on the olecranon tip.

Specific instruments can be used for removal of loose bodies or debridement.

Closure

Non-absorbable suture is used to close the skin defects. Occlusive dressings are applied. A wool and crepe bandage pressure dressing is used.

Postoperative care and instructions

The pressure dressing is removed at 48 hours. The patient mobilises the elbow fully following a diagnostic arthroscopy.

Recommended references

Kelly EW, Morrey BF, O'Driscoll SW. Complications of elbow arthroscopy. *J Bone Joint Surg Am.* 2001;**83-A(1)**:25–34.

Steinmann SP. Elbow arthroscopy: Where are we now? *Arthroscopy.* 2007;**23(11)**:1231–1236.

Viva question

1. Could you inform us of how many questions are required and the format of the questions? It would be helpful to see examples of questions from other chapters in order to keep the style consistent.

8 Surgery of the Wrist

Ramon Tahmassebi, Sirat Khan and Kalpesh R Vaghela

Wrist arthroscopy	159	Distal radio ulnar joint arthrodesis (Sauve-Kapandji procedure)	182
First extensor compartment (De Quervain's) release	162	Distal ulna hemi-resection (Bowers' procedure)	183
Ganglion excision at the wrist	165	Ulnar shortening osteotomy	183
Wrist arthrodesis	169	Trapeziectomy	186
Total wrist arthroplasty	176	Surgery for scaphoid non-union	189
Proximal row carpectomy	178	Viva questions	191
Excision of the distal ulna	180		

Wrist arthroscopy

Preoperative planning

Indications

Assessment and treatment of radiocarpal and mid-carpal joint problems to include:

- Chondral surfaces and debridement of lesions
- Triangular fibrocartilage complex (TFCC) assessment and treatment
- Assessment and assistance of fracture reduction (distal radius, scaphoid)
- Carpal instability diagnosis and treatment
- Kienbock's disease assessment and treatment
- Dorsal wrist ganglion excision
- Septic arthritis irrigation and debridement
- Removal of loose bodies
- Synovectomy

Contraindications

- Persistent infection of overlying skin
- Lack of appropriate instrumentation
- Caution in cases where shoulder or elbow stiffness is present

Operative planning

History, clinical examination and recent radiology investigations should guide the clinical questions and indications. Appropriate equipment must be available, usually a 2.4–3 mm,

30°-angled arthroscope, a traction tower or similar device and any specific additional procedure-specific equipment.

> ## Consent and risks
>
> - Nerve injury – superficial radial nerve branches, dorsal cutaneous branch of ulnar nerve
> - Infection
> - Haematoma
> - Vascular injury (usually dorsal venous branches)
> - Extensor tendon injury
> - Postoperative stiffness

Anaesthesia and positioning

Anaesthesia is general or regional in a supine position. An above-elbow tourniquet is recommended and inflated to 250 mm Hg. The shoulder is abducted to 90°, placing the arm on a side extension. Ideally a wrist arthroscopy traction tower is used. Finger traps are applied to the index and middle fingers. The arm is anchored to the base of the tower by means of a strap attached proximal to the elbow. The elbow joint is flexed to 90° and traction of up to 4.5 kg is applied through the finger traps (**Figure 8.1**).

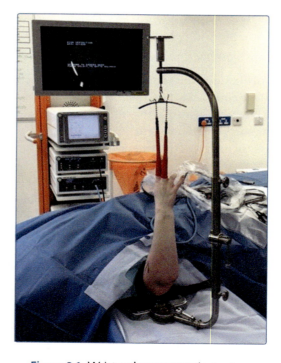

Figure 8.1 Wrist arthroscopy patient setup.

Landmarks and surgical technique

Marking the tips of the radial and ulnar styloids allows initial referencing and rough approximation of radiocarpal and mid-carpal joint levels. Saline is injected to distend the joint capsule although the procedure can be performed dry. The site or method of saline injection corresponds to the method of portal placement. The arthroscopic portals are named according to the wrist extensor compartments they lie between.

The 1–2 portal lies between the abductor pollicis longus (APL) and extensor carpi radialis brevis (ECRB) tendons. This portal is used less often due to the increased risk of injury to the radial artery and branches of the superficial radial nerve.

Lister's tubercle is the landmark for the 3–4 viewing portal which is usually placed first. The tubercle is palpated with the thumb which is then gently rolled distally, over the distal rim of the radius and into a soft spot between the extensor pollicis longus (EPL) tendon and the radial border of the fourth compartment. This point corresponds with the level of the scapholunate joint. A 1 or 2 mm incision is made in the skin only – deeper passage of the knife may risk injury to cutaneous nerves or underlying tendons. A blunt trocar or small curved haemostat is used to access the joint by applying gentle pressure and puncturing the dorsal capsule. The surgeon must account for the volar inclination of the radius in order to access the joint with minimal trauma. After placement of the 3–4 viewing portal, all subsequent portals are placed under direct vision. To facilitate ideal incision placement, a needle is placed intra-articularly in the proposed portal location before the skin incision is made.

The distal radio ulnar joint (DRUJ) is usually easily identified by palpation alone, but the joint line can be confirmed by dorsal/volar translation of the ulna respective to the radius. The tendon of extensor digiti minimi (EDM) overlies the joint, making the DRUJ a useful reference point for the 4–5 portal.

The ulnar head and base of the ulnar styloid are used to reference the level of the ulnocarpal joint. The extensor carpi ulnaris (ECU) can be palpated along the radial border of the styloid allowing placement of the 6R portal. The author's preference is to use the 6R portal for initial saline injection as the space between the triquetrum and the distal ulna is often easier to initially access. In-flow is simply established using a large syringe and simple tubing connected to the viewing portal. An assistant can apply gentle pressure and maintain a sufficient volume of fluid within the joint to maintain a good view. The surgeon must be mindful that in the presence of tears affecting the deep attachment of the TFCC, excessive volumes of fluid can transfer into the tissues of the distal forearm. Similarly, the use of high pressure during saline in-flow can cause swelling of the subcutaneous tissues around the portal sites thus hampering insertion of instruments. The 6U portal can be placed ulnar to the ECU tendon. Care must be taken to avoid iatrogenic injury to the TFCC or to the dorsal sensory branch of the ulnar nerve during placement of ulnar-sided portals.

There are two mid-carpal (MC) portals. The radial MC portal lies 2 cm distal to the 3–4 portal and can often be palpated as a soft spot. The ulnar MC portal lies 2 cm distal to the 4–5 portal, again palpable as a soft spot. Due to the oblique inclination of the scapho-capitate joint, the ulnar MC portal is often easier to access first. The radial MC portal can be placed under accurate direct visualisation (**Figure 8.2**).

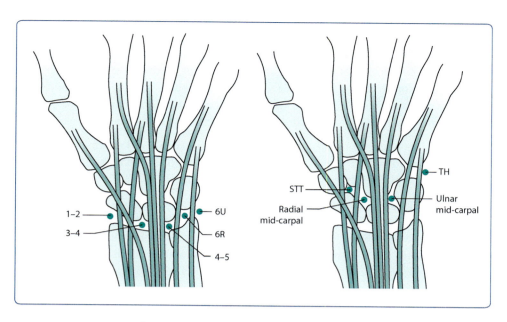

Figure 8.2 Radiocarpal and mid-carpal portals.

Procedure

The procedure is dependent on the indication. As always, a reproducible, structured approach ensures that all essential structures are adequately visualised and relevant pathology is readily identified.

Closure

Steri-Strips are sufficient to close the skin defects, and a compression bandage is then applied.

Postoperative care and instructions

The patient is usually advised to mobilise as pain allows; however, this will be dependent on the underlying pathology treated.

Recommended references

Ahsan ZS, Yao J. Complications of wrist arthroscopy. *Arthroscopy*. 2012;28(6):855–859.
Michelotti B, Chung K. Diagnostic wrist arthroscopy. *Hand Clin*. 2017;33(4):571–583.
Wagner J, Ipaktchi K, Livermore M, Banegas R. Current indications for and the technique of wrist arthroscopy. *Orthopedics*. 2014;37(4):251–256.
Wolf JM, Dukas A, Pensak M. Advances in wrist arthroscopy. *J Am Acad Orthop Surg*. 2012;20(11):725–734.

First extensor compartment (De Quervain's) release

Preoperative planning

Indications

- Stenosing tenovaginitis of the APL and extensor pollicis brevis (EPB) in the first extensor compartment
- Failure of conservative measures

Contraindications

- Infection of overlying skin or inadequate skin cover

Consent and risks

- Nerve injury and/or neuroma formation: Superficial radial nerve branches
- Failure of symptomatic relief
- Tendon instability, subluxation or adhesions

Operative planning

Confirmation of the diagnosis and exclusion of other sources of pain are essential. Other conditions that may mimic De Quervain's include the following:

- Flexor carpi radialis (FCR) tenosynovitis
- Trapezio-metacarpal joint injury, synovitis or degeneration
- Radioscaphoid impingement or degeneration
- Second or third compartment tenosynovitis
- Intersection syndrome – inflammation between the intersection of the first dorsal compartment (APL and EPB) and second dorsal compartment (extensor carpi radialis longus and extensor carpi radialis brevis).

Anatomic variations in this compartment are common, and this may play a major role in the disease process. Knowledge of this variability is important for adequate surgical decompression and prevention of postoperative complications (**Figure 8.3**).

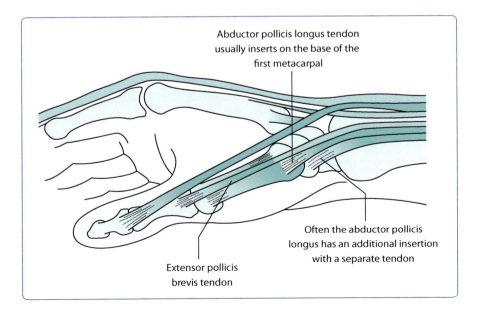

Figure 8.3 First dorsal compartment anatomy.

Anaesthesia and positioning
General, regional or local anaesthesia can be used. A bloodless field is recommended in order to adequately visualise the structures at risk and to readily identify anatomic variants. Local anaesthesia with adrenaline can be used as an alternative to use of a tourniquet. The supine position is used with a hand table.

Surgical technique
Landmarks
- Bone: Radial styloid, Lister's tubercle
- Tendon: APL and EPB – lie over the lateral aspect of the distal radius; represent the radial border of the anatomic snuffbox

Incision
Longitudinal: 2–3 cm incision based over the radial styloid and in line with the first metacarpal. A degree of obliquity can be incorporated in order to provide adequate exposure along the direction of the tendons. This can be extended proximally or distally if required. A transverse incision can be used, but this is associated with a higher rate of iatrogenic nerve injury and extension of the incision is more difficult.

Dissection

> **Structures at risk**
> - Branches of superficial radial nerve (SRN)
> - Superficial veins

In most cases, a branch of the SRN lies immediately under the skin within the subcutaneous fat. Therefore, careful skin incision and meticulous dissection technique are required to identify and protect the nerve. Care must be taken and use of retractors with sharp hooks or teeth should be avoided if possible. Any dorsal vein branches are mobilised and retracted.

Procedure
Identification of the extensor retinaculum is made easier by use of a sweeping motion with a wet swab. Passive movement of the thumb and first metacarpal will help identify the first extensor compartment and the boundary of the second compartment located dorsally. The proximal and distal margins of the retinaculum should be identified, but clear visualization can sometimes be made difficult due to adjacent connective tissue. A longitudinal incision is then made in a dorsal position along the first compartment, and the retinaculum is opened leaving a volar flap of retinaculum to prevent subluxation. The compartment is carefully explored for the single tendon of the EPB, and the multiple tendon slips of the APL. The fibro-osseous canal is then examined for septation and extra or aberrant tendons. If present, an intracompartmental septum containing additional tendon slips is usually located on the volar aspect of the compartment and must also be released. Failure to recognise and decompress this sub-sheath is a common cause of persistent pain after surgery.

If the procedure is done under local anaesthesia, the tendons are replaced and the patient asked to move the thumb to demonstrate adequate decompression and independent movement. Instability is checked for and corrected, if necessary, by loosely opposing the edges of the tendon sheath (**Figure 8.4**).

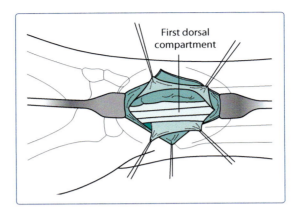

Figure 8.4 First dorsal compartment.

Closure

The tourniquet is deflated, and haemostasis is obtained. The skin is closed with a subcuticular suture. Bulky compressive dressing is applied. No splint is used for immobilisation, and early motion is encouraged.

Postoperative care and instructions

The pressure dressing is removed after 48 hours. Thumb and hand movements are initiated and increased according to comfort. Hand therapy is occasionally needed and recommended on an as-needed basis.

Recommended references

Adams J, Habbu R. Tendinopathies of the hand and wrist. *J Am Acad Orthop Surg*. 2015;23(12):741–750.

Gundes H, Tosun B. Longitudinal incision in surgical release of de Quervain disease. *Tech Hand Up Extrem Surg*. 2005;9(3):149–152.

Scheller A, Schuh R, Hönle W, Schuh A. Long-term results of surgical release of de Quervain's stenosing tenosynovitis. *Int Orthop*. 2008;33(5):1301–1303.

Ganglion excision at the wrist

A ganglion is a mucin-filled cyst which may be uni- or multi-lobulated. It is the most common soft tissue tumour of the hand, representing up to 70% of all such lesions. Dorsal wrist ganglia represent over 70% of all ganglia and most frequently arise from the scapholunate ligament (SLL). Volar wrist ganglia account for up to 20% of all ganglia and commonly arise from the scapho-trapezial joint. Many ganglia are asymptomatic and are incidental findings at the time of magnetic resonance imaging (MRI) or ultrasound investigation.

Others however are symptomatic, especially dorsal scapholunate ganglia that typically cause dorsal impingement pain when weightbearing through the extended wrist.

Preoperative planning

Indications

- Pain
- Interference with activity
- Nerve compression
- Enlarging
- Failed aspiration (success rate approximately 50% with needle aspiration)

Consent and risks

- Numbness and scar sensitivity
- Recurrence
- Nerve injury and neuroma formation: Superficial branch of radial nerve in dorsal ganglia
- Vascular injury: Radial artery injury requiring repair with volar ganglia
- Postoperative stiffness
- Scapholunate instability: Rare

Anaesthesia and positioning

General anaesthesia, regional anaesthesia or wide awake local anaesthesia no tourniquet (WALANT) are preferred. Local anaesthesia without adrenaline or tourniquet is possible, but a bloodless field is preferred and allows accurate visualisation of the neck of the ganglion and structures at risk. The patient is positioned supine and the hand positioned on a hand table.

Surgical technique

The technique described is dorsal scapholunate ganglion excision. Arthroscopic excision and open excision have similar recurrence rates. However, arthroscopic resection can be technically more challenging and requires the surgeon to be comfortable with arthroscopic procedures. However, it can lead to a quicker postoperative recovery. Both techniques aim to excise the neck or the origin of the ganglion as it arises from the dorsal ligament fibres and adjacent capsular attachment.

Arthroscopically it is performed according to the techniques described earlier by excising the dorsal capsule overlying the scapholunate articulation with use of an arthroscopic shaver. An open excision is more often used.

Incision

A transverse or longitudinal incision can be used. Transverse incisions can be placed along Langer's lines or existing skin creases, but care must be taken to avoid injury to dorsal nerves, veins and tendons. Longitudinal incisions can be more easily extended but perhaps less cosmetic (**Figure 8.5**).

Ganglion excision at the wrist

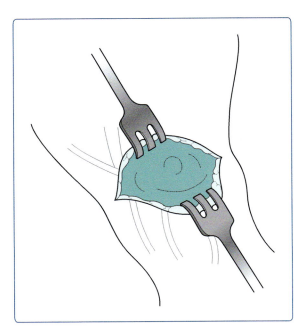

Figure 8.5 Skin incision for dorsal ganglion excision.

Structures at risk

- Dorsal sensory branches of radial (or ulnar) nerve – these must be identified and protected
- Dorsal veins
- EPL and extensor digitorum communis (EDC) tendons

Procedure

The cyst usually lies between the third and fourth extensor compartments but variability exists. Large ganglia will grow between extensor tendons and herniate through the extensor retinaculum to lie under the skin. Their position relative to the boundaries of the retinaculum must be appreciated as a retinacular release is often needed to visualise the neck. Care must be taken to identify the EPL tendon to avoid iatrogenic injury. The EPL and ECRB tendons are retracted radially and EDC tendons retracted ulnarly. Careful deep dissection around the borders of the ganglion will allow location of its neck. The ganglion must be resected at its base from the level of the capsule. A small capsular resection at this site will allow for visualisation of the dorsal SLL which is then gently curettaged. Again, care must be taken not to damage ligament fibres during the resection (**Figure 8.6**).

Closure

Avoid closure of the capsule to prevent joint stiffness. Haemostasis is achieved after tourniquet release. Vicryl is used to close the retinaculum and subcuticular suture to close the skin. A volar splint is applied in neutral.

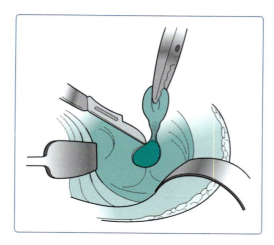

Figure 8.6 Excision of the ganglion and its stalk from the scapholunate ligament.

Surgical technique – ganglion of the scapho-trapezial joint

Structures at risk

- The palmar cutaneous branch of the median nerve
- The radial artery: Identification and mobilisation are vital; ganglion and artery are often closely associated

Landmarks

- Scaphoid tubercle
- Flexor carpi radialis tendon
- Radial artery

Incision

A longitudinal incision is created over the ganglion.

Dissection and procedure

The radial artery and vein are identified and retracted radially, taking care to cauterise any small side branches. If needed the FCR can be mobilised and retracted in an ulnar direction. The ganglion is dissected down to its origin (usually the scapho-trapezial joint) and is excised with a small portion of surrounding capsule which is left open.

Recommended references

Angelides AC, Wallace PF. The dorsal ganglion of the wrist: Its pathogenesis, gross and microscopic anatomy, and surgical treatment. *J Hand Surg Am*. 1976;1:228–235.

Finsen V, Håberg O, Borchgrevink GE. Surgery for wrist ganglia: One-hundred and twenty-two patients reviewed 8 years after operation. *Orthop Rev*. 2014;6(1):5162.

Lidder S, Ranawat V, Ahrens P. Surgical excision of wrist ganglia; literature review and nine-year retrospective study of recurrence and patient satisfaction. *Orthop Rev.* 2009;1(1):e5.

Mathoulin C, Mathilde Gras M. Arthroscopic management of dorsal and volar wrist ganglion. *Hand Clin.* 2017;33(4):769–777.

Wrist arthrodesis

Preoperative planning

Indications

- Osteoarthritis
- Rheumatoid or inflammatory arthritis
- Joint destruction secondary to infection or tumour resection
- Failed arthroplasty or limited fusion
- Neuromuscular flexion contracture
- Kienbock's disease and pancarpal arthritis

Cautions and contraindications

- Skeletal immaturity (open distal radius physis)
- Relative contraindication where the contralateral wrist has already been fused
- Caution advised in heavy smokers or those with multiple comorbidities that may hinder fusion

Consent and risks

- Residual pain
- Non-union
- Extensor tenosynovitis
- Loss of grip strength
- Subsequent re-operation
- Complex regional pain syndrome
- Nerve injury and neuroma formation
- DRUJ pain
- Carpal tunnel syndrome
- Ulnar abutment

Operative planning

The surgeon must decide between full and partial wrist fusion based on the pathology and pattern of degeneration. Partial fusions such as radioscapholunate or a 'four-corner' arthrodesis may be good motion-preserving options, but each has specific procedural indications and technique. A 'standard' total wrist fusion includes radiocarpal, mid-carpal and carpometacarpal arthrodesis using an implant spanning the distal radius, across the carpus and fixed to the third metacarpal.

Consider the need for bone grafting – autologous bone from the distal radius is not usually possible due to the necessity for placement of the plate over the site of harvest. Iliac crest harvest can be used if necessary and is usually sufficient unless there is severe bone loss. The pathologic process necessitating wrist arthrodesis may have resulted in distal radius or carpal collapse and resultant ulnocarpal impaction. This should be addressed at the time of operation in order to avoid ongoing causes of pain. Management options include a restoration of length or, more feasibly, an ulna resection or shortening osteotomy (described later).

The position of fusion is 10°–20° of dorsiflexion and 0–10° of ulna deviation. This allows for functionality and preservation of grip strength. Maximum grip is generated in 35° of dorsiflexion, but this is less functional. In rheumatoid arthritis, a more neutral position may be preferred depending on how the disease process has affected the metacarpophalangeal joints. Bilateral wrist fusions should be considered very carefully due to the accompanying restrictions in function. In cases where one wrist has already been fused, a motion-preserving procedure is often preferred for the contralateral side. This may be in the form of a partial wrist fusion or a total wrist arthroplasty. If bilateral wrist fusions are to be undertaken, both wrists can be fixed in neutral or alternatively one in slight flexion and the other in slight extension depending on functional requirements.

The choice of implant is dependent on patient anatomy, pathology and surgeon preference. Many manufacturers now provide a range of options including

- Radiocarpal fusion with no additional metacarpal fixation
- Radio-carpo-metacarpal fixation to either second or third metacarpals
- Neutral or extended positions
- Short and long bends to accommodate anatomy
- Variable screw diameters to accommodate smaller metacarpal bones
- Locking and non-locking screw options

Anaesthesia and positioning

Anaesthesia is general or regional, and the supine position is used; a hand table, tourniquet and image intensifier are also required for the procedure.

Surgical technique – dorsal approach to the wrist

Landmarks
- Radial styloid process
- Lister's tubercle
- DRUJ
- Third metacarpal

Incision

This surgical approach can be applied to a multitude of procedures. For the purposes of a wrist fusion, it can be extended distally to allow for adequate exposure of the metacarpal if desired. A dorsal longitudinal incision (or 'lazy S') is used in line with the third metacarpal, Lister's tubercle and distal radius (**Figure 8.7**).

Dissection

Proximally, full-thickness skin flaps are raised allowing exposure of the underlying extensor retinaculum. Distal to the retinaculum the extensor tendons of the third and

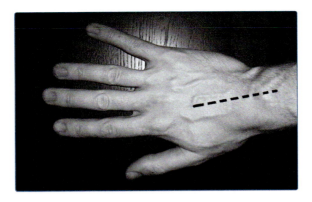

Figure 8.7 Dorsal skin incision for wrist arthrodesis.

fourth compartments (EPL and EDC) are identified. Several methods of negotiating the extensor retinaculum have been described and can be utilised including the following:

- A longitudinal incision overlying the fourth compartment, elevation of the retinaculum and sequential releases of adjacent septations between compartments with retraction of tendons. Two flaps are created on either side of the fourth compartment for later repair. These can be elevated radially and ulnarly as far as necessary for adequate exposure.
- An incision over EPL that exposes the tendon and allows it to be retracted. Subperiosteal resection of second and fourth compartments starting from the floor of the third allows them to remain unbreached within their retinacular sleeves.
- A radially based retinacular flap extending from the second to fifth compartments which gives good exposure of radial and ulnar sides of the distal radius.
- A step-cut incision that allows for lengthening if needed at the time of closure. Alternatively, one of the transverse limbs can be used to cover a dorsally placed implant, thus protecting the overlying extensor tendons (**Figure 8.8**).

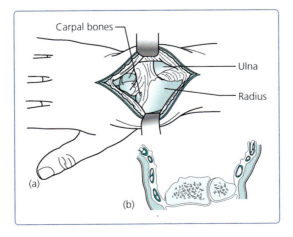

Figure 8.8 (a) Approach to the wrist joint. (b) Axial view showing the approach between the third and fourth compartments.

> ### Structures at risk
> - Dorsal veins
> - Superficial nerves – superficial radial nerve and dorsal cutaneous branch of ulnar nerve
> - Posterior interosseous nerve – see later

With any of these approaches, the dorsal surface of the distal radius must be adequately exposed at both its radial and ulnar margins. Lister's tubercle is excised (a rongeur is sufficient) to allow flat plate apposition. The posterior interosseous nerve is identified just proximal to the extensor retinaculum as it enters the radial side of the fourth compartment (it sits just ulnar to Lister's tubercle), and a 2 cm segment is excised and the ends diathermied. The ECRB tendon may need to be released off the third metacarpal for plate apposition.

To access the carpus, several capsulotomies have been described. For the purposes of a wrist fusion, these do not need to be anatomic (i.e. there is no ambition to mobilise the wrist and therefore anatomic repair of wrist ligaments or capsule is not necessary). Options for capsulotomy include the following:

- A simple midline capsulotomy with elevation of radial and ulnar flaps.
- A 'Mayo' capsulotomy – this is a ligament-preserving radially based flap with extensions along the dorsal radiocarpal and dorsal intercarpal ligaments. Provides good exposure and is easy to close. Care must be taken when exposing the ulnar aspect of the joint not to injure the dorsal limb of the TFCC.
- A distally based flap initially elevating the capsule off the radiocarpal joint and extending distally – this is a good flap to consider when undertaking carpal surgery, but a further central split would need to be undertaken to accommodate plate placement.

Arthrodesis procedure

After inspecting for arthritic lesions and making an assessment of the extent of their effects, the surgeon can sequentially perform the following:

- Excision of the cartilage and the subchondral bone in the radioscaphoid and radiolunate joints and the intercarpal joints (scaphocapitate, lunocapitate and triquetrohamate) until the cancellous bone of each carpal bone is reached. To achieve this, a small burr (with irrigation), rongeur, curette or osteotome is sufficient.
- Temporary fixation using K-wires, trying if possible to align the central axis between radius, lunate, capitate and third metacarpal.
- Filling of any gaps or defects with bone graft of adequate quality and size. Bone from the distal radius may possibly be used but is often insufficient in terms of volume, and harvest may create a cortical defect that interferes with plate fixation.
- The third carpometacarpal joint must be considered. Ideally, this should also be at least partially excised and grafted so as to remove any movement and provide a continuous bridge of bone across the fusion mass.

In this case, a precontoured plate is applied, and an intraoperative decision can be made regarding size, length or bend. Most modern plates have oval hole options that allow initial plate adjustment as well as a later option to apply compression. The distal end of the plate should reach the mid-shaft or two-thirds of the metacarpal (**Figure 8.9**). After placing two bicortical non-locking screws proximally and distally to secure the plate, a combination of screws can be used according to requirements including the option of fixation into the carpus. If possible, compression of the fusion mass should be incorporated to promote union. Specific attention should be paid to the relationship between the implant and the extensor tendons as this is a well-recognised cause of postoperative morbidity and re-operation (**Figure 8.10**).

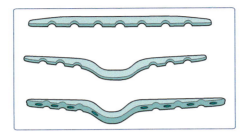

Figure 8.9 AO Wrist fusion plates.

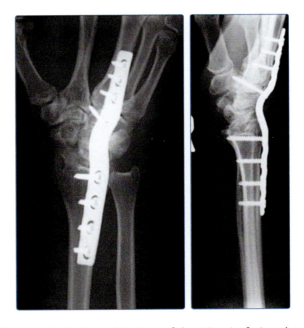

Figure 8.10 Radiographic views of the AO wrist fusion plate.

Closure

The capsule is approximated as far as possible and closed with an absorbable suture. The extensor retinaculum is closed over the plate if possible – but is not essential. Here, use of the step-cut retinacular exposure is useful. Bowstringing of the extensor tendons due to deficiency in the retinaculum should not be problematic as the wrist is now fixed in a static position. A volar splint is used for 2–6 weeks. Union is usually achieved by 3 months.

Surgical technique – partial fusion

The 'four-corner' fusion (capitate–hamate–triquetrum–lunate fusion) is indicated in scapholunate advanced collapse (SLAC) wrist, scaphoid non-union advanced collapse (SNAC) wrist or mid-carpal instability. The procedure includes a scaphoidectomy and a fusion of the capitate, lunate, hamate and triquetrum. It is vital that the radiolunate joint remains in good condition and capable of function without pain. This should be carefully evaluated preoperatively either radiographically or using wrist arthroscopy. The landmarks, basic approach and structures at risk are similar to those of full wrist fusion.

Incision

A straight or 'lazy S' incision is made over the dorsum of the wrist, again using Lister's tubercle and the third metacarpal as reference points, although the length of the incision is shorter than that required for a total wrist arthrodesis.

Dissection

The extensor retinaculum is exposed in the same way as described for total wrist arthrodesis. Capsulotomy again should allow for visualisation of the radial and ulnar sides of the carpus. A radially or distally based capsulotomy will work well (**Figure 8.11**).

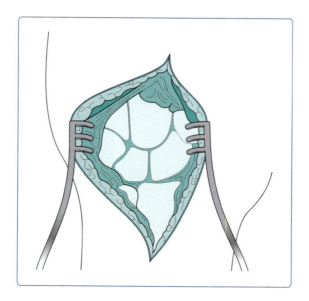

Figure 8.11 Exposure of the carpal bones.

Procedure

The soft tissue attachments to the scaphoid are first divided using sharp dissection. The scaphoid is very well attached to soft tissue on its volar and distal aspect. It may be possible to access this from a dorsal approach and undertake a piecemeal scaphoid excision using a joystick K-wire, osteotome and rongeurs. However, a small volar hockey stick incision based over the scaphoid tubercle can facilitate excision of the distal pole and often saves time. Preservation of the excised scaphoid for use as bone graft is possible, but in many cases, the scaphoid is in poor condition and does not provide good quality graft material.

The mid-carpal joint is exposed by flexing the wrist, and all cartilage surfaces and sclerotic bone are debrided until healthy cancellous bone is seen. Again, the need for bone graft must be considered especially if a significant resection is needed and there is a risk of reducing the carpal height excessively. Excision of the scaphoid renders the remaining components of the carpus unstable, most notably the mid-carpal joint. There may well also be a degree of pre-existing carpal malalignment. The lunate and mid-carpal joint can be reduced to neutral position using temporary K-wires to maintain the corrected position until definitive fixation is achieved. A range of fixation methods have been described including multiple K-wires and compression staples, but the two most commonly used forms of fixation are either dorsal 'spider' plates or intramedullary headless compression screws placed centrally along the axes of the luno-capitate and triquetro-hamate joints.

If a spider plate is being used, the four bones are reduced with temporary wires, and a reamer is used to create a dorsal trough in which the plate will sit and be recessed so as not to cause impingement. Cortical and/or locking screws are used to create compression and stable fixation of the four bones. If headless screws are being used, the mid-carpal joint must be denuded of all articular cartilage until bleeding cancellous bone is seen. Strong ligamentous attachments between capitate and hamate mean that this joint does not necessarily need preparation or stabilization with an implant. If the lunotriquetral ligament remains intact, the same rationale can be applied. Bone graft can be used to fill defects and to maintain carpal height. Again, temporary K-wire stabilization allows placement of guide wires along the central axes of the two columns. Note must be taken of the obliquity of the triquetro-hamate joint in relation to the more horizontally orientated luno-capitate joint. Screw lengths are determined ensuring that the heads are sufficiently buried so as not to cause injury to the surfaces of the lunate fossa or TFCC (**Figure 8.12**).

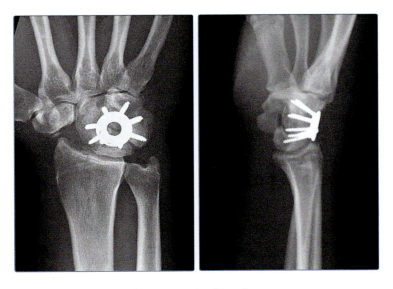

Figure 8.12 A spider plate.

Closure
See 'Surgical technique – full fusion'.

Postoperative care and instructions
- Below-elbow cast immobilisation is recommended for 6 weeks following partial and total wrist fusion.
- Hand therapy and finger exercises are commenced 1 week after surgery.
- Union is usually achieved by 3 months.

Initially, active mobilisation is undertaken under supervision only. When movement has maximised, strengthening exercises can begin.

Recommended references
Hooved P. Intercarpal fusions: Indications, treatment options and techniques. *EFORT Open Rev.* 2016;1:45–51.
Stewart DT, Froelich JM, Shin AY. Intercarpal arthrodeses. *J Hand Surg Am.* 2014;39(2):373–377.
Trail IA, Murali R, Stanley JK et al. The long-term outcome of four-corner fusion. *J Wrist Surg.* 2015;4(2):128–133.

Total wrist arthroplasty
Total wrist arthroplasty (TWA) is a motion-preserving treatment for pancarpal wrist arthritis. Modern fourth-generation TWA designs are modular, cementless and preserve bone stock with semi-constrained or constrained geometry.

Indications
- Rheumatoid or inflammatory arthritis
- Osteoarthritis

Contraindications
- Active infection
- Young, high-demand patients

Preoperative planning
Plain radiographs including AP and lateral views to assess the wrist. A computed tomography scan is useful for quantifying the bone stock available, the calibre of the metacarpal shafts and the overall alignment of the radial-carpal-metacarpal axis.

Consent and risks
- Periprosthetic fractures
- Loosening
- Osteolysis (subsequent requirement for revision)
- Infection
- Subluxation/dislocation
- Complex regional pain syndrome

Anaesthesia and positioning

General anaesthesia is used. Patient is supine on a radiolucent arm table with application of a tourniquet. Antibiotic prophylaxis is administered. An image intensifier is used.

Surgical technique

Incision

A dorsal longitudinal skin incision is preferred, and the approach to the carpus is in the same manner as described for wrist arthrodesis.

Procedure

The specific procedure performed is dependent on the implant design and can be variable, however there are some common principles. The proximal row is excised and the surfaces of the distal radius and distal row are prepared. Surfaces are resected using jigs and cutting blocks based on guide wires placed along the axis of the distal radius and on the opposite side, along the second or third metacarpals. The implant is fixed distally with screws into the carpus and metacarpals. Proximally a press-fit porous coated implant is seated. A polyethylene bearing surface is then implanted forming a semi-constrained, ellipsoidal articulation. Alternative constrained designs are based on intramedullary hydroxyapatite stems in the radius and in the capitate/third metacarpal. These are then connected via a metal on metal bearing surface. In rheumatoid patients, consideration must again be given to the position of the ulna in relation to the carpus and the DRUJ – a distal ulna resection procedure may be required (**Figure 8.13**).

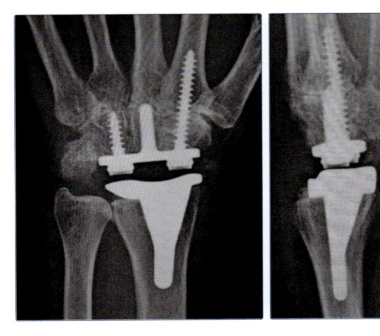

Figure 8.13 Postoperative radiographs of a total wrist arthroplasty.

Closure

The capsular flap is closed, and the extensor retinaculum is repaired. The image intensifier is used to confirm the position implants. The skin is closed with a subcuticular absorbable monofilament suture.

Postoperative care and instructions

The wrist is initially splinted for comfort, but the aim should be to commence active movements under the supervision of a hand therapist as soon as pain or soft tissue healing allow.

Recommended reference

Halim A, Weiss A-P. Total wrist arthroplasty. *J Hand Surg Am.* 2017;42(3):198–209.

Proximal row carpectomy

Proximal row carpectomy is a salvage procedure for degenerative conditions affecting the radiocarpal joint such as SNAC and SLAC. It involves excision of the proximal row of the carpus – the scaphoid, lunate and triquetrum. The capitate then moves proximally to articulate in the lunate fossa on the distal radius. It has the advantage of being motion sparing, and its success does not rely on the fusion of carpal bones. Its main disadvantages relate to the loss of carpal height which in turn leads to a reduction in grip strength. Also, the radii of curvature of the proximal capitate and proximal lunate are not the same. Therefore, late-stage radiocapitate arthritis is a potential hazard. Prerequisites for this procedure are intact cartilage surfaces of the proximal capitate and lunate fossa of the distal radius. However, if there is doubt regarding the quality of the articular surface, the capsulotomy can be modified to allow for placement of a capsular interposition graft within the lunate fossa.

Indications

- SNAC
- SLAC
- Kienbock's disease (contraindicated if the proximal capitate or lunate fossa are affected by significant degenerative change)

Contraindications

- Active infection
- Presence of advanced degenerative changes in the lunate fossa or on the proximal pole of capitate

Preoperative planning

Plain radiographs are taken including AP and lateral views to assess the joint surfaces. Magnetic resonance imaging and computed tomography are helpful, but arthroscopic assessment of the wrist provides the most definitive information. Depending on the indication, patient factors and pattern of wear inside the wrist, radioscapholunate fusion and scaphoidectomy with four-corner fusion may also be considered as part of preoperative planning.

Consent and risks

- Injury to superficial radial nerve and dorsal cutaneous branches of the ulnar nerve
- Loss of grip strength
- Stiffness and loss of range of movement
- Arthritis of the capitate and/or lunate fossa of the distal radius

Anaesthesia and positioning

General anaesthesia is used. Patient is supine on a radiolucent arm table with application of a tourniquet. Antibiotic prophylaxis is administered. An image intensifier is used.

Surgical technique

Incision and surgical approach

The approach is the same as per total wrist fusion.

Procedure

When the carpus has been adequately exposed, any remnants of the scapholunate and lunotriquetral ligaments are divided allowing the bones of the proximal row to dissociate from one another. While excising each bone, care must be taken to preserve the volar extrinsic ligaments, and in particular the radioscaphocapitate ligament. This will minimise the risk of ulnar drift of the capitate. Furthermore, iatrogenic injury to the cartilage of the proximal capitate and distal radius must be avoided. The pisiform is not removed. The capitate is guided into its new position in the lunate fossa, and the capsule is closed and tensioned accordingly (**Figure 8.14**).

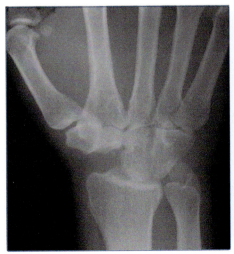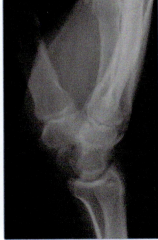

Figure 8.14 Postoperative radiographs of a proximal row carpectomy showing docking of the capitate into the lunate fossa of the distal radius.

Postoperative care and instructions

The wrist is immobilised in a cast for 3–4 weeks. A further 2 weeks of immobilisation in a removable thermoplastic splint are recommended, and subsequent range of motion exercises are supervised by a hand therapist.

Recommended references

Berkhout MJL, Bachour Y, Zheng KH, Mullender MG, Strackee SD, Ritt MJPF. Four-corner arthrodesis versus proximal row carpectomy: A retrospective study with a mean follow-up of 17 years. *J Hand Surg Am*. 2015;40(7):1349–1354.

Green DP, Perreira AC, Longhofer LK. Proximal row carpectomy. *J Hand Surg Am*. 2015;40(8):1672–1676.

Excision of the distal ulna

Indications

Pain arising from the DRUJ as a result of

- Malunion of distal radius or ulna
- Ulnocarpal impaction
- Rheumatoid or osteoarthritis affecting the DRUJ
- Salvage procedure following previously failed DRUJ operative interventions
- Reserved for patients with low functional demands

Contraindications

- Younger and high-demand patients

Distal ulna excision can take one of three different forms:

A. Distal ulna resection (Darrach's procedure)
B. DRUJ arthrodesis (Sauve-Kapandji procedure)
C. Distal ulna hemi-resection (Bowers' procedure) (**Figure 8.15**)

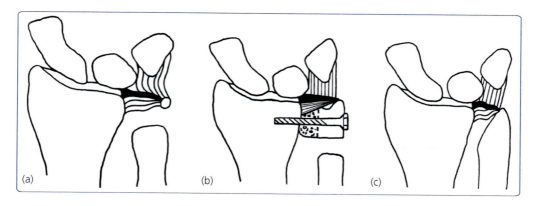

Figure 8.15 Distal ulna excision procedures: (a) Darrach's procedure, (b) Sauve-Kapandji procedure and (c) Bowers' procedure.

Preoperative planning

Consent and risks

- Outcomes are dependent on primary pathology and operative indication
- Radioulnar impingement
- Reduced grip strength
- Non-union
- Residual symptoms of pain

Surgical approach to the distal ulna and distal radio ulnar joint

Structures at risk

- Dorsal sensory branch of ulnar nerve
- Ulnar artery and nerve

Several approaches to the DRUJ and distal ulna have been proposed. The one described later has the following advantages:

- Allows minor modifications that preserve the radioulnar ligaments and minimise the risk of TFCC injury
- Allows good visualisation of the sigmoid notch of the distal radius and thus the DRUJ
- Allows a DRUJ capsular flap to be raised that can later be used for closure, stabilisation or interposition
- Preserves the attachment of the ECU subsheath, minimising the risk of instability
- Provides an exposure suitable for most DRUJ or distal ulna procedures

Patients were placed in a supine position with the limb on a hand table. An above-elbow tourniquet is used. A longitudinal dorsal incision is made between the fifth (EDM) and sixth (ECU) extensor compartments. As the superficial dissection is undertaken, care must be taken not to injure the dorsal sensory branch of the ulnar nerve. The fifth extensor compartment is opened, and the tendon of EDM is retracted. The exposure can be extended by dividing the septa separating the fourth and sixth compartments. This allows the extensor retinaculum to be elevated in both directions, thus exposing the DRUJ capsule and ulnar head below. The capsule is opened by creating a capsular flap that is ulnar based, radially based or oblique. Care must be taken when creating the distal limb of either flap as the dorsal radioulnar ligament and TFCC are at risk (**Figure 8.16**).

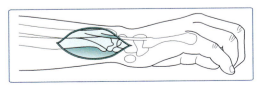

Figure 8.16 Approach to the distal ulna.

Darrach's procedure

A radially based capsular flap should be used with subperiosteal dissection to expose the ulnar head. The base of the ulnar styloid is osteotomised to allow preservation of the attachment of the TFCC and the dorsal radioulnar ligament. The ulna is osteotomised at its neck and the head excised. The remnant capsule and soft tissues around the distal ulna can then be utilised to stabilise the shaft by use of drill holes or suture anchors. The overlying retinaculum is then closed, but consideration must be made to the tendon of ECU. It may be inherently unstable now that the subsheath is no longer attached to the ulnar head. If this is the case, a slip of extensor retinaculum can be used to fashion a sling, keeping the ECU tendon located dorsally.

Postoperative care and instructions

Postoperative immobilisation with a wrist splint is maintained for 6 weeks. Early active exercises are encouraged at 2 weeks.

Recommended references

Darrach W. Partial excision of lower shaft of ulna for deformity following Colles fracture. *Ann Surg*. 1913;57:764–765.

De Witte PB, Wujffels M, Jupiter JB, Ring D. The Darrach procedure for post-traumatic reconstruction. *Acta Orthop Belg*. 2009;75(3):316–322.

Grawe B, Heincelman C, Stern P. Functional results of the Darrach procedure: A long-term outcome study. *J Hand Surg Am*. 2012;37(12):2475–2480.

Mansat P, Bonnevialle N, Ayel J et al. Long-term outcome of distal ulna resection-stabilisation procedures in post-traumatic radio-ulnar joint disorders. *Orthop Traumatol Surg Res*. 2010;96(3):216–221.

Distal radio ulnar joint arthrodesis (Sauve-Kapandji procedure)

Indications

These are the same as per Darrach's procedure.

Surgical technique

The DRUJ is exposed in the same way as previously described via the fifth compartment. Here, exposure of the fourth compartment and retraction of the tendons may facilitate a better view of the sigmoid notch of the distal radius. Also, the ulnar dissection need not be as extensive. And in particular, the TFCC and subsheath attachment of ECU to the ulnar head should be preserved. A capsulotomy is made as before, and the ulnar head is delivered to allow preparation of the articular surfaces. Chondral surfaces are debrided. Use of a small power burr ensures accurate excision of cartilage while preserving bone stock – care must be taken not to over-resect the underlying cancellous bone from both surfaces which may necessitate additional bone grafting. Ensure debris is washed out from the joint surfaces.

Under fluoroscopy, compress the prepared ulnar head into the sigmoid notch, and from the lateral subcutaneous border of the ulna pass two percutaneous guide wires for either partially threaded cannulated screws or headless compression screws (of approximately 3 mm diameter). Measure and insert the screws maintaining neutral rotation and good compression of the surfaces. Next, expose the ulnar neck and resect approximately 1 cm of the subcapital bone using an oscillating saw. Protect the surrounding soft tissues throughout. The resulting pseudarthrosis will allow rotational movements to occur below the level of the arthrodesis so that pronation and supination are maintained. Persistent instability of the ulnar shaft is a recognised complication. Several additional procedures have been described that can be undertaken at the same sitting or as late-stage procedures if required. These include stabilising the shaft using a section of mobilised pronator quadratus muscle attached by an anchor or by using a distally based strip of flexor carpi ulnaris tendon that is passed through a drill hole in the shaft and secured. The capsulotomy and retinaculum are closed. The tendon of EDM can be left outside of the retinaculum if the capsule is thin and there is a risk of impingement against the arthrodesis.

Postoperative care

Keep in an above-elbow cast in neutral rotation for 6 weeks and then in a below-elbow cast until union is achieved.

Distal ulna hemi-resection (Bowers' procedure)

Indications

These are the same as discussed earlier.

Surgical technique

Expose the DRUJ and ulnar head via the floor of the fifth extensor compartment as described earlier. Again, care must be taken to preserve the attachment of ECU, the dorsal limb of the radioulnar ligament and the attachments of the TFCC to the fovea of the distal ulna. An oblique resection of the articular portion of the ulnar head is made, extending from the medial aspect of the head towards the base of the styloid which should be preserved. The edges of the resected ulna should be beveled and smoothed off. The ulnar-based capsular flap can again be sutured to the volar aspect of the sigmoid notch using bone anchors, thus creating a sling that can reduce subsequent ulnar instability. Equally, pronator quadratus can be mobilised from its ulnar insertion and used as an interposition. Wound closure is as previously discussed.

Postoperative care

Place in an above-elbow cast for 3 weeks in neutral rotation followed by a further 3 weeks in a below-elbow cast before mobilising.

Ulnar shortening osteotomy

Preoperative planning

Indications

Ulnar positive variance

- Acquired
  - Distal radial fracture
  - Essex-Lopresti-type injury
  - Traumatic distal radial growth arrest

- Congenital
  - Idiopathic ulnar impaction syndrome
  - Madelung deformity (often in conjunction with other procedures)
  - Development of degenerative changes in the TFCC, DRUJ, ulnar head and articular surfaces of the lunate and triquetrum owing to ulnar abutment

Cautions and contraindications

- Malalignment with respect to ulnar inclination and the sigmoid notch
- DRUJ dysplasia
- Advanced osteoarthritis or significant malalignment of the DRUJ
- Smokers (higher incidence of delayed union and non-union)

Consent and risks

- Non-union
- Delayed union
- Prominent metalwork and tendonitis from hardware irritation necessitating removal
- Reduced grip strength: Variable depending on the primary pathology
- Nerve injury, commonly dorsal sensory branch of the ulnar nerve
- Compartment syndrome

Preoperative planning

'90/90' radiographs are obtained (an AP and lateral wrist X-ray taken with the shoulder in 90° abduction and the elbow in 90° flexion). This allows the most accurate estimation of true radioulnar variance. Usually the contralateral side is referred to for comparison. A measurement is made to indicate the amount of shortening required to achieve a final ulnar variance of neutral or −1 mm. A wrist arthroscopy may be performed before an ulnar shortening osteotomy to identify chondral lesions on the proximal lunate or TFCC tears that may benefit from debridement or may guide postoperative recovery.

Anaesthesia and positioning

Anaesthesia can be general or regional. Use of a tourniquet is recommended. Intravenous antibiotics are administered on induction of anaesthesia. The patient is positioned supine, with a hand table. An image intensifier is used.

Surgical technique

Incision

A longitudinal incision is made along the subcutaneous ulnar border of the ulna starting 3–4 cm proximal to the ulnar styloid. This is extended proximally for approximately 10 cm.

Structures at risk

- The dorsal sensory branch of the ulnar nerve is present at the distal extent of the incision.

Dissection

The fascia and muscle fibres of flexor carpi ulnaris (FCU) and ECU blend over the subcutaneous border of the ulna. This interval is incised, and a subperiosteal elevation is undertaken, predominantly on the volar side to mobilise FCU and expose the ulnar shaft. Care must be taken as the ulnar neurovascular bundle lies on the radial side of the tendon and is at risk. Hohmann retractors are placed around the ulna to retract the muscle of FCU and expose the volar side of the ulnar shaft. This will allow placement of the plate on the flat surface of the ulnar shaft and ensure that it remains flush with the lateral border of the bone. The plate will sit under the muscle of FCU, and the likelihood of painful metalwork prominence will be reduced (**Figure 8.17**).

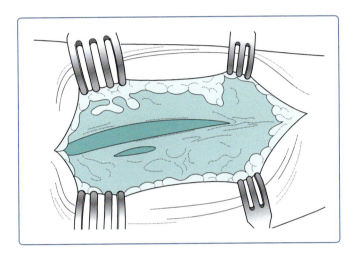

Figure 8.17 Approach between the extensor carpi ulnaris and flexor carpi ulnaris.

Procedure

Numerous ulnar shortening systems are available. Each manufacturer and implant has a recommended technique, but they share common principles. The ulnar plate is positioned, initial screw holes are drilled and cortical screws are used to secure the plate to the bone. A cutting block is then applied through which an initial oblique cut is made with an oscillating saw while the plate remains *in situ*. This ensures that control and stability of the bone can be maintained throughout the procedure. The cutting block can then be accurately advanced by a predetermined distance according to the length of resection required. A second parallel bone cut is made, and a wedge of ulnar shaft is excised. Care must be taken to protect the soft tissues when using the saw. Copious irrigation must also be used to reduce the risk of thermal injury to the bone surfaces. The osteotomy system will then allow the gap to be closed and the ends of the bone compressed. An oblique lag screw and additional shaft screws ensure compression and rigid fixation (**Figure 8.18**).

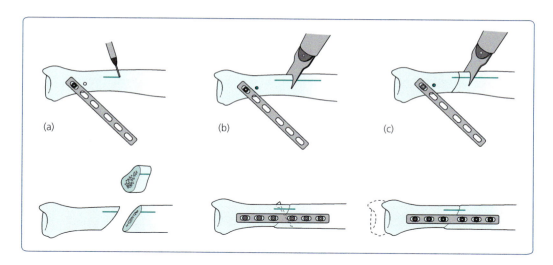

Figure 8.18 Surgical technique for ulnar shortening using a dynamic compression plate.

Closure
Avoid a tight closure of the fascia overlying the flexor compartment. Standard closure of the skin in layers is undertaken. A cast is not required but may be applied for comfort.

Postoperative care and instructions
The fixation is strong enough to support early active movement within the limits of the patient's comfort with no specific restrictions in terms of forearm rotation or wrist or elbow movement.

Recommended references
Chen NC, Wolfe SW. Ulna shortening osteotomy using a compression device. *J Hand Surg Am*. 2003;28:88.

Chun S, Palmer AK. The ulnar impaction syndrome: Follow up note of ulnar shortening osteotomy. *J Hand Surg Am*. 1993;18:46–53.

Fulton C, Grewal R, Faber KJ, Roth J, Gan BS. Outcome analysis of ulnar shortening osteotomy for ulnar impaction syndrome. *Can J Plast Surg*. 2012;20(1):e1–e5.

Nagy L, Jungwirth-Weinberger A, Campbell D, Pino JG. The AO ulnar shortening osteotomy system indications and surgical technique. *J Wrist Surg*. 2014;3(2):91–97.

Tatebe M, Nishizuka T, Hirata H, Nakamura R. Ulnar shortening osteotomy for ulnar-sided wrist pain. *J Wrist Surg*. 2014:3(2):77–84.

Trapeziectomy
The first carpometacarpal joint (CMCJ) is a biconcave saddle joint and can be considered to be composed of several joints forming a complex articulation – the trapezium-metacarpal, trapezium-trapezoid and scapho-trapezium-trapezoid (STT) joints. Basilar thumb arthritis is common and is thought to be caused by a combination of anatomic and biologic factors. Trapeziectomy is a well-described procedure that is essentially an excision arthroplasty. The trapezium in its entirety may be excised leading to an improvement in pain. There is no single best technique, and a multitude of variations have been proposed. The greatest controversy surrounds the use of additional procedures to

augment the stability of the first metacarpal. These 'ligament reconstruction' procedures aim to restore the subluxed and adducted first metacarpal to a more functional position after the trapezium has been excised. In theory, they also aim to provide a greater restraint to axial loading of the first metacarpal. However, their effectiveness is much debated. The following description is an overview of a simple trapeziectomy undertaken through a dorsal approach. A volar approach has also been described and may be used, again with a multitude of variations.

Indications
- Severe CMCJ arthritis
- Pain refractory to analgesics, corticosteroid injections, hand therapy and splintage

Contraindications
- Active infection
- Uncertain diagnosis – consider other causes of radial-sided wrist/hand pain including de Quervain's tenosynovitis

Preoperative planning
Clinical examination demonstrates CMCJ swelling, crepitus on movement and first metacarpal adduction with compensatory development of metacarpophalangeal joint hyperextension resulting in a Z-thumb posture. In cases where there is pan-trapezial arthritis and STT involvement, residual pain from the arthritic scapho-trapezial joint may persist after the trapezium has been excised.

Consent and risks
- Superficial radial nerve injury
- Radial artery injury
- Flexor carpi radialis tendon injury
- Shortening of the thumb
- Infection
- Persistent pain
- Loss of grip strength

Anaesthesia and positioning
General or regional anaesthesia is used. The patient should be in supine position, hand placed on an arm extension with application of an above-elbow tourniquet.

Surgical technique
Landmarks for the dorsal approach are identified. The subluxed base of the first metacarpal is often easily identified, especially when passively moved. However, the metacarpal base overhangs the trapezium which is not readily palpated. The next identifiable bony structure

is the tip of the radial styloid. The tendons of the first extensor compartment may be palpable between the two. A skin incision is made centered over the trapezium. Branches of the superficial radial nerve are identified, mobilised and protected throughout.

The APL and EPB tendons are mobilised and retracted. At this stage the surgeon may choose to identify and protect the radial artery to avoid injury during further exposure of the joint. This lies dorsally and may be retracted with use of a vessel loop taking care to cauterise any side branches. The presence of significant degenerative change may hamper easy identification of the trapezio-metacarpal joint. One way to overcome this is to apply axial traction to the metacarpal in order to correct the subluxation and uncover the joint that may be obscured by the metacarpal base. Again, a multitude of capsulotomies have been described, but a simple longitudinal capsulotomy is described here. Begin the capsulotomy with subperiosteal dissection at the metacarpal base – this will allow easier confirmation of the joint location. Continue the longitudinal capsulotomy to the level of the scapho-trapezial joint so that the proximal and distal margins of the trapezium are under direct vision. A combination of sharp dissection and the use of a periosteal elevator can allow for capsular flaps to be raised on either side of the arthritic joint. In order to aid this, a K-wire or corkscrew device may be placed into the trapezium in order to allow it mobilisation and retraction. The FCR tendon is well attached to the trapezium as it passed through a fibro-osseous tunnel on its volar aspect. Care must be taken during the dissection and during trapezial excision not to injure the FCR.

The trapezium may be excised as a single piece or more commonly piecemeal by fracturing it into halves or thirds with an osteotome. It is particularly important to remove the dorsal osteophyte between the first and second metacarpals. This may not be readily visible within the wound and so the surgeon must take steps to identify and excise this fully. The stability of the first metacarpal may then be assessed. Many ligament reconstruction techniques utilise the nearby tendons of FCR or APL which can be easily harvested. Increasingly, synthetic tape, bone anchors, biotenodesis screws or tightrope devices are also used in the ligament reconstruction or 'suspensionplasty' process. Wound washout is important to ensure that joint debris is not retained. The capsule is closed and a final check is made of the radial artery and its branches.

Postoperative care and instructions

Immobilise the wrist in a thumb spica for 2–4 weeks. The patient may benefit from further support in a thermoplastic splint as range of motion exercises are commenced under the supervision of a hand therapist.

Recommended references

Croog A, Rettig M. Newest advances in the operative treatment of basal joint arthritis. *Bull NYU Hosp Jt Dis*. 2007;65(1):78–86.

Gangopadhyay S, McKenna H, Burke FD, Davis TRC. Five- to 18-year follow-up for treatment of trapeziometacarpal osteoarthritis: A prospective comparison of excision, tendon interposition, and ligament reconstruction and tendon interposition. *J Hand Surg Am*. 2012;37(3):411–417.

Vermeulen GM, Slijper H, Feitz R, Hovius SER, Moojen TM, Selles RW. Surgical management of primary thumb carpometacarpal osteoarthritis: A systematic review. *J Hand Surg Am*. 2011;36(1):157–169.

Surgery for scaphoid non-union

The scaphoid is particularly susceptible to fracture and subsequent non-union due to a range of biologic and anatomic factors. Fractures of the scaphoid waist are most common and therefore waist non-union is the most prevalent. However, proximal pole fractures although seen less commonly have a higher incidence of progression to non-union. This section focuses on the surgical treatment of a recognised, established scaphoid non-union using non-vascularised bone graft.

Indications
- Established scaphoid non-union recalcitrant to non-operative treatments
- Lack of radiographic union after 6 months' post-fixation

Contraindications
- Development of SNAC wrist and widespread arthritis
- Non-reconstructable scaphoid

Preoperative planning

History and clinical examination will lead the surgeon to suspect a scaphoid fracture or non-union, but confirmation of the diagnosis will come from imaging. Scaphoid series X-rays are an essential starting point. However, CT and MRI can provide additional information. The surgical plan will be affected by several key factors.

Distal pole fractures are best approached from the volar side. If a tubercle fracture remains non-united it may be excised, whereas larger distal fragments may be fixed internally. In the acute setting, scaphoid waist fractures may be approached from either a volar or dorsal approach. However, when considering non-union surgery, a volar approach is recommended. The classic 'humpback' deformity occurs as the non-united scaphoid fragments flex and collapse. This is often associated with osteolysis and cavitation on the volar surface that will need to be adequately visualised and corrected – something that is rarely possible from a dorsal approach.

Consent and risks
- Delayed union
- Persistent non-union
- Wrist stiffness and loss of range of movement
- Vascular injury – radial artery
- Neurologic injury – palmar cutaneous branch of the median nerve (runs along the ulnar side of FCR)

Anaesthesia and positioning

General or regional anaesthesia is used. Patient is supine on a radiolucent arm table with application of a tourniquet. Antibiotic prophylaxis is administered. An image intensifier is used.

Surgical technique

Landmarks
- Scaphoid tubercle
- Tendon of FCR

Incision
A hockey stick incision is made centred on the scaphoid tubercle. Proximally the incision follows the line of the FCR tendon. On reaching the tubercle it is angled along the line of the first metacarpal. If a distal radius bone graft is planned, the proximal limb is lengthened.

Procedure
Develop an interval between the FCR tendon the radial artery. Retract the FCR in an ulnar direction and the artery radially. Incise the floor of the sheath. Identify the tubercle again and expose the radioscaphocapitate (RSC) and long radiolunate (LR) ligaments. These are essentially condensations in the fibres of the volar capsule. Distally, origins of thenar muscle can be divided to allow exposure of the scapho-trapezial joint. This must be adequately exposed to allow for accurate placement of the guidewire for headless screw fixation. In this 'ligament splitting' technique, the volar capsule and hence the RSC and LR ligaments are divided longitudinally. More recently, ligament-preserving techniques have also been described that essentially take a zigzag path across these structures to expose the volar scaphoid.

The scaphoid non-union is identified and cleared of fibrous tissue. Numerous techniques have been described for volar wedge grafting of a non-united scaphoid, but they all share common themes. Sclerotic bone must be excised, cavitation must be curettaged and debridement must be taken back until healthy punctate bleeding points are seen within the bone. The length and alignment of the scaphoid are restored – either joystick K-wires or a small laminar spreader are used to maintain the corrected position and an estimation is made of the size of graft required. The most common donor sites are the distal radius and iliac crest. If the distal radius is to be used, the dissection between FCR and the radial artery is continued proximally, and the pronator quadratus is elevated off the volar surface of the radius. Four points of a square or rectangle matching the shape of the graft required are marked on the volar radius. Each of these points is then drilled using a small-diameter drill bit or a K-wire to prevent crack propagation. A fine sagittal saw or small sharp osteotome is used to fracture the volar cortex. If care is taken, a cortico-cancellous wedge can be removed as a single piece. Using a gauge, additional cancellous bone can be harvested. Cavities in either end of the scaphoid are packed with graft, and the cortico-cancellous wedge is impacted into the central defect. A trough is made in the volar aspect of the trapezium at the level of the scapho-trapezial joint. This will allow better exposure of the central point of the distal scaphoid that marks the ideal entry point for the guide wire. The wire is passed along the central axis of the scaphoid and checked with fluoroscopy. This is measured and a screw inserted. As a rule of thumb, the length of screw used is approximately 4 mm shorter than the length measured. This allows for the screw to be buried under articular cartilage, accounts for a degree of compression and minimises the chance of screw prominence.

Closure

Haemostasis is achieved after tourniquet release and closure of the volar capsule using interrupted Vicryl sutures. The skin is closed with a subcuticular absorbable monofilament suture.

Postoperative care and instructions

The wrist is immobilised in a cast, with or without thumb spica for 6–8 weeks. Follow-up radiographs or CT are used to assess progression of healing.

Recommended references

Moon ES, Dy CJ, Derman P, Vance MC, Carlson MG. Management of nonunion following surgical management of scaphoid fractures: Current concepts. *J Am Acad Orthop Surg*. 2013;21(9):548–557.

Pinder RM, Brkljac M, Rix L, Muir L, Brewster M. Treatment of scaphoid nonunion: A systematic review of the existing evidence. *J Hand Surg Am*. 2015;40(9):1797–1805.e3.

Viva questions

1. Give a histologic definition of a cyst.
2. What are the other sites for cystic swellings in the wrist and hand?
3. Talk through an excision of a ganglion cyst.
4. What is the risk of recurrence post-excision?
5. How many dorsal compartments are found at the wrist and what are their contents?
6. Which nerve and artery are at risk during surgical release of the first dorsal compartment?
7. What is the optimal position for wrist arthrodesis?
8. Between which dorsal wrist compartments do you classically approach through to access the wrist joint?
9. What is a 'four-corner' fusion?
10. Name and describe the common wrist arthroscopy portals.
11. Dorsal wrist ganglions usually arise from which ligament?
12. Describe the radiographic features of a wrist with scapholunate advanced collapse.
13. What is the non-union rate in total wrist fusions?
14. What are the main functional disadvantages with Darrach's procedure?
15. What alternatives are there to Darrach's procedure in younger and higher-demand patients?
16. What is complex regional pain syndrome? What is the incidence after wrist or hand procedures?
17. When should an ulnar shortening osteotomy not be performed?

18. What is the most significant factor influencing the rate of non-union in an ulnar shortening osteotomy?
19. What is the significance of the posterior interosseous nerve in wrist procedures?
20. Where is the posterior interosseous nerve identified at the wrist?
21. What is a proximal row carpectomy?
22. What is the pathophysiology of CMCJ arthritis?
23. Describe the volar approach to the scaphoid.

9 Surgery of the Hand

Norbert Kang, Ben Miranda and Dariush Nikkhah

Dupuytren's surgery	193	Tendon transfers	224
Synovial cyst treatment	201	Soft tissue reconstruction	228
Arthrodesis in the hand	203	Trigger finger surgery	234
Arthroplasty in the hand	209	Trigger thumb surgery	235
Extensor tendon repair	213	Viva questions	237
Flexor tendon repair preoperative planning	219		

Dupuytren's surgery
Preoperative planning
Indications
Dupuytren's surgery is indicated in patients with a flexion deformity that interferes with their activities of daily living. Using the 'table-top test' (i.e. an inability to get the hand flat on the table) or specific degrees of flexion deformity (e.g. 30° at the proximal interphalangeal [PIP] joint) as an indication for surgery is unhelpful as this may over- or underestimate the need for surgery. The best indication is to intervene only if the patient requests it – regardless of the degree of the deformity.

Operative planning
It is vital to record the range of movement, vascularity and sensation in the digit(s) preoperatively so that a comparison can be made with the postoperative outcome.

There are three common procedures:

- Fasciotomy (open, needle or enzymatic) or segmental fasciotomy
- Fasciectomy
- Dermofasciectomy

Fasciotomy
This is a procedure to divide rather than excise the Dupuytren's cord tissue. It can be performed under direct vision (open fasciotomy), percutaneously (needle fasciotomy),

enzymatically or by excising a short segment of cord tissue – also under direct vision (segmental fasciotomy).

Indications

- Discrete Dupuytren's cord at any level in the finger or hand.
- Metacarpophalangeal (MCP) joint flexion deformity.
- PIP joint flexion deformity. Although there is a greater risk of neurovascular injury after both needle and enzymatic fasciotomy at this level, no complications should be encountered if appropriate techniques are used.
- Patients unwilling to undergo or unsuitable for a major operative procedure or wishing to avoid general anaesthesia.
- Needle fasciotomy is performed under local anaesthesia or regional block, while it is recommended that enzymatic fasciotomy be performed without anaesthesia to maintain awareness of the digital nerves.

Contraindications

- Diffuse Dupuytren's disease can be difficult to treat with fasciotomy but this is only a relative contraindication.
- Patients unable or unwilling to comply with indefinite postoperative night-time splintage with the digit(s) in full extension. If they fail to comply with splintage post-operatively, recurrence of the flexion deformity may be rapid (within a few weeks).

Consent and risks

- Injury to the neurovascular bundle. (This risk is reduced with open/segmental fasciotomy.)
- Skin tears are common after needle and enzymatic fasciotomy. These heal rapidly (within 2–3 weeks) by secondary intention (McCash technique).
- Tendon ruptures have been infrequently reported after enzymatic fasciotomy.
- Chronic regional pain syndrome Type 1.
- Short procedure (takes 5–10 minutes to treat a single digit).

Anaesthesia and positioning

Local anaesthesia, upper limb blockade or general anaesthesia can be used. The arm should be placed supine on an arm table or arm board. It is helpful to use a tourniquet for open and segmental fasciotomy; no tourniquet is required for needle or enzymatic fasciotomy.

Surgical technique

Landmarks

The cord(s) to be divided are palpated and marked.

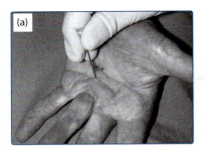 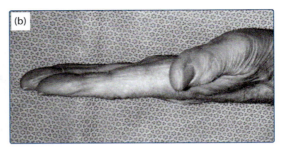

Figure 9.1 Needle fasciotomy: (a) needling of fascia and (b) postoperative appearance.

Needle fasciotomy

A white-hubbed (16G) hypodermic needle is held in a tripod grip using the thumb, index and middle fingers of one hand (**Figure 9.1**). The orientation of the needle tip is important – the bevel should face proximally – allowing the needle tip to be used like the blade of a very fine scalpel. The first 2–3 mm of the tip of the needle are inserted vertically through the skin and into the cord with the digit held in full extension to make the cord easy to palpate and to facilitate division of the cord tissue. Small, sweeping movements are now made at right angles to the cord using the needle tip to divide the cord tissue. Simultaneously, the digit is pushed into extension. If successful, a tearing sound is often heard as the weakened cord tissue is torn in half allowing the finger to extend. If this does not happen, then repeat the process to divide and weaken more of the cord tissue. Now, repeat the process of gentle passive manipulation of the finger to see if it will extend. Be wary when doing this not to overdo the manipulation as this can result in fracture of the phalanges – especially in older, female patients with osteoporosis. If the finger will still not extend, it may be necessary to convert to an open procedure to release the volar plate under direct vision.

Skin tears are very common, especially when there has been a long-standing and significant flexion deformity (e.g. PIP joint flexion of >60°). However, the surgeon can be assured that even when the tendon or neurovascular bundles are exposed, all wounds on the volar aspect of the hand and digit can be left to heal by secondary intention within 2–3 weeks. While healing is taking place it is critical to keep the digit in full extension at rest to prevent rapid recurrence of the flexion deformity. After releasing the digit(s), the hand is placed in a plaster of Paris splint with all the digits in full extension and the wrist in neutral for 10 days. The plaster splint is then removed and the hand is mobilised as quickly as possible.

Enzymatic fasciotomy

Collagenase is isolated from the gram-negative bacterium clostridium histolyticum and acts to lyse collagen (peptide bonds) resulting in disruption of Dupuytren's cords. After carefully following the manufacturer's reconstitution guidelines, a 26/27G hypodermic needle may be used to infiltrate the diseased cord percutaneously using a three-step approach (initial injection, just distal and just proximal). This is performed in an outpatient setting. Care must be taken not to infiltrate the underlying flexor tendon since this will then be at increased risk of rupture during subsequent passive manipulation. Passive manipulation of the finger is performed 24 hours later (also within an outpatient setting) by firmly and vigorously pushing the flexed digit into extension. If successful, a 'carrot snap' sound is heard as the enzymatically treated diseased cord 'breaks suddenly'.

Open fasciotomy

A longitudinal incision is made over the course of the cord tissue. The incision is made sufficiently long to allow direct visualisation of the cord and adjacent structures. The cord tissues are divided with a scalpel while forcibly extending the digit. If successful, the cord tissues are torn in half allowing the finger to extend.

Segmental fasciotomy

The procedure is the same as for open fasciotomy but, in addition, a short segment (approximately 1 cm) of cord tissue is excised in the belief that this reduces the risk of recurrence.

Closure

After needle or enzymatic fasciotomy, the puncture wounds and skin tears are allowed to heal by secondary intention. This takes 2–3 weeks with simple dressings. For open and segmental fasciotomy, the skin is closed with absorbable sutures (e.g. using 5-0 Vicryl rapide).

Postoperative care and instructions

All patients undergoing fasciotomy of any type should be able to mobilise their digits freely after treatment. For patients where there has been a long-standing flexion deformity, a period of static splintage (e.g. 7–14 days) in extension may also be helpful. However, in order to decrease the recurrence of a significant flexion deformity in the long term, patients should be advised about the advantages of using a thermoplastic splint at night – indefinitely. The splint should hold the treated digit(s) in full extension.

Fasciectomy

Consent and risks

- 'White finger' due to vascular injury followed by finger necrosis
- Paraesthesiae or anaesthesia due to digital nerve injury (10% risk after a redo procedure)
- Infection
- Skin flap necrosis
- Flexion loss
- Recurrence of Dupuytren's followed by recurrence of the flexion deformity
- Chronic regional pain syndrome Type 1
- Lengthy procedure (typically takes 30–45 minutes for single digit)

Indications

Any degree of Dupuytren's contracture. This includes recurrent disease and MCP, PIP and distal interphalangeal (DIP) joint flexion deformities.

Contraindications

- Diffuse Dupuytren's disease with extensive skin involvement (pits and fixed skin over cords) can be difficult to address with a fasciectomy. However, this is only a relative contraindication.
- Multiple previous fasciectomies with subsequent recurrence of flexion deformities. Scarring from previous surgery can make a redo procedure very challenging.
- Patients with a severe Dupuytren's diathesis (males, onset <50 years, Garrod's pads, ectopic disease, bilateral disease, strong family history, e.g. a sibling or parent).
- Patient unwilling or unable to comply with hand therapy postoperatively.
- Heavy smoker and unwilling to stop smoking preoperatively.

Anaesthesia and positioning

Fasciectomies can be performed under local anaesthesia (maximum of two digits), upper limb block or general anaesthesia. The arm should be held supine on an arm table with a lead hand. All surgery should be carried out under tourniquet with loupe magnification.

Surgical Technique

Landmarks

A straight-line incision is marked over the midline on the volar aspect of the affected digit, beginning at the distal finger crease. An alternative is the Bruner zigzag pattern. A straight-line incision allows the surgeon to perform Z-plasties when there is a volar skin shortage, recruiting skin from the sides of the finger. However, Bruner incisions can also recruit extra skin onto the volar side of the finger by converting each flap into 'Y to V' plasties, and this approach has the added advantage of avoiding the need to design Z-plasties. All incisions are extended proximally to the mid-palmar crease. A further transverse incision is marked across the palm following the line of the mid-palmar crease. The length and position of the transverse incision are determined by the position and number of digits which are to be treated (**Figure 9.2**).

Incision

For fingers with significant flexion deformities, it is often helpful to carry out a fasciotomy to gain access to the volar side of the finger and palm before starting the dissection. Having an extended finger at the start of the procedure makes marking and surgical access much simpler.

The transverse incision is created before proceeding into the digits. All incisions should be full thickness.

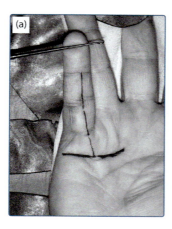 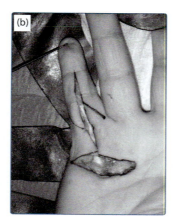 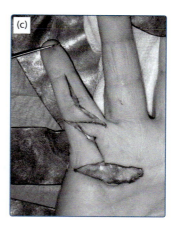

Figure 9.2 Fasciectomy. (a) Skoog's straight-line incision. (b,c) Z-plasty marked out and performed.

Dissection

> ### Structures at risk
> - Neurovascular bundles
> - Skin flap tip necrosis
> - Flexor sheath (loss of pulleys)

Thin skin flaps should be developed above the cords. Particular care must be taken to avoid buttonholing the skin when there is significant pitting or skin involvement. Ensure that the skin flaps are thick enough to be viable (ideally just thicker than subdermal) but thin enough so that minimal amounts (ideally none) of the diseased cord tissue is left in the hand – in the hope that this will avoid a recurrence.

Any longitudinal cord tissue should be excised, leaving the transverse fibres of the palmar aponeurosis in place wherever possible. The neurovascular bundles should be visualised in the palm on either side of the flexor tendon. The rest of the dissection is directed at freeing the neurovascular bundles from the cord tissue on both sides of the finger by a combination of blunt and sharp dissection. Once both bundles have been skeletonised as far as the DIP joint, any soft tissues remaining between the skin and the tendon sheath can be excised and discarded.

Any remaining flexion deformity must now be assessed (e.g. due to a Boutonniere deformity, volar plate contracture, shortening of the flexor sheath or volar skin shortage). In many cases, it is due to a combination of all of these factors. Boutonniere deformities sometimes respond to static splintage in full extension for 1 week – but only if the flexion deformity has not been long-standing (i.e. <6 months). Volar plate contractures require either passive manipulation of the PIP joint or sharp release of the volar plate/check-rein ligaments.

Any 'white fingers' must be noted. The tourniquet must be released before skin closure to check the perfusion of the digit and to carry out haemostasis. If the finger fails to perfuse, then both vessels need to be visualised to ensure that they are in continuity. You only need one intact artery to perfuse the digit. If the vessels are intact but the digit is still white, the digit is allowed to flex to its former position for 5–10 minutes. If this fails, the surgeon can try bathing the vessels in a few drops of verapamil (2.5 mg/mL) or glyceryl trinitrate (5 mg/mL). It is important to tell the anaesthetist before doing this. If the vessels have been divided, they will require someone experienced in microvascular techniques to restore circulation to the finger.

Closure

Treatment of any skin shortage in the digit may require closure of the skin with a Z-plasty. The ideal Z-plasty for closure in the digit has a 30° angle and is as large as possible. It is not necessary to locate the transverse limb of the Z-plasty at a flexor crease. This simply makes planning difficult. Often, only one Z-plasty is required to allow sufficient lengthening of the volar incision to allow closure with minimal skin tension. The skin of the finger is closed with interrupted or continuous absorbable sutures (e.g. 5/0 Vicryl rapide).

Any transverse palmar incisions should be left open. As long as the maximum width of the incision does not exceed 1.5 cm it will heal by secondary intention within 2 weeks, without contracting. Leaving the palm open also simplifies closure and reduces the risk of a haematoma by allowing free drainage from the dissected areas.

Postoperative care and instructions

All patients undergoing fasciectomy should be allowed to mobilise their digits freely after treatment unless they have a significant Boutonniere deformity and/or needed significant manipulation/release of the PIP joint intraoperatively. This later group of patients should be splinted continuously in full extension for 1–2 weeks. Thereafter, all patients must use a splint at night for at least 3 months to keep the treated digit(s) in full extension.

Dermofasciectomy

This is a fasciectomy combined with excision of the skin of the proximal digit (**Figure 9.3**). All the soft tissues on the volar side of the proximal part of the digit are excised, down to the mid-lateral line, with the exception of the tendon/tendon sheath and the neurovascular bundles. The resulting defect is then resurfaced with a full-thickness skin graft. The aim is to remove any tissue that may result in subsequent recurrence of a longitudinal cord volar to the axis of flexion of the digit.

Consent and risks

- Full-thickness graft loss
- Loss of flexion
- Scarring from harvest of graft
- Injury to neurovascular bundles
- 'Hairy' digit – from failure to remove hair follicles in the graft
- Chronic regional pain syndrome – Type 1

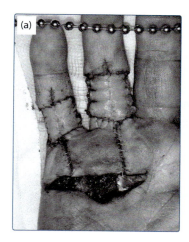 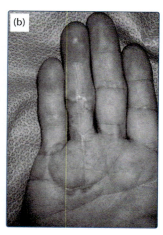

Figure 9.3 (a) Dermofasciectomy of little and ring fingers and (b) 3 months postoperatively with healed graft.

Correction of the flexion deformity is now checked – as for a fasciectomy (p. 196). Haemostasis and digital perfusion are also checked – as for a fasciectomy (p. 196). Then a full-thickness graft of appropriate size is harvested from the forearm or groin and secured to the finger with 4/0 or 5/0 Vicryl rapide. The authors' preferred approach is to anchor the four corners of the graft and to then secure all the edges of the graft with a continuous (over and over) suture of 5/0 Vicryl rapide. The middle of the graft is then secured to the tendon sheath with two or three quilting sutures of 5/0 Vicryl rapide to reduce the tendency for the graft to slide, thereby improving graft take.

Postoperative care and instructions

The hand should be splinted continuously with the digits in full extension for 1 week to help the graft take. The splint and dressings are then removed, and the graft is checked. Regardless of whether the graft has taken, the patient should mobilise the digit with the assistance of a hand therapist. Patients will still need to splint the digit in full extension at night for 3 months.

Recommended references

Hall PN, Fitzgerald A, Sterne GD et al. Skin replacement in Dupuytren's disease. *J Hand Surg Br.* 1997;**22**:193–197.

Hindocha S, Stanley JK, Watson S, Bayat A. Dupuytren's diathesis revisited: Evaluation of prognostic indicators for risk of disease recurrence. *J Hand Surg Am.* 2006;**31**:1626–1634.

Hueston JT. Recurrent Dupuytren's contracture. *Plast Reconstr Surg.* 1963;**31**:66–69.

Hurst LC, Badalamente MA, Hentz VR et al.; CORD I Study Group. Injectable collagenase clostridium histolyticum for Dupuytren's contracture. *N Engl J Med.* 2009;**361(10)**:968–979.

McFarlane RM. Patterns of the diseased fascia in the fingers in Dupuytren's contracture. Displacement of the neurovascular bundle. *Plast Reconstr Surg.* 1974;**54**:31–44.

Nikkhah D, Kang N. Percutaneous needle fasciotomy – Further insights. *JPRAS.* 2017;**70(1)**:144–146.

Peimer CA, Blazar P, Coleman S et al. Dupuytren's contracture recurrence following treatment with collagenase clostridium histolyticum (CORDLESS study): 3-year data. *J Hand Surg Am.* 2013;**38(1)**:12–22.

van Rijssen AL, Werker PM. Percutaneous needle fasciotomy in Dupuytren's disease. *J Hand Surg Br.* 2006;**31**:498–501.

Synovial cyst treatment

Preoperative planning

Ganglia are the result of mucoid degeneration of fibrous connective tissue and are most frequently encountered arising dorsally associated with the scapholunate joint (in 70% of cases) or at the DIP joint. Volar wrist ganglia are rarer and constitute 10% of cases. Long-term follow-up of ganglia has demonstrated that the majority should be treated non-surgically in the first instance because 50% will resolve spontaneously within a few years and the morbidity of surgical excision is significant. This does not mean that ganglia should never be treated but patients should be advised appropriately and over-enthusiastic reliance on surgical excision should be avoided. In specific cases, simultaneous treatment of the underlying pathology (e.g. arthrodesis of a DIP joint for osteoarthritis) will remove the ganglion and the underlying cause – permanently.

Indications
- Pain (may be caused by underlying pathology – e.g. arthritic joint)
- Impaired function (if a ganglion is large enough, it may catch on clothing)
- Cosmesis: This is probably the most common reason for patients to seek help

Contraindications
There are no absolute contraindications for treating a ganglion.

Consent and risks
- Bleeding
- Infection
- Recurrence
- Joint instability
- Stiffness
- Troublesome scars
- Accidental nerve injury

Anaesthesia and positioning

This depends on the location of the ganglion and the preference of the patient. Anaesthesia is unnecessary for simple aspiration of a ganglion. For excision of a ganglion in the digit, most cases can be treated under local anaesthesia. However, excision of a ganglion at the wrist should be treated under regional block or general anaesthesia as deep dissection is often necessary. A tourniquet should be used in the majority of volar wrist ganglions where the radial artery is in close proximity.

Surgical technique

Aspiration of ganglia

The largest gauge needle compatible with comfort for the patient is attached to a 2 mL syringe – typically, a blue hubbed (23G) needle. The needle is inserted into the ganglion with one swift movement and aspiration begins immediately. If the contents do not enter the syringe, the needle is extracted, and the contents manually expressed through the small puncture hole. Injecting a small amount of Adcortyl (5 mg) into the ganglion/adjacent tissues reduces post-treatment inflammation and discomfort. Ultrasound may also be used for diagnostic and therapeutic purposes.

Flexor sheath ganglia

Landmarks and incision

Typically, these ganglia arise from the A2 pulley at the level of the proximal finger crease and can easily be ruptured with a needle. For excision, a transverse incision, directly over the ganglion, is used.

Dissection and procedure

> **Structures at risk**
> - Neurovascular bundles
> - Flexor tendon

The ganglion is excised *en bloc* with (if necessary) a small cuff of the flexor sheath.

Closure

The skin is approximated with interrupted 5/0 Vicryl rapide sutures. A light dressing is applied, which will not impede movement and allows immediate mobilisation.

Mucous cysts

As it enlarges, it emerges on either the ulnar or radial side of the joint at the interval between the terminal extensor tendon and the collateral ligament of the joint (**Figure 9.4**). The

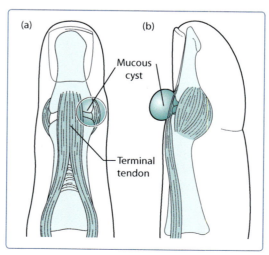

Figure 9.4 A mucous cyst.

skin over the mucous cyst is often very thin. Therefore, attempts to separate the skin from the ganglion wall are fruitless. The surgeon can decide to either excise the skin with the ganglion or simply make a longitudinal incision over the ganglion knowing that it will burst.

Dissection and procedure

Structures at risk

- Terminal extensor tendon – injury may cause mallet deformity
- Germinal matrix of nail complex – injury may result in notching of the nail plate

---

Whether or not an ellipse of skin was excised with the ganglion, excision of the rest of the ganglion wall is often an academic exercise because the remnant is usually so flimsy. Excise whatever remains of the ganglion wall (piecemeal if necessary) down to the DIP joint. Any obvious osteophytes should also be removed with a bone nibbler as this improves cosmesis.

Closure

The skin is closed with interrupted 5/0 Vicryl rapide sutures. If an excessively large area of skin has been excised, it will be difficult to close the wound directly. The options then are to use a small split-thickness skin graft or a local rotation flap – converting an operation of dubious value (excising a mucous cyst) into an operation with a multitude of potential complications. If the defect is very small and no important structures are exposed, then allowing the wound to heal by secondary intention is more acceptable. The finger is dressed lightly, which allows immediate mobilisation.

Postoperative care and instructions

The hand is elevated to reduce pain and swelling. Any bulky dressings are removed after 48–72 hours. The hand/finger is mobilised with the help of a hand therapist, as quickly as possible.

Recommended references

Dias JJ, Dhukaram V, Kumar P. The natural history of untreated dorsal wrist ganglia and patient reported outcomes 6 years after intervention. *J Hand Surg Eur.* 2007;**32**:502–508.

Green DP, Hotchkiss RN, Pederson WC eds. *Green's Operative Hand Surgery.* 5th ed. Edinburgh, Scotland: Elsevier, 2005.

Arthrodesis in the hand

Preoperative planning

Indications

An arthrodesis is a very reasonable salvage operation for certain joints and for certain situations. It can restore its pain-free form and function in one operative step. Indications include:

- Pain
- Instability

- Deformity
- Failed arthroplasty
- Joints where arthroplasty is not desirable/possible

Certain joints respond particularly well to arthrodesis because of the functional requirements of the hand. Others do less well (see 'Operative planning' later).

Contraindications

- Poor skin cover over the joint.
- Active infection in the upper limb – inserting metalwork should be avoided.
- Non-compliant patient – the joint needs to be immobilised for 8 weeks after surgery to allow bony union.
- Smoking is a contraindication due to poor wound healing.

Consent and risks

- Damage to any of the adjacent structures (e.g. tendons, neurovascular bundles, damage to the nail bed in DIP joint fusion)
- Infection
- Malunion
- Non-union (up to 10% – especially the DIP joint) – more frequent in smokers
- Stiffness of adjacent joints and fingers
- Flexor and/or extensor adhesions

Operative planning

Distal interphalangeal joint
Patients do very well after arthrodesis of this joint because the loss of range of movement at the DIP joint has relatively little effect on overall hand function. DIP joint arthrodesis is particularly useful in cases of delayed presentation after flexor digitorum profundus (FDP) tendon rupture, chronic mallet deformity or painful arthritis of the DIP joint (with or without deformity) and chronic mucous cysts.

Proximal interphalangeal joint
Arthrodesis of the PIP joint results in significant impairment of hand function because the PIP joint accounts for up to 40% of total active flexion of the finger. However, it is still a reasonable option to deal with chronic pain and instability, especially for the little and ring fingers. This is because PIP joint replacements do particularly badly in the little and ring fingers.

Interphalangeal joint of the thumb
The IP joint of the thumb responds very well to arthrodesis. The thumb, in contrast to the fingers, is used as a pillar for opposition, and (therefore) loss of active range of motion at the IP joint and MCP joint do not affect function as much.

Metacarpophalangeal joint
The MCP joints of the fingers should not be arthrodesed as this results in significant impairment of function. In contrast, arthrodesis of the MCP joint of the thumb is an excellent procedure that significantly enhances hand function.

Carpometacarpal joint
The first carpometacarpal (CMC) joint should not be fused, as this will result in significant impairment of hand function. The second and third CMC joints normally behave as if they are fused; therefore, arthrodesis of these joints is seldom necessary. In contrast, the fourth and fifth CMC joints are surprisingly mobile, even in normal hands. Nevertheless, arthrodesis of these joints remains a reasonable solution in cases of chronic pain and instability (typically after trauma).

Anaesthesia and positioning
Local anaesthetic digital block is suitable for IP joint, DIP joint or PIP joint arthrodesis. Regional block (wrist or axillary) or general anaesthesia with arm tourniquet may be more suitable for arthrodesis of the thumb MCP joint or CMC joints. Use of local anaesthetic with adrenaline should also be considered in order to minimise or avoid the need to use a tourniquet.

Surgical technique
Several different techniques are available for arthrodesis of a joint (e.g. K-wires, interosseous wires, screws, plates and staples). Different methods of fixation are more or less suitable for particular joints and in particular situations. Regardless of the technique, the usefulness of the arthrodesis is determined by the final position of the bones after fusion (*Table 9.1*). Also, the arthrodesed digit will be shorter by the amount of bone that needs to be removed to allow the arthrodesis to be performed.

Table 9.1 Arthrodesis positions in the hand

	Thumb	Index	Middle	Ring	Little
DIP joint	N/A	0°–10°	0°–10°	0°–10°	0°–10°
IP joint	0°–20°	N/A	N/A	N/A	N/A
PIP joint	N/A	30°	30°–40°	40°–50°	50°
MCP joint	0°–20°	Do not fuse	Do not fuse	Do not fuse	Do not fuse
CMC joint	Do not fuse	N/A	N/A	0°	0°

Abbreviations: CMC, carpometacarpal; DIP, distal interphalangeal; IP, interphalangeal; MCP, metacarpophalangeal; N/A, not applicable; PIP, proximal interphalangeal.

Fusion techniques
This depends on the joint. Image intensifier guidance (preferably using a mini-C-arm) is essential in ensuring that any metalwork is correctly positioned.

Landmarks and incisions

- *DIP and thumb IP joint*: An 'H'- or 'Y'-shaped incision over the dorsum of the joint or a mid-lateral incision for plating (**Figure 9.5**).
- *PIP joint*: Longitudinal incision over the dorsum of the joint.
- *Thumb MCP joint*: Longitudinal incision over the dorsum of the joint.
- *CMC or intercarpal arthrodesis*: Longitudinal incisions over the dorsum of the relevant joint.

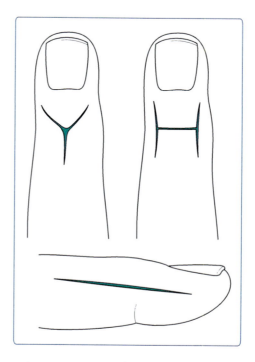

Figure 9.5 Incisions for access to DIP joint.

Distal interphalangeal joint

The terminal extensor tendon is detached from the base of the distal phalanx, exposing the joint. The collateral ligaments are excised, and the volar plate detached from the base of the distal phalanx. This allows the joint to be disarticulated completely. The joint surfaces are removed with a saw or bone nibbler to expose the cancellous bone with the intention of creating two flat surfaces with the correct angulation (i.e. 0°–10°). For fixation, 90°–90° wiring is probably the easiest technique to understand and perform. Tension band wiring is also acceptable but technically more challenging (**Figure 9.6**). Other acceptable alternatives include the use of a Lister loop (although the K-wire then needs to be removed at 8 weeks), Herbert or cannulated screw fixation and plating.

Proximal interphalangeal joint

A longitudinal split in the extensor tendon or a Chamay approach (distally based 'V'-shaped incision in the central slip; **Figure 9.7**) can be used for PIP joint exposure. The joint is

Arthrodesis in the hand 207

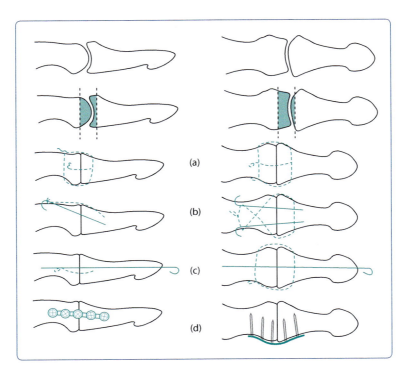

Figure 9.6 Methods of distal interphalangeal (DIP) joint fusion. (a) '90–90' wiring. Two interosseous wires of 0.35 to 0.45 gauge dental wire passed at 90° to each other. (b) Tension band wiring using two 1.1 mm K-wires and a 0.35–0.45 gauge dental wire. (c) Lister loop with a single 1.1 mm K-wire and a 0.35–0.45 gauge dental wire. The K-wire must be removed at 4 weeks. (d) Plating of the DIP joint with a mini-plate (the most difficult technique).

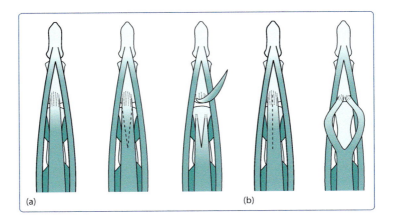

Figure 9.7 (a) Chamay approach. (b) Longitudinal split.

disarticulated by excising the collateral ligaments and detaching the volar plate. The joint surfaces are removed with a saw or a bone nibbler to create two flat surfaces with the correct angulation (*Table 9.1*). As for the DIP joint, there is no preferred method of fixation. Any techniques which are appropriate for DIP joint fusion are also suitable for PIP joint fusion. The senior author's preference is to use a tension band technique – because the metalwork is easy to insert and remove.

Metacarpophalangeal joint of the thumb

The joint is exposed through a longitudinal split in the extensor tendon and disarticulated by dividing the collateral ligaments and detaching the volar plate. The joint surfaces are excised. The senior author's preference for arthrodesis of the thumb MCP joint is a tension band wire technique.

Carpometacarpal joint

The extensor tendons are retracted from over the CMC joints and soft tissue excised to expose the specific joint. Use of an image intensifier confirms that the correct joint has been identified. The joint surfaces are excised, and bone graft is inserted. The graft is harvested from the distal radius. Bone substitute (e.g. hydroxyapatite) can also be used. The joint is secured with an oblique K-wire passed through the base of the respective metacarpal and the corresponding trapezoid, capitates or hamate. The wire is buried and removed after 8 weeks.

Closure

Any extensor tendons that have been split to approach the joints should be repaired with 4/0 or 5/0 PDS interrupted or continuous sutures. The tourniquet is then released and haemostasis achieved with bipolar diathermy. All wounds should be washed out with saline to remove any loose particles of bone. Incisions are closed with interrupted, absorbable 4/0 or 5/0 Monocryl sutures for the dermis followed by a subcuticular 5/0 Monocryl or 4/0/5/0 Vicryl rapide suture. Surgeons should avoid using interrupted, non-absorbable sutures on the dorsum of the hand and fingers as they leave very unsightly suture marks which may require scar revision at a later stage.

Postoperative care and instructions

A light dressing is applied and removed after 48–72 hours to allow active joint mobilisation on either side of the treated joint. A splint must be used to immobilise the joint for 8 weeks. Scars are massaged from 2 weeks onwards. Coban elastic bandage should also be applied to reduce soft tissue swelling from 2 weeks after surgery. A removable thermoplastic splint should be supplied to support the relevant joint for 6–8 weeks while the bone heals.

Recommended references

Allende BT, Engelem JC. Tension band arthrodesis in the finger joints. *J Hand Surg Am.* 1980;**5**:269–271.
Green DP, Hotchkiss RN, Pederson WC, eds. *Green's Operative Hand Surgery.* 5th ed. Edinburgh, Scotland: Elsevier, 2005.
Lister G. Intraosseous wiring of the digital skeleton. *J Hand Surg Am.* 1978;**3**:427–435.
Pechlaner S, Hussl H, Kerschbaumer F. *Atlas of Hand Surgery.* Stuttgart, Germany: Thieme, 2000.
Sennwald G, Segmuller G. The metacarpophalangeal arthrodesis of the thumb according to the tension-band principle: Indications and technique. *Ann Chir Main.* 1983;**2**:38–45.

Arthroplasty in the hand

Preoperative planning

The decision to operate must not be made purely on the basis of the X-ray appearances. However, function is not always the only consideration. Although it is generally not a good idea to perform an arthroplasty in patients who have good function, many patients still ask for surgery to 'improve' the appearance of their hands.

Indications

- Painful or stiff joints unresponsive to medical treatment
- Deformity and/or loss of range of movement affecting activities of daily living
- Failure of conservative measures; however, before this can be said, patients must have had an adequate trial of
  - Regular non-steroidal anti-inflammatory drugs (NSAIDs) and splintage
  - Steroid injections (administer at least one or two of these)
  - Using home or work aids
  - Appropriate alterations to their home or work circumstances
- To 'improve' the appearance of the hand
- MCP joint in preference to PIP joints
- Index or middle finger PIP joints

Contraindications

- Absent or poor flexor or extensor tendon function
- Absent or poor nerve function (e.g. peripheral neuropathy)
- Patients with significant vascular compromise (e.g. scleroderma, Raynaud's phenomenon)
- Patients with poor skin cover over the joint
- Patients unwilling or unable to comply with postoperative hand therapy
- Heavy smoker and unwilling to stop preoperatively
- DIP joint – an arthrodesis is recommended instead
- PIP joint of ring and little fingers – joint instability is often worse after arthroplasty in these digits

Artificial joints fare better in older/lower-demand patients. A resurfacing/interposition arthroplasty is less destructive and tries to restore the normal shape of the joint using either autologous or artificial materials and is more suitable for young or active patients.

In general, replacement arthroplasty works best for the MCP but not for the PIP or DIP joints. If PIP joint arthroplasty is contemplated, then this is best performed in the index and middle fingers only. Although DIP joint arthroplasty (e.g. with a Swanson's replacement) has been reported to be successful in post-traumatic osteoarthritic joints, arthrodesis is a more reliable option in patients who are not concerned about preserving movement.

A variety of artificial materials has been described for replacement arthroplasty. However, silicone is the only material that has withstood the test of time (e.g. Swanson's implant; **Figure 9.8**). The technique for insertion is described here.

> **Consent and risks**
>
> - Flexor tendon/neurovascular injury
> - Instability (only for PIP joint arthroplasty)
> - Recurrent deformity (affects one-third of arthroplasties)
> - Dislocation, loosening or fracture of the implant (implant failure affects one-third of implants)
> - Infection necessitating implant removal
> - Range-of-motion loss
> - Ongoing pain
> - Dislocation, fracture or implant extrusion (7%–15%)
> - Silicone synovitis

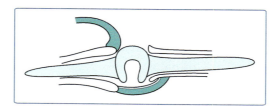

Figure 9.8 Swanson's implant in place.

Operative planning

The choice is between a replacement arthroplasty or a resurfacing/interposition arthroplasty. A replacement arthroplasty excises the joint completely and replaces it with an artificial or autologous joint (usually taken from the foot).

Anaesthesia and positioning

Local, regional or general anaesthesia can be used. The position is supine with the hand on an arm table.

Surgical technique

Metacarpophalangeal joint

Landmarks and incision

A longitudinal incision (straight or curvilinear) is made over the dorsum of the joint. Any curvature in the incision is usually towards the radial side. This makes it easier to access and reef the radial sagittal bands of the extensor hood. Reefing of the extensor hood allows ulnar subluxation of the extensors to be corrected in cases with rheumatoid arthritis.

Dissection

The skin and subcutaneous fat are widely degloved over the joint to expose the extensor tendons and the sagittal bands. The sagittal bands are divided longitudinally on the radial side, leaving a minimum 2–3 mm fringe along the extensor tendon edge: this allows the bands to be reefed at a later stage. The extensor mechanism is now freed from the underlying capsule and retracted ulnarly. The joint capsule is often flimsy in these patients, and it is often easier to simply excise it together with any synovial proliferations. After excising the capsule and any associated synovial tissue, any remnants of the collateral ligaments can also be excised.

Procedure
The volar plate must be freed from the neck of the metacarpal to allow the base of the proximal phalanx to align correctly with the metacarpal. The metacarpal head is excised with an oscillating saw. In the rheumatoid patient, the metacarpal head is often excised with a slight radial tilt to help correct any ulnar drift. The amount of bone that should be excised is determined by the requirement to accommodate any pre-existing intrinsic muscle tightness: the tighter the intrinsics, the more bone that needs to be excised (up to a limit). However, excessive bone shortening should be avoided, and intrinsic release considered instead. (This simply means dividing the intrinsic tendons until the IP joints are able to flex easily with the MCP joint in hyperextension.) The base of the proximal phalanx is not excised unless there is a severe deformity. However, any osteophytes must be removed with bone nibblers since these may interfere with flexion. The base of the proximal phalanx is now pierced with an awl. This opening is enlarged, and the medullary cavities of the proximal phalanx and metacarpal are now reamed by hand using progressively larger reamers. Sizers are used to determine the correct size of Swanson's implant which should be used. In general, the largest implant which fits should be selected. The implant fits when the long stem fits snugly in the metacarpal and the short stem fits snugly in the proximal phalanx. There should be no compression of the midsection with the fingers in extension. Generally, size 3 or 4 implants are used for the MCP joints. The sizer is removed, and the wound is washed with saline to remove any bone particles. The appropriate permanent implant is now inserted using a 'no-touch' technique. The implants are usually supplied with stainless steel 'grommets'. These should not be used.

Closure
It is not necessary to formally repair the collateral ligaments – scar tissue forms rapidly around the implant and confers stability to the joint – especially if the patient mobilises quickly after surgery. The sagittal bands are repaired with 4/0 or 5/0 PDS and are reefed as necessary if there is significant subluxation of the extensor tendons into the ulnar gutters. The skin is then closed with absorbable sutures. The senior author recommends using interrupted 5/0 Monocryl for the dermis (to approximate the wound edges) and then a running subcuticular 5/0 Monocryl or 5/0 Vicryl rapide suture for final closure.

Proximal interphalangeal joint
Landmarks and incision
A longitudinal incision (straight or curvilinear) is made over the dorsum of the joint.

Dissection
After the incision is made, the skin and subcutaneous fat are widely degloved over the joint to expose the extensor tendon and lateral bands. To reach the joint, the central slip of the extensor tendon can be split longitudinally or a Chamay approach can be used (see **Figure 9.7**). It is important to preserve the central slip insertion whichever method is used.

As for the MCP joint, the capsule of the PIP joint is usually very flimsy and should be excised together with any associated synovial proliferations. If possible, the collateral ligaments and volar plate are preserved to maintain joint stability. However, sometimes these structures are grossly damaged and it is necessary to excise/detach them to restore the correct alignment of the proximal and middle phalanges.

Procedure

> **Structures at risk**
>
> - Flexor tendon
> - Neurovascular bundles

The head of the proximal phalanx is now excised at neutral, using an oscillating saw. Care is taken not to damage the flexor tendon on the volar side of the joint. The base of the middle phalanx is not usually resected except in cases of severe deformity. However, osteophytes must be nibbled away as these may interfere with flexion. Sizing and reaming of the middle and proximal phalanges are performed in the same way as for the MCP joint. For the PIP joint a size 1 or 2 implant is usually used.

Closure

The longitudinal split in the extensor tendon or the Chamay flap is repaired with a continuous 4/0 or 5/0 PDS suture. In all other respects, closure is the same as described for MCP joint arthroplasty.

Distal interphalangeal joint

Landmarks and incision

The procedure is performed under ring block anaesthesia. An 'H'- or 'Y'-shaped incision is used to access the DIP joint.

Dissection

Dissection involves division of the collateral ligaments and removal of all tissue lateral to the extensor tendon. The extensor tendon can be divided and later repaired once the Swanson implant is fitted. Another approach is to preserve the extensor tendon by removing the damaged joint and osteophytes with a Ronguer. Once the extensor has been divided, an oscillating saw is used to remove bone.

Procedure

After excision of bone, the joint is irrigated with sterile saline and a size 1 or size 0 implant is inserted with a no-touch technique. The extensor apparatus is now repaired with 5/0 PDS sutures and the skin closed with interrupted 5-0 Vicryl rapide.

> **Structures at risk**
>
> - Extensor tendon
> - Flexor tendon
> - Nail complex

Postoperative care and instructions

- *MCP joint*: Patients are placed in a resting splint (volar plaster of paris [POP] or thermoplastic) or bulky bandage for 3–5 days. This is then replaced with alternate-day flexion (MCP joints at 70°–90°) and then extension (MCP joint at neutral) splints for 24-hour periods. After 4 weeks these splints are worn at night only and the patient mobilises the hand during the day with protective splinting only.
- *PIP joint*: The digit is placed in a T-bar (thermoplastic) splint. This maintains the PIP joint in full extension with the MCP joint flexed at 60° for 6 weeks at night and at rest. During the day, the patient is encouraged to begin immediate, regular, active mobilisation of the PIP joint out of the splint.
- *DIP joint*: Immediately after surgery, a Zimmer splint is applied to immobilise the DIP joint. Active mobilisation begins as soon as possible. For rehabilitation, patients are taught to carry out active flexion and extension exercises of the DIP joint(s) of the involved finger(s) themselves five times per day. A thermoplastic splint is used at night for 8 weeks to protect the DIP joint.

The emphasis in therapy for MCP, PIP and DIP joint arthroplasty is early supervised, active and passive movement.

Recommended references

Sierakowski A, Zweifel C, Sirotakova M, Sauerland S, Elliot D. Joint replacement in 131 painful osteoarthritic and post-traumatic distal interphalangeal joints. *J Hand Surg Eur*. 2012;**37(4)**:304–309.

Swanson AB. Silicone rubber implants for replacement of arthritic or destroyed joints in the hand. *Surg Clin North Am*. 1968;**48**:1113–1127.

Swanson AB. Flexible implant arthroplasty for arthritic finger joints: Rationale, technique and results of treatment. *J Bone Joint Surg Am*. 1972;**54**:435–437.

Takigawa S, Meletiou S, Sauerbier M et al. Long-term assessment of Swanson's implant arthroplasty in the proximal interphalangeal joint of the hand. *J Hand Surg Am*. 2004;**29**:785–795.

Extensor tendon repair

Injuries to the hand extensor apparatus are common. Non-surgical intervention is the best treatment for some of the more common injuries – especially in the finger, e.g. mallet deformity. The key to a successful outcome is recognition of the specific injury and implementation of appropriate surgical repair, splintage and/or early mobilisation to deal with the particular problem (**Figure 9.9**; *Table 9.2*). This will be influenced by whether the patient presents early (within a few days) or late (weeks or months later). In all cases, appropriate hand therapy and splintage are more important than any surgery to restore full function.

Indications and operative planning

- *Zone 1*: A mallet deformity. If it is open, the wound should be washed out as the DIP joint is often opened as well. The skin is then closed (converting an open mallet injury into a closed mallet injury) but the extensor tendon should not be repaired. Surgical repair is usually fruitless and leaves sutures close to the skin where they often extrude. If 12 weeks of dedicated and consistent splintage fails, then the patient should either accept the

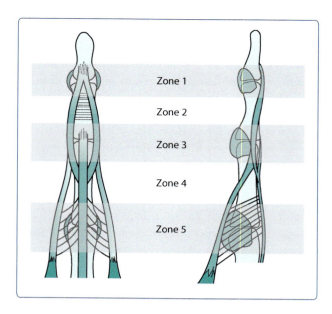

Figure 9.9 The zones of the extensor tendon.

Table 9.2 Anatomy of the extensor tendon

Zone	Description of tendon anatomy
1	The terminal tendon formed from the convergence of the two lateral bands
2	Lateral bands held together by the triangular ligament
3	Insertion of the central slip into the proximal phalanx
4	Central slip and intrinsic tendons
5	Extensor hood
6	Over the metacarpals
7	Over the wrist
8	In the forearm

position or consider arthrodesis of the DIP joint. An avulsion fracture of the insertion of the terminal extensor tendon also results in a mallet deformity. This fracture does not need surgical fixation regardless of the size of the fragment and the appearances on an X-ray. Very, very rarely, percutaneous fragment reduction under image intensifier guidance may be necessary to improve the position of the avulsion fragment.

- *Zone 2*: Injuries to the extensor apparatus in zone 2 result in a mallet deformity and are treated as for injuries in zone 1.
- *Zone 3*: Injury to the central slip results in a Boutonniere deformity, and this is often a late presentation. If it is an open injury and the damage to the central slip is recognised acutely, then it may be worth considering surgical re-insertion or repair of the central slip. The lack of soft tissue for reattachment means a mini-Mitek bone anchor or a 'washing-line' will often be needed to suture the tendon to the bone (see later for details of the surgical technique). Even if the central slip is reinserted surgically, the

patient will need the same splintage and hand therapy postoperatively as for a closed injury. So, there is a strong argument for not doing anything other than closing the skin as for injuries in zones 1 and 2. If the presentation is delayed or chronic, the PIP joint is statically splinted in full extension for 3 weeks followed by application of a Capener (dynamic) splint for another 3 weeks. Only if this fails, should surgery be considered to reinsert/reef the central slip and/or to mobilise the lateral bands which will have slipped volar to the axis of movement of the PIP joint.
- *Zone 4*: Injuries in zone 4 behave like zone 3 injuries. However, there is now sufficient tendon material to consider surgical repair using interrupted horizontal mattress sutures of 4/0 PDS.
- *Zone 5*: Injuries in zone 5 result in an extensor lag which can be debilitating. However, patients usually do very well after surgical repair of tendons in this zone followed by early active mobilisation (see later for mobilisation regimen).
- *Zones 6–8*: In these zones, the extensor tendons are more rounded, making a surgical repair much easier.

Contraindications

- *Active infection*: The repair may rupture and the tendon may become adherent.
- *Skeletal instability*: Unstable fractures must be fixed at the same time as any tendon repair.
- *Fixed joints*: There is no point in repairing a tendon injury.
- *Delayed presentation* (more than 6–8 weeks) of extensor ruptures in zones 6, 7 and 8 can rarely be repaired primarily as the tendon ends will have retracted and shortened.
- *Attrition ruptures*: Tendon grafts or transfers are required and may or may not be possible.
- *Smokers*: Because the tendon repairs are more likely to fail and the soft tissues may not heal.
- Poor social or psychological circumstances.
- Patients who do not understand their injury and cannot or do not comply with the hand therapy that is required after a tendon injury seldom regain full function of the affected part. This often includes very young children.
- If there is 20% (or less) division or loss of the extensor apparatus at any level then the skin should be closed and the tendon injury ignored.

Consent and risks

- *Scars*: It is often necessary to extend the wounds to gain access to the tendon ends.
- *Splintage and physiotherapy*: The patient will not have full use of the affected hand for 8–10 weeks. This may have significant economic consequences. The importance of compliance with the postoperative physiotherapy must be stressed.
- Infection.
- Rupture: 5%.
- *Adhesions*: A particular problem if there is an underlying fracture.
- *Bow stringing*: In zone 7 injuries.

Anaesthesia and positioning

For finger injuries up to zone 5, a ring block is sufficient. For more proximal injuries, in zones 6–8, a general anaesthesia or regional block is used. Positioning is supine with an arm table and a tourniquet appropriate to the part affected.

Surgical technique

Landmarks and incisions

If there is a skin laceration over the injured extensor tendon then it can be incorporated into any incision after suitable debridement of the wound edges. Incisions are extended proximally and distally as needed to gain access to the tendon ends. This is particularly necessary in zones 6, 7 and 8 where the proximal ends may have retracted a considerable distance. 'Zigzag' or 'lazy-S' incisions are preferred since these heal better when making long incisions over the dorsum of the hand and wrist.

Dissection

> #### *Structures at risk*
> - Necrosis of skin flaps – especially in smokers
> - Injury to dorsal veins and nerves

Skin and subcutaneous fat are incised and then skin flaps are elevated. These can be retracted with skin hooks or held in place with 'stay' sutures. The dorsal veins and nerves should always be preserved wherever possible. The extensor tendons are identified and care is taken to preserve the paratenon.

Procedure

- *Zones 1 and 2*: The tendon injury is usually treated non-operatively.
- *Zone 3*: Where appropriate, the central slip can be reinserted using a mini-Mitek bone anchor or a 'washing-line' (**Figure 9.10**). Two mini-Miteks are inserted into the base of the middle phalanx. The PIP joint is fully extended, and the central slip is secured

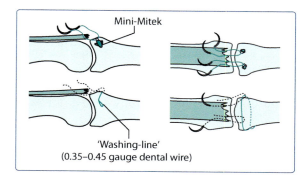

Figure 9.10 Reinserting the central slip with mini-Mitek anchors or a 'washing-line'.

with the two strands of suture. Alternatively, a 0.35–0.45 gauge dental wire is inserted across the base of the middle phalanx. The wire is formed into a loop close to the bone, leaving enough of a gap to allow the passage of multiple sutures (PDS preferred) under the wire. The whole wire acts as a suture anchor allowing multiple sutures to be passed into the central slip and under the 'washing-line'.

- *Zones 4 and 5*: The extensor tendons are flat, so horizontal mattress sutures using 5/0 or 4/0 PDS are best for any repair. The repair is augmented with a continuous, over-and-over suture of 5/0 PDS to keep the tendon ends tidy (**Figure 9.11**). In zone 5, any lacerations to the sagittal bands must be repaired with 5/0 PDS to prevent the extensor tendon subluxing into the radial or ulnar gutters.
- *Zones 6–8*: The ends of the tendon are minimally trimmed and repaired with a modified Kessler core suture, using a 3/0 or 4/0 PDS. If necessary, the core suture can be further augmented with a single horizontal mattress suture of 4/0 PDS. A continuous epitendinous suture is then placed around the circumference of the repair using 5/0 or 6/0 PDS (**Figure 9.12**). This also augments the repair and helps to keep the tendon ends tidy. A round bodied needle is preferred for both core and epitendinous sutures to reduce the chance of cutting the core suture accidentally. If a primary repair of the extensor tendon cannot be performed (e.g. delayed presentation or loss of tendon substance) an interposition tendon graft or tendon transfer must be used, e.g. with palmaris longus tendon. A Pulvertaft weave (**Figure 9.13**) must be used to secure the tendon graft to the ends of the tendon as this is strong enough to allow early mobilisation.
- *Zone 7*: Free excursion of the repaired extensor tendon must be confirmed under the retinaculum. If necessary, the retinaculum is divided to allow free movement of the tendon but preserving as much of it as possible intact prevents later bow-stringing. The repair is now tested by passively flexing and extending the finger. There must be no gapping of the repair and it must glide freely through the full excursion of the tendon.

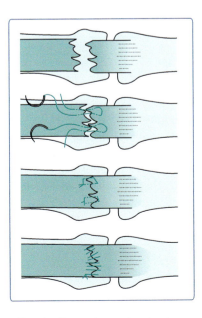

Figure 9.11 Repair of an extensor tendon in zones 4 and 5.

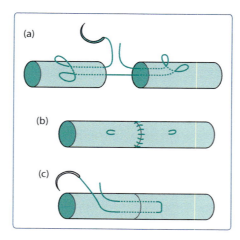

Figure 9.12 Zones 6–8 extensor tendon repair. (a) Kessler stitch, (b) epitendinous suture and (c) augmentation with a horizontal mattress suture.

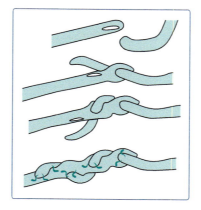

Figure 9.13 A Pulvertaft weave.

Closure

The tourniquet is released and haemostasis achieved. The wound is washed out with saline and closed with interrupted absorbable 4/0 or 5/0 Monocryl sutures and a subcuticular 5/0 Monocryl suture. Interrupted, non-absorbable sutures are avoided on the dorsum of the hand and fingers as this leaves very unsightly suture marks. Mepitel or non-adherent silicone dressings are applied to the wound together with dressing gauze and Velband padding before placing the hand and forearm in a volar plaster of Paris splint with the fingers in full extension and the wrist at neutral. The plaster should be allowed to set before the patient comes off the operating table.

Postoperative care and instructions

The senior author recommends the Norwich regimen for injuries in zones 5–7. The plaster of Paris is replaced with a thermoplastic splint the day after surgery. Passive and active extension are commenced straight away, protected in the splint for 4 weeks. For a further 4 weeks, the patient removes the splint for active extension and active flexion of the IP/MCP joints but wears it at all other times. For central slip injuries (zones 3 to 4) the finger is placed in a cylinder splint (PIP joint static in extension, DIP joint free) for 3 weeks and then 3 further weeks in a Capener splint.

Recommended references

Abouna JM, Brown H. The treatment of mallet finger. The results in a series of 148 consecutive cases and a review of the literature. *Br J Surg.* 1968;**55**:653.

Lange RH, Engber WD. Hyper-extension mallet finger. *Orthopaedics.* 1983;**6**:1426.

Newport ML, Williams CD. Biomechanical characteristics of extensor tendon suture techniques. *J Hand Surg Am.* 1992;**17**:111.

Newport ML, Pollack GR, Williams CD. Biomechanical characteristics of suture techniques in extensor zone IV. *J Hand Surg Am.* 1995;**20**:650–656.

Stuart D. Duration of splinting after repair of extensor tendons in the hand. A clinical study. *J Bone Joint Surg Br.* 1965;**47**:72.

Sylaidis P, Youatt M, Logan A. Early active mobilisation for extensor tendon injuries. The Norwich regime. *J Hand Surg Br.* 1997;**22**:594.

Wehbé MA, Schneider L. Mallet fractures. *J Bone Joint Surg Am.* 1984;**66**:658.

Flexor tendon repair preoperative planning

Indications and operative planning

- *Zone 1*: The technique for flexor repair in zone 1 depends on how close to the insertion the FDP has been divided. If the tendon is divided close to the bone (e.g. FDP avulsion) then it may be necessary to use a suture anchor (such as a mini-Mitek) to secure the tendon end.
- *Zone 2*: Proximal zone 1 and zone 2 repairs of the FDP tendon are treated in a similar way. The aim is to repair the tendon but to avoid any bulkiness at the repair site to allow the tendon to glide within the flexor sheath. If the repair is done badly it will be too bulky and may trigger, rupture or jam in position unless the flexor sheath is opened. Special care must be taken with repairs of FDS in this zone (see later).
- *Zone 3*: Zone 3 repairs are easier to perform because there is no tight flexor sheath to contend with and the tendon ends are larger. Distal zone 3 repairs may catch on the A1 pulley, which may need to be divided.
- *Zones 4–5*: Repairs in these zones are the same as repairs of the extensor tendons in zones 6–8.
- *Complete division*: Primary repair of a flexor tendon should be performed as soon as possible. Unlike extensor tendons, surgical intervention in some form is always necessary when the flexor tendons have been divided.
- *Timing of repair*: There is good evidence that the outcome of primary repair is superior when carried out as quickly as possible (within 72 hours). There is a particular urgency in carrying out a repair of the flexor tendons (as compared to the extensor tendons) because the flexor pulleys will eventually collapse/fill with scar tissue after 3–4 weeks. Any tendon repair will then need to reconstruct the pulleys and make surgery more complicated than necessary.
- *Particular tendons*: The flexor muscle bellies (especially flexor pollicis longus, FPL) have a tendency to shorten quickly. This may make primary repair of a tendon

impossible. The ring and middle fingers are particularly prone to avulsion injuries of the FDP tendon. Repair of combined injuries of flexor digitorum superficialis (FDS)/FDP tendons in the little and ring fingers are particularly prone to form adhesions to the surrounding tissues. **Therefore, consideration should be given to repairing just the FDP tendon in these digits**.

- *Zone of injury*: As for extensor tendons, the surgical technique for repair of flexor tendons varies depending on the zone of injury (**Figure 9.14**).
- *Partial division of flexor tendons*: There is good evidence that inserting sutures into a tendon results in necrosis of the tendon substance. Therefore, the use of sutures should be avoided for any partial tendon injury involving less than 50% of the diameter of the tendon. Instead, we recommend trimming the edges of the tendon laceration to prevent triggering (if any is present) followed by supervised mobilisation in a splint for a complete flexor tendon division for the next 8 weeks.

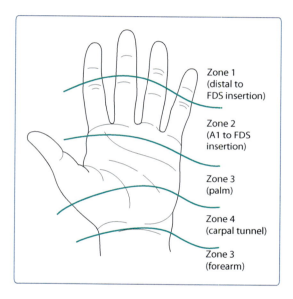

Figure 9.14 The zones of flexor tendon injury. FDS, flexor digitorum superficialis.

Contraindications

- Active infection
- Skeletal instability
- Fixed joints
- Delayed presentation (more than 3–4 weeks) can rarely be repaired primarily as the tendon ends will have retracted and shortened and the flexor pulleys will have collapsed
- Attrition ruptures
- Smokers
- Poor social or psychological circumstances
- Partial tendon rupture of less than 50% should not be repaired
- Delayed presentation

Consent and risks

- *Scars*: It is often necessary to extend the wounds to gain access to the tendon ends.
- *Splintage and physiotherapy*: Patients will not have full use of the affected hand for 12 weeks. The importance of compliance with the postoperative physiotherapy must be stressed.
- Infection.
- *Adhesions*: A particular problem when there is an underlying fracture. Overall, there is a 5% tenolysis rate.
- *Rupture*: Zone 2 finger flexors – 5%, FPL repair – 12%.
- *Bow stringing*: May not be evident for some years after the original event. It may occur if it proves necessary to divide the flexor sheath completely in order to repair the tendons. A subsequent pulley reconstruction will then be required.
- Neuroma formation.

Anaesthesia and positioning

For isolated FDP injuries, it is usually possible to perform a repair under digital nerve block with a finger tourniquet. For FPL, FDS and more proximal flexor injuries, general anaesthesia or a regional block may be necessary because of the need for an arm tourniquet. To avoid the need for a tourniquet, surgeons should consider using local anaesthetic with adrenaline. This 'wide-awake' approach has many additional advantages. The arm is positioned in the supine position with an arm table.

Surgical technique

Landmarks and incisions

The Bruner (zigzag) incision (**Figure 9.15**) is preferred. If there is a laceration, then it can be incorporated into the incision after suitable debridement of the wound edges.

Dissection

Structures at risk

- Edges of the skin flaps
- Neurovascular bundles

The flaps can be retracted with skin hooks or held in place with 'stay' sutures. A 'window' is opened in the flexor sheath by creating zigzag flaps or by lateral 'venting' of the pulley on one side. Ideally, the window should be as small as possible and should be positioned only between the annular pulleys to allow maximum preservation of the pulley system. If the flexor sheath is opened with zigzag flaps, it is usually possible to repair the sheath with a slightly larger diameter by approximating the tips of the flaps. This will allow any

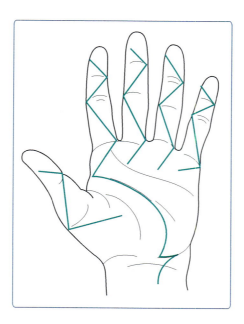

Figure 9.15 Suggested Bruner incisions to approach the flexors.

reconstructed pulley system to accommodate a bulkier, less than perfect, tendon repair. However, it is also worth noting that there is good evidence that division of the A4 pulley does not cause significant bow stringing of the flexor tendon if the distal part of the A2 pulley remains intact. Therefore, consider leaving the A4 pulley completely open to avoid any concerns about snagging of the repair in the sheath once the patient starts to mobilise.

Tendon retrieval

If a tendon has been fully divided, flexion of the finger or thumb normally delivers the distal end into the wound. If the proximal end of the tendon has retracted it can sometimes be retrieved by passing a small curved artery clip or skin hook into the flexor sheath. If this method is not successful, then the palm of the hand must be opened, and the tendon(s) pushed up into the finger with forceps. In exceptional cases, it may be necessary to use a paediatric feeding tube or dental wire to retrieve the FDP or FPL tendon. If the laceration is in the wrist or palm, it may be necessary to extend the incisions more proximally to find the tendon ends. Once retrieved, a 20G (blue-hub) needle can be passed through the tendon ends to prevent them from retracting again until the repair is complete.

Tendon suture technique

Zone 1. If there is a very short stump of tendon (<1 cm), then it is possible to repair the tendon by inserting 4/0 or 5/0 PDS sutures as a half-Kessler proximally and as a horizontal mattress distally. Multiple sutures can be inserted to increase the strength of the repair since there is no concern about the bulk of the repair getting caught in the flexor sheath. When the tendon is avulsed and/or there is a fracture of the distal phalanx, then alternative methods of fixation must be considered, e.g. suturing the tendon to the remnants of the periosteum or using a suture anchor (such as a mini-Mitek). If there is a fracture, then a mini-plate can be used to fix the fracture, and the plate can also be used as a suture anchor.

Flexor digitorum superficialis distal to the metacarpophalangeal joint

If the FDS is injured where it is beginning to flatten out or after it has split into its two terminal slips, then horizontal mattress sutures must be used to repair the tendon because there will not be enough tendon substance for a modified Kessler core suture. Each terminal slip must be repaired separately. If there is room for it, an epitendinous suture using 5/0 or 6/0PDS can be used to tidy the ends of the repair. Note that in combined FDS/FDP injuries of the little and ring fingers there is an argument for not repairing the FDS tendon to avoid creating two bulky tendon repairs, both of which will be unable to glide in the flexor sheath.

Flexor digitorum superficialis, flexor pollicis longus and flexor digitorum superficialis proximal to metacarpophalangeal joint

The tendon ends are approximated and held in position by transfixing them with a 20G needle. The ends of the tendon are trimmed, and the back wall of the repair is started with a continuous 5/0 or 6/0 PDS 'over-and-over' or Silfverskiold-pattern epitendinous suture. A four-strand, core suture (e.g. 2 × modified Kessler, 1 × modified Kessler with 1 × horizontal mattress or 1 × cruciate) is now inserted using 4/0 or 3/0 PDS, taking particular care to bury the knot(s) in the middle of the repair. The anterior part of the epitendinous suture is then completed (**Figure 9.16**). The core suture should always be over-tightened to prevent gapping when early active mobilisation is started postoperatively. Only round-bodied needles should be used - to reduce the risk of cutting the core suture accidentally. There must be no gapping of the repair and it must glide freely through the full excursion of the tendon when the repair is complete. Active testing of the repair is easy to achieve using the 'wide-awake' approach. Any pulleys restricting gliding of the tendon should be divided in a zigzag fashion or excised altogether.

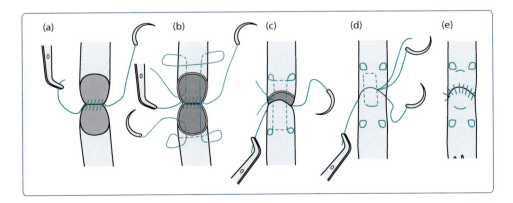

Figure 9.16 (a–e) Steps in the repair of flexor tendons.

Closure

All wounds are washed out with saline and closed with interrupted, absorbable 4/0 or 5/0 Vicryl rapide sutures. Unlike the dorsum of the hand, suture marks are not so much of a problem on the volar side because of the thicker epidermis. Therefore, subcuticular sutures do not have to be used. Mepitel or other non-adherent, dressings, gauze and Velband bandage are applied and the hand and forearm are placed in a dorsal plaster of Paris with the fingers flexed at 90° at the MCP joint and the wrist in neutral. The plaster should be set before the patient comes off the operating table.

Postoperative care and instructions

Early active mobilisation begins on day 1 following the Belfast regimen. The plaster of Paris is replaced with a thermoplastic splint the following day. Full passive flexion is commenced in all digits. The repaired tendon is allowed to commence immediate, controlled, active flexion and extension. All exercises are performed in the splint for the first 4 weeks. After 4 weeks, the patient can remove the splint, but only to do exercises. At all other times, the splint must remain in place. No passive extension is permitted for 8 weeks.

Recommended references

Kessler I, Nissim F. Primary repair without immobilisation of flexor tendon division within the digital sheet. *Acta Orthop Scand.* 1969;**40**:587–601.

Kleinert HE, Kutz JE, Ashbell TS et al. Primary repair of lacerated flexor tendons in 'No Man's Land'. Proceedings, American Society for Surgery of the Hand. *J Bone Joint Surg Am.* 1967;**49**:577.

Lalonde DH. Reconstruction of the hand with wide awake surgery. *Clin Plast Surg.* 2011;**38(4)**:761–769.

Silfverskiold KL, Anderson CH. Two new methods of tendon repair: An *in vitro* evaluation of tensile strength and gap formation. *J Hand Surg Am.* 1993;**18**:58–65.

Sirotakova M, Elliott D. Early active mobilisation of primary repairs of the flexor pollicis longus tendon with two Kessler two-strand core sutures and a strengthened circumferential suture. *J Hand Surg Br.* 2004;**29**:531–535.

Small JO, Brennan MD, Colville J. Early active mobilisation following flexor tendon repair in Zone 2. *J Hand Surg Br.* 1989;**14**:383–391.

Sourmelis SG, McGrouther DA. Retrieval of the retracted flexor tendon. *J Hand Surg Br.* 1987;**12**:109–111.

Tang JB. Release of the A4 pulley to facilitate zone II flexor tendon repair. *J Hand Surg Am.* 2014;**39(11)**:2300–2307.

Wong J, McGrouther DA. Minimizing trauma over 'no man's land' for flexor tendon retrieval. *J Hand Surg Eur.* 2014;**39**:1004–1006.

Tendon transfers

Preoperative planning

Tendon transfers are useful to restore hand function in patients where primary tendon repair is difficult or impossible. The essence of a good transfer is to keep it simple and to plan carefully. The senior author recommends listing all the functions (absent and present) to allow formulation of a plan. An example is given in *Table 9.3*.

Indications

- *Nerve palsies*: Tendon transfers are particularly useful for isolated nerve palsies. For a transfer to be possible, the hand or upper limb must have sufficient numbers of functioning tendons which can be used for the transfer without adversely affecting

Table 9.3 Example: Planning for an anterior interosseous nerve injury

Tendons present	Tendons absent	Suggested options
All extensors + brachioradialis (BR)	Flexor pollicis longus (FPL)	FDS from ring to FPL BR to FPL Arthrodesis interphalangeal joint
Pronator teres	FDP to index	Suture FDP middle to FDP index
Flexor carpi ulnaris (FCU)	Pronator quadratus	Do not replace
Flexor digitorum profundus (FDP) to little, ring and middle		Do not replace
Flexor digitorum superficialis (FDS)		Do not replace
Flexor carpi radialis (FCR)		Do not replace

overall hand function. Therefore, patients with a global loss of nerve function (e.g. cerebral palsy) will always do less well.
- *Delayed presentation of a tendon rupture*: Tendon transfers may be necessary to restore function even in cases of delayed presentation because of shortening of the muscle bellies after rupture.

Contraindications

- The joint which the tendon is intended to move is not fully supple.
- The part of the hand/upper limb which is to be moved by the tendon is not fully sensate.
- The soft tissue bed through which the transfer will pass is poorly vascularized and/or heavily scarred (e.g. under a skin graft).
- The transfer results in loss of an essential function.
- The power of the transferred muscle is less than 5 (Medical Research Council [MRC] grade). This is because any transferred muscle loses at least one MRC grade after the transfer.
- If the amplitude of the transferred muscle is not similar to that of the muscle which it is replacing. For example, finger flexors have an excursion of about 70 mm. Wrist extensors/flexors have an excursion of only 30–40 mm. This is not a good match.
- Before 9–12 months have elapsed after any motor nerve repair. If motor recovery has not occurred by this time, then it is very unlikely to occur, and a tendon transfer is then justified.
- Where other procedures would be more beneficial, e.g. for delayed presentation of an FDP laceration or avulsion, a tendon graft or an arthrodesis of the DIP joint may be the preferred options. Similarly, a flexor rupture in zone 1 and 2 for patients with rheumatoid arthritis is usually better treated with a tendon graft.

Consent and risks

- *Donor site morbidity*: Patients may experience weakness or some loss of function after harvest of a tendon. For example, after harvest of the extensor indicis proprius (EIP), patients may experience an extensor lag at the index finger MCP joint.

- *Additional scarring*: After harvest of the tendons/grafts.
- *Rupture*: To reduce this risk, the senior author recommends using a Pulvertaft weave or a side-to-side repair with multiple horizontal mattress sutures. It is a particular risk after interposition tendon grafting with two repairs.
- Patients must be warned of the prolonged rehabilitation which must be followed after any tendon transfer (8–12 weeks) during which they will be unable to use their hand normally.
- Infection.
- *Neuromas*: The superficial branch of the radial nerve is a particular problem because of its propensity for neuroma formation after even minor trauma.
- Recurvatum deformity (essentially a swan-neck posture of the donor finger) due to hyperextension of the PIP joint after harvest of the FDS in patients with hyperextensible joints.
- Damage to adjacent tendons or pulleys.
- Imbalance of the transfer (i.e. too tight or too loose).
- Tendon imbalance due to spontaneous recovery of normal functions if the tendon transfers were performed too early (i.e. before 9–12 months after repair of a motor nerve).

Anaesthesia and positioning

Most transfers are performed under general or regional anaesthesia. However, there is an increasing trend to perform tendon transfers using the 'wide-awake' approach which allows the tension in any transfer to be assessed more accurately with the cooperation of the patient. Patients should be supine, and the arm should be placed on a hand table. Use of an arm tourniquet is essential.

Surgical techniques

Over many years, hand surgeons have developed standard combinations of transfers to deal with specific nerve palsies. In all cases, the assumption is made that only one nerve is injured, and the rest of the hand forearm is 'normal'.

- For a high radial/posterior interosseous nerve palsy
  - Palmaris longus (PL) to extensor pollicis longus (EPL) to restore thumb extension.
  - Flexor carpi radialis (FCR) or flexor carpi ulnaris (FCU) to extensor digitorum communis (EDC) to restore finger extension. For posterior interosseous palsy, FDS from ring or middle finger to EDC is preferred instead.
  - Pronator teres (PT) to extensor carpi radialis longus or brevis (ECRL/ECRB) to restore wrist extension.
- For a low median nerve palsy
  - FDS from ring finger or EIP or abductor digiti minimi (ADM) (Huber) to abductor pollicis brevis (APB). Palmaris longus can also be used to improve abduction (Camitz transfer).
  - Loss of the lumbricals may result in clawing of the index and middle fingers. The best solution is a dynamic transfer using FDS from the ring finger split into two slips inserted into the A2 pulleys of index and middle fingers (i.e. a Zancolli 'lasso').

- For a high median palsy
  - FDS from ring finger or EIP or ADM to APB for an opponensplasty as in a low median palsy.
  - The FDP from ring or little fingers can be sutured side-to-side to the FDP of the index and middle fingers to restore finger flexion.
  - BR or FDS from ring or little finger to FPL to restore thumb flexion.
  - If clawing is present, then a Zancolli lasso as for a low median palsy. Alternatively, a PL free tendon graft from the transverse carpal ligament to the radial lateral bands of the index and middle fingers for a static extension block.
- For a low ulnar palsy
  - The best solution for clawing (which is passively correctible) is a Zancolli lasso.
  - FDS from the middle or index finger to adductor pollicis for weak adduction.
  - EIP to extensor digitorum minimi (EDM) corrects Wartenberg's deformity.
- For high ulnar palsy
  - Suture of FDP middle and index side to side to FDP for the little and ring fingers.
  - FDS from middle or index to adductor pollicis if adduction is weak.

Other technical aspects of tendon transfers

When measuring the length of donor tendon required for transfer, remember that 2–3 cm of tendon are required to perform a Pulvertaft weave. A Pulvertaft weave is one of the keys to a good transfer because the repair is sufficiently strong to allow early mobilisation. Getting the correct tension in the transferred tendon is another key point. The joint should be positioned where the transfer will be at its maximum length and the tendon is then sutured under maximum tension. Unfortunately, this is not always possible if the donor tendon is too short. Therefore, it is important to carry out a tenodesis test to ensure that an overly tight transfer has been avoided. Having said that, all repairs should be 'over-tensioned' on the table to allow for a small amount of subsequent 'stretching' of the tendon.

Closure

All wounds are closed in layers with absorbable sutures using interrupted 4/0 or 5/0 Monocryl to dermis and 4/0 or 5/0 Vicryl rapide as a subcuticular stitch. Mepitel, dressing, gauze and Velband bandage are applied as needed and the hand and forearm are placed in a resting volar plaster. The plaster should be set before the patient comes off the operating table.

Postoperative care and instructions

After 24–48 hours, the plaster of Paris splint is removed, and the patient can be placed in an appropriate thermoplastic resting splint which can be removed by the patient and therapist to allow early mobilisation to begin. The precise rehabilitation regimen depends on the tendons which have been transferred. However, in all cases, one of the keys to a successful outcome is the ability to begin early active mobilisation. In order for this to happen, any tenorrhaphy must be sufficiently strong to allow this mobilisation to occur.

Nerve transfers

A nerve transfer is a surgical technique that involves the transfer of redundant or expendable nerves to restore muscle function and/or sensation after nerve injury. With appropriate planning, a nerve transfer can be as good as a tendon transfer in patients with isolated nerve palsies and has additional advantages over traditional tendon transfers. Nerve transfers use nerves (or branches of nerves) that perform redundant or less important roles and then uses them to restore function to muscles which are normally innervated by the injured nerve. Surgeons aim to carry out the nerve repair as close to the target muscle as possible to shorten the re-innervation time (i.e. before the motor end plates degenerate after the muscle is denervated). Interestingly, nerves whose original function was entirely outside the limb (e.g. intercostal nerves) can be used to restore function in the limb (e.g. to re-innervate biceps). Initially, the patient may have to breathe in to make the muscle contract, but brain plasticity eventually allows the patient to move the limb just by thinking about it. Another example of a nerve transfer is in proximal ulnar nerve injuries. The anterior interosseous nerve (AIN) is the nerve transfer of choice for recovering ulnar nerve motor function after a proximal ulnar nerve transection where repair of the ulnar nerve is difficult or impossible. The AIN is transferred end to side to the ulnar nerve in the forearm. This has the effect of transferring the motor functions of one of the terminal branches of the median nerve to the (normally) ulnar innervated muscles.

Recommended references

Davidge KM, Yee A, Moore AM, Mackinnon SE. The supercharged end-to-side anterior interosseous-to-ulnar motor nerve transfer for restoring intrinsic function: Clinical experience. *Plast Reconstr Surg.* 2015;**136(3)**:344e–352e.

Green DP, Hotchkiss RN, Pederson WC, eds. *Green's Operative Hand Surgery.* 5th ed. Edinburgh, Scotland: Elsevier, 2005.

Lalonde DH. Wide-awake extensor indicis proprius to extensor pollicis longus tendon transfer. *J Hand Surg Am.* 2014;**39(11)**:2297–2299.

Tang JB. Wide-awake primary flexor tendon repair, tenolysis, and tendon transfer. *Clin Orthop Surg.* 2015;**7(3)**:275–781.

Soft tissue reconstruction

Preoperative planning

For the purposes of this handbook, the focus is on three areas:

- The operative correction of aberrant scarring
- The use of split-thickness skin grafts
- The use of full-thickness skin grafts

Indications

- Primary wound closure cannot be achieved.
- Primary wound closure can be achieved but may result in functional impairment.
- Allowing a wound to heal by secondary intention will result in functional impairment. For example, leaving tendons exposed which would result in their desiccation and necrosis.
- There is aberrant scarring. Examples include webbed volar scars from poorly placed incisions, burns or other traumatic scarring (**Figure 9.17**).

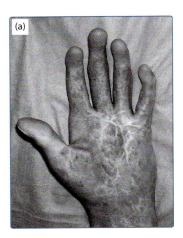 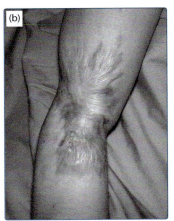 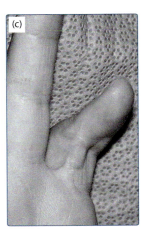

Figure 9.17 Soft tissue reconstruction needed for (a) skin loss after sepsis, (b) burns or (c) a poor volar scar.

Contraindications

- *Active infection*: Beta-haemolytic streptococci in particular will dissolve any graft. Other bacteria will reduce the likelihood of the graft taking and can result in patchy graft take.
- *Smoking*: Expect a 40% increase in wound healing complications in any patient who smokes.
- *Long-term steroid use*: Particularly in rheumatoid arthritis (relative contraindication).
- Peripheral vascular disease or similar, e.g. Buerger's disease, scleroderma or severe Raynaud's.
- Previous radiotherapy to the hand.
- *Recipient site unsuitable*: Grafts will not take on bare bone or tendon unless these areas are very small (<5 mm diameter) in which case the grafts may survive by 'bridging'.
- Donor site problems.

Consent and risks

- *Scarring*: Particularly with split skin grafting which leaves large, unsightly scars.
- Infection.
- *Flap necrosis*: This is nearly always the result of technical error (e.g. flaps too narrow, closure too tight) but may also be a consequence of infection.
- Graft loss.
- *Prolonged healing*: A split skin graft (SSG) donor site may take months (or even years) to heal if the patient and donor site are poorly selected.

Operative planning

There are three main techniques to master:

- *Z-plasty*: An operation that involves the transposition of two triangular skin flaps of equal dimension to lengthen a scar or change its direction. There is a risk of necrosis of the flaps if they are poorly designed.

- *Split-thickness skin grafts*: If an SSG is used, it is often used as a temporary biological dressing rather than for definitive skin cover.
- *Full-thickness skin grafts* (FTGs): These can be used for definitive skin cover anywhere on the hand except the pulps of the fingers and thumb.

Anaesthesia and positioning

The form of anaesthesia depends on the size of graft that needs to be harvested and the area where it is needed. Local anaesthesia is suitable for harvesting small grafts and for surgery to the digits. However, patients may be more grateful for a general anaesthetic when harvesting large grafts and operating on multiple areas (e.g. harvest a FTG from the groin for use in the hand) and on the palm of the hand. The hand is placed in the supine position on an arm table. A tourniquet is extremely useful during surgery involving the use of flaps or grafts in the hand.

Surgical technique

Z-plasties are used when there is a need to change the direction and/or length of a scar. The best example of their use is to correct a webbed volar scar. Z-plasties can also be used to lengthen a scar after Dupuytren's fasciectomy (see **Figure 9.2**, p. 198).

Landmarks and incisions

In most cases, a 30° or 60° angle is used for the Z-plasty design. A 60° angle achieves more lengthening of the scar, but a 30° angle is often easier to transpose. The width of the base of each flap in relation to its length is important in determining flap survival. The longer and narrower the flap, the less likely it is to survive. The flaps are marked out as shown in **Figure 9.2** (p. 198).

It is a myth that the limbs of the Z-plasty must be aligned to fall in skin crease. Skin creases exist because the fingers flex. When a finger ceases to flex (e.g. after an arthrodesis) the creases eventually disappear. The Z-plasty should be placed where it is needed.

Superficial dissection

The flaps are raised with a small amount of subcutaneous fat to ensure the subdermal plexus is uninjured. When raising the flaps, the underlying anatomy must be considered. For example, it is very easy to divide the neurovascular bundle when raising the Z-plasty flaps after a Dupuytren's fasciectomy.

Procedure

- The first stage is to raise one flap and transpose it across the scar. This ensures that the design is right for the second flap before you commit yourself to raising it.
- If the design is correct, then the two flaps should automatically transpose themselves across the scar when the finger straightens.
- The flaps are now tacked into the correct corners and any dog-ears ignored. (These will flatten in a few weeks anyway.)

Closure

Interrupted or continuous, absorbable, 4/0 or 5/0 Vicryl rapide sutures are used for closure. Do not use non-absorbable sutures in the hand. There is no difference in wound healing and scar quality comparing absorbable and non-absorbable sutures in the hand, and patients find it very painful to have them removed.

Split-thickness skin grafts

A small SSG (<3 cm × 3 cm) can be harvested with a handheld knife (e.g. Watson). The description of the technique given below assumes a hand-powered knife is being used. However, ideally, a powered dermatome (air or electric) should be used to harvest all SSGs (**Figure 9.18**). The technique for harvesting a graft with a powered dermatome is similar to that using a handheld knife.

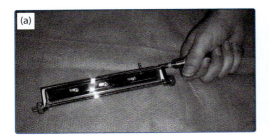
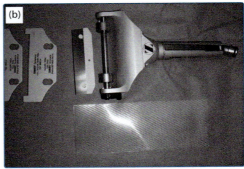

Figure 9.18 A Watson hand knife (a) and an air-powered dermatome (b) for harvesting split skin grafts.

Landmarks and incisions

The first decision is to determine the amount of SSG needed. This is best worked out in terms of the length and width of the defect which needs to be covered. A marginally larger area than you think you will need should always be taken (approximately 1 cm beyond is 'about right'). It is easy to trim the SSG down to size, but harvesting more graft is always a problem. Ensure the correct settings are selected on the hand knife or dermatome. Typically, the SSG should be between 0.2 and 0.4 mm thick. The thicker the SSG, the less it will contract, but the longer it will take for the donor site to heal and the more obvious the donor site scar.

Harvesting

Liquid paraffin (or Hibiscrub cleaning solution) is applied to the skin and the knife. This acts as a lubricant and prevents the blade from catching on the skin. If the blade catches rather than cuts, it will tear the SSG or result in holes where you do not want them. It is also critically important to ensure that the skin at the donor site is under tension while the skin is being harvested. The best way to do this is to have an assistant who can squeeze the thigh or arm while you concentrate on harvesting the skin. A rapid sawing motion is used to harvest the skin with a hand knife, keeping the blade flat with respect to the skin and not pressing too hard or the graft thickness will increase. If a powered dermatome is used, the machine does the sawing for you. Regardless, the aim is to harvest the graft in one smooth action.

Meshing the skin increases the area which can be covered with a given size of SSG. It also increases the take rate by allowing free drainage of haematoma and seroma. It is possible to mesh skin by hand but using a skin mesher is quicker and neater. However, once it has taken, meshed skin contracts even more than a sheet graft. An alternative is to perforate it with multiple stabs using a number 15 blade. The perforations allow haematoma and seroma to ooze through.

The donor site is dressed with Mefix adhesive dressing applied directly to the wound. Gauze, Velband and crepe bandages are applied over this to absorb any exudate.

Grafting

The SSG is applied shiny side down onto a prepared wound bed and secured with absorbable 4/0 or 5/0 Vicryl rapide either as interrupted or continuous sutures. The same sutures are used to 'quilt' the SSG onto the wound bed to reduce shearing movements, improve contact with the wound bed and improve haemostasis under the graft. The SSG is dressed with Jelonet and a layer of gauze. A bulky bandage (Velband and crepe) is applied and the hand immobilised in a plaster of Paris. The graft should be reviewed in 2–3 days.

Full-thickness graft

The best donor sites for a FTG are the groin and postauricular sulcus because these areas are well hidden. However, skin taken from these sites is usually a poor colour match for the skin of the hand. Therefore, a FTG applied to the hand will always be obvious as a darker area with a different texture. In males, a FTG from the groin is also likely to be hairy resulting in obvious problems when it is applied to any part of the hand unless a concerted effort is made to remove the hair follicles before the FTG is used.

Landmarks and incisions

An assessment of the area of FTG needed is made, using a piece of paper as a template. The template is transferred to the donor site to mark out a similar area of skin. If harvesting a FTG for a case of Dupuytren's dermofasciectomy, multiple small pieces of FTG may be needed (**Figure 9.19**).

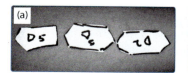
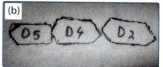
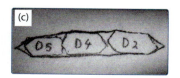

Figure 9.19 (a) Templating, (b) marking and (c) planning incision for multiple full-thickness grafts for Dupuytren's dermofasciectomy.

Harvesting

The outlines of the pieces of skin that you intend to take are scored with a number 15 scalpel blade. This ensures that you do not lose the outline of the individual pieces of skin. Lift up one corner of the ellipse that you intend to raise and grip this with an artery clip. This saves your hand from getting tired and allows the graft to be held firmly over your index finger while harvesting the graft. Fat should be removed from the graft as it is harvested. This avoids the need to de-fat the graft after it has been detached from the donor site.

The donor site can now be closed with a couple of interrupted 4/0 Monocryl sutures in the dermis. Final closure is completed with a continuous suture of 4/0 Monocryl into the dermis which is locked at both ends with a buried knot. Once the dermal suture is complete, final closure continues with a 4/0 Monocryl subcuticular suture.

Grafting

Any remaining fat on the graft is removed using a pair of tenotomy scissors. This is a very tedious but very important step. The more fat there is on your FTG, the less likely it is to take. The FTG is secured to the recipient site with a couple of interrupted 4/0 or 5/0 Vicryl rapide sutures. Securing the graft is now completed with a continuous over-and-over suture at the edge, using 4/0 or 5/0 rapide. It is important to add quilting sutures to the center of the graft to prevent haematoma formation and reduce shearing movements. Copious quantities of Vaseline ointment are now spread onto the graft and a Jelonet and gauze dressing is applied. The graft should be reviewed in 5–7 days.

Postoperative care and instructions

- *Z-plasty*: The patient can mobilise their hand immediately unless a graft was also used. Even if the last 2–3 mm of the tips of the flaps do not survive, the wound will go on to heal by secondary intention without compromising the final outcome. Therefore, mobilise the hand since mobility is more important than any concern about the wounds.
- *SSG*: The graft is left undisturbed for 48–72 hours. If it is pink after that, then it has taken and gentle mobilisation can begin. The donor site on the thigh or arm is left undisturbed until 10–14 days have passed, and the patient says it is no longer painful. If the dressing is taken off too early, newly formed epithelium will be ripped off with the dressing. Once a continuous layer of epithelium is present at both recipient and donor sites, the patient applies a thick layer of Vaseline to both areas. The SSG has no sweat or sebaceous glands and will quickly dry out, crust, flake and crack if it is not protected in this way.
- *FTG*: The hand is immobilised for 1 week in a plaster of Paris splint to further minimise shearing forces that would interfere with graft take. At 5–7 days, all the dressings are removed, and the graft can be inspected. If graft take is complete, then copious quantities of Vaseline ointment must be applied daily for the next 3 months after which the glands in the graft will have started to function and it can self-moisturize.

Recommended references

McGregor AD, McGregor IA. *Fundamental Techniques of Plastic Surgery and Their Surgical Applications.* 10th ed. Edinburgh, Scotland: Churchill Livingstone, 2000.

Thorne CH, Bartlett SP, Beasley RW et al. (eds). *Grabb and Smith's Plastic Surgery.* 5th ed. New York, NY: Lippincott-Raven, 1997.

Trigger finger surgery

Preoperative planning

The diagnosis of triggering is normally easy to make but overt triggering is sometimes absent, and the patient only gives a history of pain on flexion of the digit which may be confused with or concurrent with arthritis. Trigger finger is common in patients over the age of 50 years, patients with diabetes and patients with rheumatoid arthritis. Where overt triggering is absent, but pain is present, the use of steroid injections is particularly efficacious.

Indications

- Persistent triggering (not relieved by steroid injections)
- Acutely locked finger

Contraindications

- Presence of infection.
- Triggering in a patient with rheumatoid arthritis (RA). A rheumatoid patient with triggering needs steroid injections or a synovectomy. Release of the A1 pulley in RA patients may make ulnar drift worse by creating further changes in the alignment of the tendons.

Consent and risks

- Infection
- Injury to the tendon and neurovascular bundles
- Recurrence
- Stiffness/loss of flexion

Anaesthesia and positioning

Local anaesthesia is used with the patient supine and with the arm on an arm table. Use of a tourniquet is optional.

Surgical technique

Landmarks and incision

The proximal border of the A1 pulley lies at the neck of the corresponding metacarpal (**Figure 9.20**), roughly at the level of the mid-palmar crease. A 1.5 cm long, transverse, incision is made in the crease over the corresponding metacarpal.

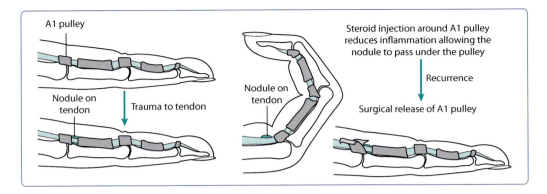

Figure 9.20 Trigger finger.

Surgical dissection

Blunt dissection is performed through the subcutaneous fat and palmar fascia, using tenotomy scissors, to expose the flexor sheath. It is rarely necessary to visualise the neurovascular bundles running parallel to the flexor tendons: in any case, these should be protected by retractors.

The proximal edge of the A1 pulley is identified, and the pulley is then divided longitudinally with a scalpel taking particular care to stay over the midline of the tendon to avoid the risk of damage to the neurovascular bundles. The patient is then asked to flex and extend the digit several times to test for any residual triggering. The arm tourniquet is released, the wound washed out with saline and haemostasis achieved.

Closure

Skin closure is with interrupted absorbable sutures. A bulky dressing is applied to the hand for 24–48 hours. This can then be de-bulked by the patient to allow the fingers to flex freely.

Postoperative care and instructions

Active mobilisation of the hand is commenced immediately. The bulky dressing should be taken down after 24–48 hours to facilitate this.

Recommended references

Doyle JR, Blythe WF. The finger flexor tendon sheath and pulleys: Anatomy and reconstruction. In: *AAOS Symposium on Tendon Surgery in the Hand*. St. Louis, MO: Mosby, 1975:81–87.
Idler RS. Anatomy and biomechanics of the digital flexor tendons. *Hand Clin*. 1985;**1**:3–11.

Trigger thumb surgery

Preoperative planning

Indications

- Persistent triggering not relieved by steroid injections. Administer at least one, sometimes two injections before going ahead with surgery and wait 3 months after each injection to assess outcome.

- Locked thumb in an adult.
- Locked thumb in a child (usually noticed at <2 years) unresolved for 12 months. Thirty percent of trigger thumbs in infants will resolve within the first year after it is noticed. Flexion contractures do occur, but these will correct themselves spontaneously if the triggering resolves or if surgical release is performed before the age of 3 years.

Contraindications

- Presence of infection

Consent and risks

- Infection
- Injury to the tendon and neurovascular bundles
- Recurrence
- Stiffness/loss of range of movement
- Bow stringing of the FPL due to accidental division of A1 pulley *and* oblique pulley (more likely if the A1 pulley is divided through its ulnar attachment)

Incision and dissection

In the thumb, the proximal border of the A1 pulley is at the level of the proximal digital skin crease over the MCP joint. A 1–1.5 cm transverse incision is created in the crease. Tenotomy scissors are used for blunt dissection through the subcutaneous fat and palmar fascia to expose the FPL tendon sheath and A1 pulley. The digital nerves and vessels running parallel to the FPL tendon are identified and protected with right-angle retractors. The A1 pulley is identified, and the radial attachment of the pulley is divided completely with a scalpel from proximal to distal. The thumb is then flexed and extended several times to test for any residual triggering. Any tourniquet is released and haemostasis is achieved. The wound is washed out with saline before closure.

Closure

The skin is closed with 5/0 Vicryl rapide interrupted or subcuticular sutures. A light bandage should be applied which does not interfere with movements of the thumb.

Postoperative care and instructions

Active mobilisation of the hand and thumb is begun immediately after surgery. Heavy use of the hand is avoided for 1–2 weeks.

Recommended reference

Ger E, Kupcha P, Ger D. The management of trigger thumb in children. *J Hand Surg Am.* 1991;**16**:944–947.

Viva questions

1. What are the theoretical advantages of dermofasciectomy compared to fasciectomy for Dupuytren's disease?
2. What is the mechanism of action of collagenase used for Dupuytren's contracture and how is it obtained?
3. How do you deal with any residual flexion deformity of a digit after excision of all diseased Dupuytren's cord tissue?
4. What are the possible complications of a fasciectomy?
5. Describe the solutions for a painful distal interphalangeal joint with mucous cyst in a 50-year-old manual worker.
6. An elderly woman with rheumatoid arthritis comes to you with a painful and unstable thumb metacarpophalangeal joint. Describe your management.
7. A man of 30 years with a history of psoriatic arthropathy attends your clinic with painful and deformed distal interphalangeal joints affecting all the fingers of both hands. How would you treat this?
8. A woman of 40 years attends your clinic with a history of an untreated pilon fracture of the PIP joint of her right little finger dominant hand 10 years ago. The finger is painful, angulated and has restricted (20°–40°) active flexion. What surgical options would you give her?
9. A 50-year-old builder attends your clinic with a painful right index finger carpometacarpal joint. He punched a fellow builder 5 years ago and heard a loud 'click' at the time. Since then, he has experienced increasing movement at the joint associated with pain on lifting heavy objects. What options would you offer him?
10. Describe the management and treatment options for a young manual worker with a painful, stiff, PIP joint after previous trauma with evidence of marked joint deformity on X-ray.
11. A young woman presents with a painless but stiff index finger MCP joint after an infection. What surgical options would you present to her?
12. Describe the surgical management of a manual worker with a laceration in zone 6 and loss of extension of the thumb and index finger of his dominant hand?
13. What is the management of a closed mallet injury in a 16-year-old rugby player?
14. A 60-year-old woman presents with a passively correctible boutonniere deformity of her index and middle fingers of her dominant hand 1 year after a fall in the street. How would you treat this?
15. A 50-year-old lawyer with rheumatoid arthritis has suddenly lost extension of his little and ring fingers of his non-dominant hand. What options can you offer him?
16. How do you manage an isolated division of the flexor digitorum profundus tendon in the little finger of a dominant hand?

17. Describe the operative steps involved in the repair of a combined FDS/FDP tendon injury in zone 2 of the ring finger of a 30-year-old painter and decorator?
18. A patient presents with a tight volar web scar after Dupuytren's fasciectomy. How would you correct this?
19. You have decided to carry out a correction of a congenital camptodactyly of the little finger. The finger is now straight, but it is obvious that there is a shortage of skin on the volar side of the finger which contributed to the flexion deformity in the first place. How would you correct this?
20. Describe the risks and pitfalls in the management of trigger finger.
21. Describe your management of an acutely locked trigger thumb.

10 Surgery of the Hip

Daud TS Chou, Jonathan Miles and John Skinner

Primary total hip arthroplasty	239	Femoroacetabular impingement surgery	268
Revision total hip arthroplasty	255	Hip arthroscopy	272
Hip resurfacing	262	Hip arthrography	275
Hip arthrodesis	264	Viva questions	277
Excision hip arthroplasty	267		

Hip	Range of motion
External rotation	60°
Internal rotation	40°
Flexion	125°
Extension	0°
Adduction	25°
Abduction	45°

Optimum position of arthrodesis
- External rotation: 0°–10°
- Flexion: 20°–25°
- Adduction: 0°–5°

Primary total hip arthroplasty
Preoperative planning
Indications
Total hip arthroplasty (THA) is indicated in painful conditions of the hip that have failed conservative management. These are too numerous to list in this book but the most frequent underlying conditions are

- Osteoarthritis
- Inflammatory arthritis and other arthropathies

- Avascular necrosis
- Trauma

Contraindications

- Infection (generalised or of the hip joint)
- Absolute dysfunction of the abductor complex, including profound neurological disease

Young age is a relative contraindication, though in the highly symptomatic patient, total hip arthroplasty should be discussed with and performed by an appropriately experienced surgeon.

Consent and risks

- Mortality: 0.3%
- Nerve injury: 1%
- Infection: 1%–2% in osteoarthritis, 5% in rheumatoid arthritis
- Thromboembolism; deep vein thrombosis: 2%
- Pulmonary embolism: 1%
- Dislocation: 3%
- Heterotopic ossification: 10% (though the majority are asymptomatic)
- Limb length discrepancy: 15%
- Loosening: Revision surgery is required for loosening in up to 10% at 15 years
- Component failure: Stem fracture, locking mechanism failure in modular uncemented cups and other failures of components are rare, but recognized, complications

Operative planning

Recent radiographs of the pelvis and hip must be available. A templating software programme or physical templates should be routinely used to indicate the appropriate site for the femoral neck cut and provide a guide to implant placement and sizing. Availability of the implants must be checked by the surgeon.

Anaesthesia and positioning

Anaesthesia is usually general, regional or combined. An initial dose of antibiotic is given intravenously. The antibiotic of choice depends upon local policy, but a common choice is a second-generation cephalosporin or a combination of gentamicin and flucloxacillin. Tranexamic acid is often administered before the skin incision is made to reduce intra-operative bleeding and the need for postoperative transfusion.

Patient positioning will depend on the surgical approach chosen by the surgeon. In the United Kingdom, the lateral position is most commonly used and requires well-fixed supports abutting the lumbo-sacral spine posteriorly and the bony pelvis anteriorly (**Figure 10.1**). The pelvis should be vertically orientated to aid cup positioning; if it is not vertical, the operating table can be tilted to properly align the pelvis.

Bony prominences must be carefully padded. The hip joint should be sufficiently mobile to allow safe dislocation and intraoperative stability assessment. The surgical field is

Primary total hip arthroplasty

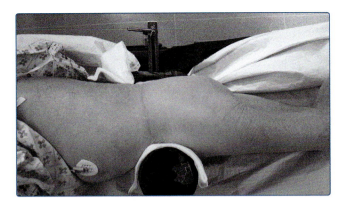

Figure 10.1 The lateral position for hip surgery.

prepared with a germicidal solution. Waterproof drapes are used with adhesive edges to provide a seal to the skin. The foot and lower leg are carefully excluded with a stockinette. If a lateral approach is to be used, a sterile 'leg bag' should be used to maintain sterility when the hip is displaced.

Surgical technique

The surgical approach may be dictated by the surgeon preference, previous surgical scars, patient body habitus, degree of bony deformity and implant selection. The two common approaches are the posterior and lateral approaches. A less commonly performed approach in the United Kingdom is the direct anterior approach to the hip (DAA) which is not described in this chapter.

Posterior approach (extensile)

Landmarks
The greater trochanter is palpated, particularly noting the tip and posterior border. The posterior superior iliac spine and femoral shaft are also useful palpable landmarks.

Incision
A 15 cm skin incision is made with its midpoint lying over the posterior half of the greater trochanter (**Figure 10.2**). The proximal extent of the incision is curved posteriorly, to lie in the line of the fibres of the gluteus maximus. The distal portion lies along the line of the femoral shaft.

Superficial dissection
The incision is continued through subcutaneous fat and down to fascia lata. Beginning distally, the fascia lata is incised in line with the skin incision, overlying the lateral femur. Proximally this continues beyond the greater trochanter, in a posterior direction, to incise in line with the underlying fibres of the gluteus maximus. The fibres of the gluteus maximus are gently split, using diathermy to coagulate bleeding vessels. The fascial incision should run from about 6 cm above the tip of the greater trochanter down to the insertion of the gluteus maximus tendon on the posterior femur (**Figure 10.3**).

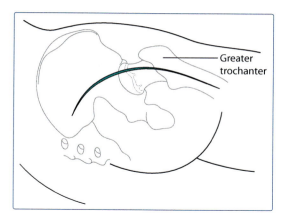

Figure 10.2 The skin incision for the posterior approach to the hip.

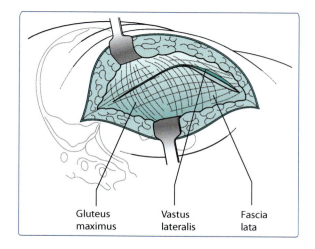

Figure 10.3 Dissection of the posterior approach to the hip.

A self-retaining retractor is carefully placed underneath the fascia to provide adequate exposure to further dissection.

Deep dissection

Structures at risk

- *Sciatic nerve*: See later.
- *Inferior gluteal artery*: Lying below piriformis. If it is cut, immediate supine repositioning of the patient and abdominal approach to tie off the internal iliac artery may be required to arrest the haemorrhage.
- *Obturator arterial branches*: Present within quadratus femoris.

The trochanteric bursa is now visible, covering the short external rotators and lying below the posterior border of gluteus medius (**Figure 10.4**). This can be swept off the short external rotators, using blunt or sharp dissection.

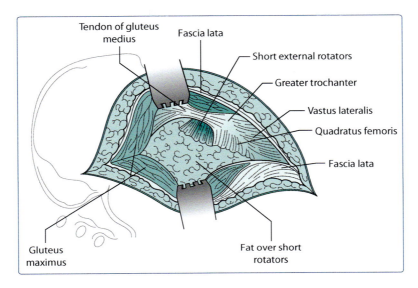

Figure 10.4 Deep dissection of the posterior approach.

At this point the sciatic nerve can be palpated and/or visualised. Aggressive dissection around the nerve is not recommended, certainly in primary arthroplasty it is unnecessary and can increase the risk of damaging the epineurial vessels, causing a haematoma and potential neuropraxia. The sciatic nerve exits the sciatic notch and passes into the posterior thigh underneath the piriformis and overlying the following short external rotator muscles (listed from cranial to caudal) (**Figure 10.5**):

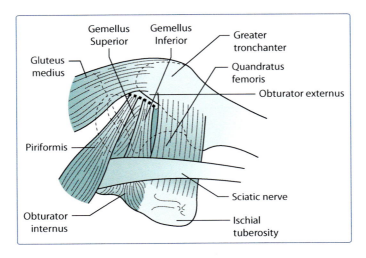

Figure 10.5 The path of the sciatic nerve over the external rotators of the hip.

- Gemellus superior
- Obturator internus
- Gemellus inferior
- Obturator externus
- Quadratus femoris

The nerve then runs down *underneath* the gluteus maximus' tendon at its femoral insertion.

An assistant now internally rotates the extended hip and flexes, stretching the short external rotators, making them easier to divide. This also increases the distance between the sciatic nerve and the site of division of these short muscles. Strong, stay sutures are inserted into the tendons of obturator internus and piriformis, just below their insertion into the femur. Visible vessels within the operative field are coagulated: typically these lie on the tendon of piriformis and within the substance of quadratus femoris. The short external rotators, from piriformis down to gemellus inferior, are divided as close to their insertion onto the femur as possible. If further access is required, the division can be carried on further distally. The muscles are allowed to rest over the sciatic nerve, providing some protection for it throughout the rest of the operation. This exposes the posterior capsule of the hip joint. To improve visibility, the interval between the superior part of the hip capsule and the gluteus minimus is identified and dissected free with blunt dissection or scissors. This view is maintained by inserting a Hohmann retractor in the interval to displace the gluteus minimus superiorly. The capsule is incised transversely to gain access. The visible portion of capsule can either be excised or preserved for later repair. The visible portion of the acetabular labrum is excised.

Lateral approach

Landmarks
- Central landmark is the greater trochanter.
- The anterior superior iliac spine (ASIS) and the femoral shaft are also palpable and act as useful reference points.

Incision
A straight 15 cm incision is created, parallel to the femoral shaft and centred on the anterior half of the greater trochanter (**Figure 10.6**).

Superficial dissection
The incision is continued through subcutaneous fat and down to fascia lata. The fascia lata is incised distally in line with the skin incision overlying the lateral femur and proximally in line with the fibres of gluteus maximus (**Figure 10.7**). At this point a self-retaining retractor is inserted.

Deep dissection

Structures at risk

Superior gluteal nerve – between the gluteus medius and minimus; this may be as close as 3 cm above the tip of the greater trochanter.

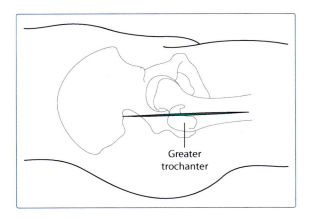

Figure 10.6 The skin incision for the lateral approach to the hip.

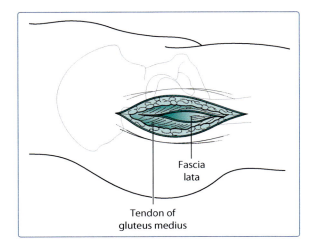

Figure 10.7 Dissection of the lateral approach to the hip.

The deep dissection continues in line with the skin and fascial incision. This begins proximally within the fibres of the gluteus medius and must be limited to a point 3 cm above the tip of the greater trochanter to avoid damage to the superior gluteal neurovascular bundle. The incision continues distally, in the line with the fibres of gluteus medius and across the greater trochanter, entering the vastus lateralis. The fibres of the vastus lateralis overlying the greater trochanter are split.

The dissection develops an anterior flap, consisting of the anterior fibres of the gluteus medius and gluteus minimus above the greater trochanter and the anterior fibres of the vastus lateralis lying over and below the greater trochanter. This is elevated off the greater trochanter subperiosteally, with either a scalpel or cutting diathermy. A cuff of gluteus medius is left posteriorly on the greater trochanter, allowing for reattachment at the time of closure.

The dissection progresses anteriorly, detaching the insertion of the gluteus medius and minimus onto the greater trochanter, to reveal the capsule of the hip. The anterior flap is retracted by placing a Hohmann retractor. The capsule is incised in a T shape, with the

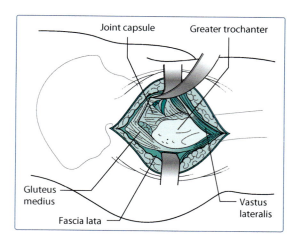

Figure 10.8 Deeper dissection of the lateral approach.

downstroke of the T lying in line with the femoral neck and the bar of the T running under the femoral head (**Figure 10.8**).

Dislocation and retractor positioning

This must be done gently as excess force can fracture the femur (typically a spiral fracture running from the subtrochanteric region down the shaft). In younger patients, the ligamentum teres can remain intact, preventing full dislocation; if this occurs it can be first divided with a scalpel. If the dislocation is difficult, further capsule can be excised, visible labrum can be removed and any acetabular osteophytes can be excised with nibblers or an osteotome. If the hip can still not be removed with minimal force, division of the femoral neck *in situ* with a double neck cut and removal of the head with a corkscrew are recommended.

- *Posterior approach dislocation and retraction*: Hip joint dislocation is performed by placing the hip in adduction and flexion then gently internally rotating it till dislocation, ending up with the calf lying vertically and the sole of the foot facing the ceiling. A bone hook can be carefully passed around the femur, at the level of the lesser trochanter, and used to ease the femoral head away from the acetabulum.
- *Lateral approach dislocation and retraction*: The hip can be dislocated with adduction, flexion and external rotation, again with a blunt bone hook around the femoral neck. The leg is then placed in the leg bag, i.e. the foot pointing to the floor, on the opposite side of the operating table.

Procedure

Structures at risk

- Femoral neurovascular bundle nerve – injudicious placement of anterior retractors
- Sciatic nerve – vulnerable posteriorly
- Obturator arterial branches – large branches are present below the transverse acetabular ligament; cutting them should be avoided

Hohmann retractors are inserted around the superior and inferior aspects of the femoral neck, supporting and stabilising the proximal femur and exposing the whole of the intertrochanteric line. Any soft tissues along this line are removed until the superior portion of the lesser trochanter is seen or at least easily palpable.

The planned femoral neck osteotomy site is marked with diathermy or an osteotome. A number of hip replacement sets have a specific instrument to aid identification of the correct site and orientation for this osteotomy; use of a trial prosthesis or a rasp as a guide is recommended in those sets without a neck cutting guide. This is particularly important with collared stems. Pre-operative templating will have provided a guide to the height above the lesser trochanter that the osteotomy should pass through the calcar. An oscillating saw is used to perform the osteotomy, with the Hohmann retractors protecting the surrounding soft tissues. If the line of the osteotomy passes into the greater trochanter, the osteotomy is stopped before entering the trochanter and a second osteotomy is performed vertically down from the piriformis fossa to meet the lateral extent of the first osteotomy (**Figure 10.9**). The femoral head is removed and can be utilised as autograft.

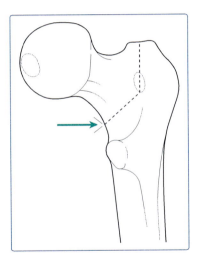

Figure 10.9 A typical neck cut.

Acetabular preparation

Any soft tissues overhanging the acetabulum around its circumference, including the labrum, are excised. It is vital to obtain a clear view around the whole acetabulum. The transverse acetabular ligament is identified, lying across the inferior boundary of the acetabulum. Any remaining ligamentum is also excised. Preservation of the transverse acetabular ligament (TAL) is advocated by most surgeons.

The TAL provides an indication of the acetabular version, and it helps to prevent inferior cement extrusion when implanting a cemented cup. If using the posterior approach, sharp Hohmann retractors are placed over the anterior wall, to lever the femur anteriorly, and under the TAL to expose the whole acetabulum for its preparation. If using the lateral approach, the proximal femur is levered posteriorly rather than anteriorly.

Within the acetabulum the medial wall or floor is defined which is sometimes visible as a flat plate of cortical bone. If it is not seen, then, it is likely to be covered in osteophytes or soft tissues, which should be removed with diathermy, an osteotome or curette to reveal the floor. This is an important step as definition of the medial wall allows proper and safe 'medialization', providing maximum cover of the cup when it is inserted.

Sharp, hemispherical, cheese-grater reamers are now used to remove the remaining acetabular cartilage and expose subchondral bone. Beginning with the smallest reamer, reaming is directed medially and checked regularly to ascertain the depth of reaming. The desired depth is up to, but not through the true medial wall (the flat cortical bone of the quadrilateral plate). The acetabulum is now enlarged with increasing sizes of reamers, not increasing the depth but just the width. This is performed in the desired alignment of the acetabular component to be inserted. The appropriate alignment is *40°–45° from the horizontal and 15°–20° of anteversion* (**Figure 10.10**). The aim is to create a hemisphere, removing all cartilage but preserving as much subchondral bone as possible.

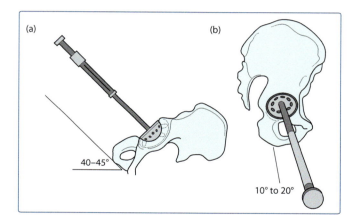

Figure 10.10 Acetabular reaming (a) 40°–45° from vertical and (b) 10°–20° of anteversion.

If the acetabular component to be used is of uncemented design, a trial cup can be inserted at the correct angle to assess the coverage and stability.

Cemented cups can also be trialled to ensure an adequate cement mantle around the implant.

At this point any osteophytes around the acetabulum (that may lead to impingement) are often apparent. These can be removed with nibblers or an osteotome. The component is inserted using the appropriate technique. It is worthwhile at the point of cup implantation, to ensure that the pelvis has remained vertical. Malposition of the patient could in turn cause angulation of the implant, with consequent risk of instability.

Technical points in uncemented cup insertion
- The uncemented cup relies on a secure fit to confer initial stability.
- In the press-fit technique an implant 1–2 mm larger than the last reamer is used. This can be augmented with screws as necessary.

- The line-to-line technique uses an implant of the same size as the last reamer and relies on augmentation with screws to obtain fixation.
- If fixation is not solid and stable, even after screws have been used, changing to a cemented cup is recommended.
- Screw holes are aligned to coincide with the safe zone, described later. Pilot holes should be drilled, their depth ascertained with an angled depth gauge and screws inserted with a universally jointed screwdriver and a screw holder to control the direction of the screw.
- Screw augmentation, if to be used, should be done with care and awareness of the safe quadrants. The safe quadrants, as depicted in **Figure 10.11**, are created by drawing two lines through the middle of the acetabulum. The first line is drawn from the anterior superior iliac spine through the centre of the acetabulum, and the second line is drawn perpendicular to this line (**Figure 10.11**).

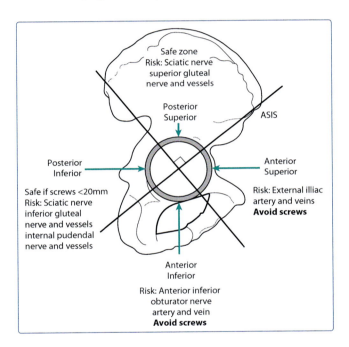

Figure 10.11 The quadrants of acetabular screw positioning. (Redrawn with permission from Miller, *Review of Orthopaedics*. Philadelphia, PA: Saunders; 2004.)

Structures at risk

Posterior superior – the safe zone

- At risk – sciatic nerve and superior gluteal neurovascular bundle

Posterior inferior – safe if screws less than 20 mm

- At risk – inferior gluteal and internal pudendal neurovascular bundles

> Anterior superior – avoid screws
> - At risk – external iliac vessels
>
> Anterior inferior – avoid screws
> - At risk – anterior inferior obturator neurovascular bundle

When all of the screws are properly seated, the liner can be inserted. If using a polyethylene liner, a 10° or 20° elevated rim can be selected and orientated as desired. It should be remembered however, that this reduces the arc of motion and therefore may negatively contribute to hip stability.

Trials are available and should be used if there is any doubt. It is usual for the elevated lip to be situated posterosuperiorly or more posteriorly if a posterior approach has been used.

Technical points in cemented cup insertion
- Many acetabular components have a lip augment, which should be correctly orientated in the posterior to superior area. If the cup has a flange (which can help to prevent cement extrusion), this will need to be trimmed to the size of the reamed acetabulum.
- Drill holes (keyholes) should be created into the ilium and ischium, but not the quadrilateral plate, to enhance the cement fixation. The bone surface is washed with pulsatile lavage and dried thoroughly. Many acetabular components have pegs on the medial surface; these are designed to ensure a uniform cement mantle of around 3 mm.
- The cement should be introduced from a cement gun with a short nozzle. It is first introduced to the keyholes in the ilium and ischium. This is done with the nozzle hard against the bone, to increase the pressure. It is then introduced to the rest of the acetabulum and pressurised with an impactor: most sets have a polypropylene impactor to pressurise the cement into the acetabular bone.
- The surgeon should be aware of the specific properties of the cement that is being used to ensure that the cement and component are inserted at the appropriate time. It is vital that the component is held perfectly still while the cement is curing. Care should be taken to ensure that the cup introducer is able to be released without undue force, to reduce the stresses on the cement to component interface.
- Any excess cement should be removed.

Femoral preparation

For the posterior approach the assistant extends and internally rotates the hip while supporting the leg with the knee flexed. For the anterior approach, the leg is maximally adducted and the hip externally rotated; the knee is flexed to position the lower leg in the leg-bag drape.

An entry point is created in the proximal femur, with a box chisel, to allow the insertion of reamers; it must be correctly situated to prevent varus malposition of the component. The starting point is further posterior than anterior, to allow for the anterior bow in the femur. It must also be lateral, so that it lies directly over the lateral margin of the medullary canal (**Figure 10.12**). This allows instruments to run towards the medial femoral condyle,

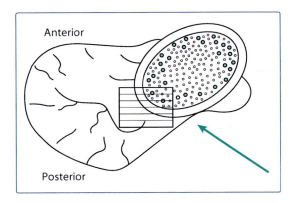

Figure 10.12 The box chisel 'starting point' in femoral preparation.

preventing varus malpositioning of the femoral component. This usually gives a starting point that enters the proximal portion of the greater trochanter.

The femur is initially prepared with a tapered reamer to remove a cone of medullary bone within which rasping can begin. The smallest reamer is first inserted into the medullary canal. The reamer is allowed to run down the lateral cortex, thus following the medullary canal, but the tip of the reamer should be angled slightly medially, as if trying to come out through the medial femoral condyle. This is, again, to prevent eventual varus malposition of the femoral component. If the reamer will not follow the canal, further bone needs to be removed from the greater trochanter. The entry point position and angle should be checked and adjusted if necessary. Sequentially larger tapered reamers are then used to increase the diameter, until contact with cortical bone is felt.

The next step is shaping of the proximal femur to receive the implant, whether it is to be cemented or uncemented, with particular care paid to the anteversion of the rasp within the proximal femur. This is performed with implant-specific rasps. The rasps are positioned to provide around 15° of anteversion. In the posterior approach, this is done by angling the medial side of the rasp downwards 15°; in the lateral approach it is angled 15° upwards.

Sequentially larger rasps are used to the point where stability can be achieved with the definitive component.

Technical points in uncemented stem insertion
- The rasps used are specific to each stem design.
- The version of the rasp must be precisely controlled throughout rasping.
- A small rasp is used to begin with and the size increased until stability is achieved.
- Impaction is with controlled hammer blows, watching the progress of the impactor.
- When the rasp stops progressing, it should not be impacted further as this may lead to proximal femoral fracture. When stable, the rasp is a tight fit within the canal and rotation of the component rotates the femur with no 'toggle' between the two.
- The templated size should be borne in mind.
- Selection of a prosthesis several sizes smaller than that achieved on templating is usually due to varus alignment of rasps or may indicate excessive anteversion.
- The depth of the rasp is noted. This should be such that the cutting teeth are at or just below the level of the neck cut.

- Trial reduction is carried out, with a variety of offset options available on most uncemented systems (see later for details).
- The rasp is removed and the definitive prosthesis can be inserted, following the version of the rasps. An attempt at changing the version of the stem at this point is likely to cause a femoral fracture.
- The canal is not washed out, as the bone swarf aids in union across the implant to bone interface.

Technical points in cemented stem insertion
- The rasps allow for a 2–3 mm cement mantle to be created between the component and bone. The technique is similar to that used for uncemented stems, with increasing rasp size until stability is achieved.
- If using a collared stem, the final broach is sunk to the required depth and the 'calcar cutter' is used. This attaches over the final rasp and provides a smooth, stable neck cut at the level upon which the collar will be supported.
- The height of the final rasp can be gauged in respect to both the greater trochanter and the medial extent of the femoral neck cut. It is vital to be able to reproduce these relationships with the definitive stem, when it is cemented *in situ*.
- Trial reduction is carried out (see later for details).
- A cement restrictor is used to occlude the medullary canal distally. The depth of insertion is obtained by measurement against the final rasp used, aiming for 1–2 cm of clearance to allow for distal cementing. The canal must now be thoroughly washed with pulse lavage, using a long nozzle and a brush to clean debris and fat from the entire length of the prepared bone. Suction is used to remove the saline cleaning solution. The canal is then dried and packed with swabs or a preformed absorbent sponge.
- Cementation is performed with a double mix of polymethylmethacrylate cement, using a cement gun with a long nozzle. The cement is introduced when it is of sufficient viscosity (when the cement does not stick to the surgeon's glove, the required viscosity has been reached – typically after around 2–3 minutes).
- The nozzle is introduced up to the cement restrictor and then cement is pumped firmly to introduce it into the canal. The cement gun is not withdrawn, rather it is allowed to be pushed out by the cement as it fills the canal. Use of suction removes the fluid extruded from the canal.
- When the cement reaches the proximal femur, the nozzle is withdrawn and cut. A proximal cement pressuriser is placed over the remaining nozzle and reintroduced into the femoral canal, occluding the proximal femur. Further cement is introduced under pressure, as the restrictor occludes the femoral cavity, for around 30 seconds.
- The definitive stem should be checked and correctly assembled on its introducer. The correct time for introduction of the stem is determined by the type of cement and ambient temperature conditions. It is usually at around 4–6 minutes. The femoral component is introduced in the correct version and manually inserted to the correct depth. The version must remain constant and the insertion manoeuvre is a smooth, even application of force. The end result should be a reproduction of the depth of the trial at time of rasping. Removing the stem introducer should be done carefully so as not to toggle the stem while the cement is still setting.
- The implant must be held perfectly still within the femur until the cement has cured, typically after 10–12 minutes.

Trialling and reduction

Trial reduction is a vital step in performing a THA. The assessment is essentially of stability, range of motion and leg length.

Reduction is carried out with appropriate trial components, usually consisting of the last rasp left *in situ* and a trial head. Reduction is via the surgical assistant applying in-line traction followed by rotation of the head into the acetabulum. The traction is assisted by the surgeon pushing on the femoral head with a conical pusher. If reduction cannot be achieved, a shorter femoral head and/or a neck with less offset is selected and the manoeuvre repeated.

The position of the head with respect to the greater trochanter is noted and compared with preoperative templating.

The hip is passed through a functional range of motion and must not dislocate in any position. The hip can then be forced into non-physiological positions to assess the point at which dislocation can occur. In the lateral approach, the hip should remain in joint even when the leg is replaced in adduction and external rotation, back into the sterile 'leg bag'. In the posterior approach, the hip is tested in flexion, slight adduction and forced internal rotation; the degree of internal rotation to dislocation should be noted and should be no less than 40°.

The tissue tension is assessed by the 'shuck test' – the femur is pulled sharply downwards and the degree of telescoping of the femoral head away from the acetabular socket is noted. Any more than a few millimetres of movement suggests that instability may be present. In this case, a longer trial femoral head may be required.

The lateral tissue tension can be assessed with the 'lateral shuck test'. A dislocation hook is passed around the femoral neck and the component sharply pulled laterally. Again, excessive movement suggests instability, and a greater amount of offset may be required.

The operated leg is placed against the opposite leg in order to compare leg length. Gross differences suggest incorrect tissue tension. Note that stability and range of motion are of higher importance than subtle differences in leg length; however, lengthening of the operated leg to greater than 1 cm longer than the other leg is associated with significant patient dissatisfaction.

If a stable hip is not achievable in a functional range of motion, consideration must be given to the following factors:

- Component position – are the stem and cup components in the correct degree of version? Is the cup sufficiently medialized? Is the stem at the correct height? Repositioning one or both components may be required to achieve stability.
- Use of a lip augment on the acetabulum. In uncemented acetabula, exchange of the liner is relatively simple. The use of a 10° or 20° lip augment can improve hip stability.
- Use of a larger femoral head will increase the stability of the hip.
- The use of a constrained prosthesis is a last resort and is not usually appropriate in primary hip surgery.

Closure of posterior approach

If the capsule has been preserved, it is sometimes possible to repair this directly, using a heavy absorbable suture. Proper repair of the short external rotators to the femur is vitally important. The rotators should be intact and easily identified by the sutures passed through their tendons prior to their division. If these sutures are left long at the time of their insertion, they can be used to reattach the muscles. If not, four sutures are secured to the cut ends of the short external rotators.

A small (e.g. 2.5 mm) drill is used to create bone tunnels through the greater trochanter, from anterior to posterior, in the line of attachment of the short external rotators (**Figure 10.13**). A suture passer can be used to pull one of the sutures through – both ends of the same suture are pulled through the one hole. Three further drill holes are created and the three remaining sutures pulled through.

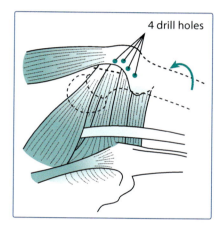

Figure 10.13 Position of drill holes for reattachment of the short external rotators.

Both ends of the upper two sutures are then tied to each other, then the same procedure is carried out with the lower two sutures. This is done with the leg in around 10° of abduction and only a few degrees of external rotation, which allows approximation of the tendon to the greater trochanter without causing a fixed rotation deformity. The split fibres of the gluteus maximus are loosely approximated with absorbable sutures.

If a surgical drain is to be used, it is inserted now. Closure of the fascia lata is performed with the hip in slight abduction. Superficial closure utilises absorbable sutures to approximate the subcutaneous fat, then cutaneous sutures or surgical staples. An occlusive dressing is applied.

Closure of lateral approach

If the capsule is repairable, this is performed first. The gluteus medius anterior and posterior flaps are approximated. These are then tightly sutured together with the leg in around 10° of abduction.

Superficial closure follows the same technique as that for the posterior approach.

Postoperative care and instructions

The patient is returned to the supine position and an abduction pillow can be inserted between the legs. Any straps present on these pillows should not be used, due to the risk of peroneal nerve damage. Precautions against thromboembolism should be used. Common options include aspirin, low molecular weight heparin, graduated compression stockings and foot or calf intermittent compression pumps. Early mobilisation should be encouraged in all patients.

Dependent on local guidelines, 24-hour antibiotic coverage can be considered. Haemoglobin levels should be monitored and transfusion considered as necessary.

In general, full weightbearing is encouraged following cemented, uncemented and hybrid THAs. Cautious weightbearing may be considered if an intraoperative fracture has occurred. The patient is asked to avoid crossing of the legs or excessive flexion of the hips. To this end, they are provided with a raised toilet seat and instructed to avoid low seats. *Particular care is recommended when putting on socks and shoes* – a common cause of early dislocation. Return to work is allowed after around 6 weeks for sedentary jobs, but may be delayed to 3 months or more in active work. Follow-up is recommended at 6 weeks, 6 months and 1 year after surgery. Continuation of follow-up is typically at 5 years, 10 years, 15 years and then at yearly intervals. The patient should be encouraged to return to clinic if they experience pain or functional deterioration.

Recommended references

Barrack RL, Mulroy RD Jr, Harris WH. Improved cementing techniques and femoral component loosening in young patients with hip arthroplasty. *J Bone Joint Surg Br.* 1992;**74**:385–389.
Charnley J. Arthroplasty of the hip: A new operation. *Lancet.* 1961;**1**:1129–1132.
Hardinge K. The direct lateral approach. *J Bone Joint Surg Br.* 1982;**64**:17–19.
Lidwell OM, Lowbury EJ, Whyte W et al. Effect of ultraclean air in operating rooms on deep sepsis in the joint after total hip or knee replacement. *BMJ.* 1982;**285**:10–14.
Murray DW, Carr AJ, Bulstrode CJ. Which primary total hip replacement? *J Bone Joint Surg Br.* 1995;**77**:520–527.
Pellicci PM, Bostrom M, Poss R. Posterior approach to total hip replacement using enhanced posterior soft tissue repair. *Clin Orthop Relat Res.* 1998;**(355)**:224–228.
National Joint Registry. http://www.njrcentre.org.uk

Revision total hip arthroplasty

This section refers extensively to the previous section and is not intended as a stand-alone text to enable all surgeons to revise all hips. It aims to provide some useful directions as to appropriate techniques that can be applied to solve some problems, but cannot cover all potential problems.

Preoperative planning

Indications

Revision hip arthroplasty is indicated for failure of a primary hip arthroplasty. The most common causes are

- Aseptic loosening of the socket and/or stem
- Deep infection (see later section)

- Instability, resulting in recurrent dislocation
- Fracture of either the implant, proximal femur or the acetabulum

Contraindications

- Continuation of preoperative pain after hip arthroplasty (suggests that the original diagnosis may have been wrong and warrants further investigation).
- Pain-free radiographic loosening is a relative contraindication, except in cases associated with significant and progressive osteolysis.

> ### Consent and risks
>
> - Nerve injury: 3%–7%
> - Infection: Quoted up to 30%, 5% is a more commonly accepted figure
> - Thromboembolism: 3%
> - Dislocation: 7%
> - Aseptic loosening: 10%–30% at 10 years
> - Fracture
> - Limb length discrepancy

Operative planning

Revision arthroplasty is more challenging than primary hip arthroplasty, so it requires even more precise planning. Recent radiographs are essential. 'Judet views' can be very helpful in assessing acetabular bone loss. If there is significant bone loss, a fine-cut computed tomography (CT) scan can be used to assess and quantify this. The patient should have been seen in outpatients recently so that the clinical and functional status can be formally assessed. This is as vital as the osseous imaging in decision-making.

The soft tissue status must be assessed and any signs of infection warrant investigation and treatment. It is not always necessary to revise all components in aseptic failures; consideration should be given to retaining any well-fixed and functional prosthetic component. If the prosthesis is infected, usually a two-stage procedure is preferred (see later).

Templating should be carried out with great care. It is necessary to be prepared for unexpected findings at the time of surgery and a wide range of implants should be available to the surgeon.

There are a number of extra instruments and pieces of equipment which can be useful in revision procedures:

- Image intensifier
- Implant-specific extraction instruments for the existing THA
- Bone allograft, for morcellized or block grafting
- Cement removing osteotomes and ultrasonic cement removal systems
- Supplementary metalwork, including cabling systems, trochanteric fixation devices, acetabular reconstruction rings and plates, cages, mesh and even computer-aided design/computer-aided manufacturing (CAD/CAM) implants

- Universal modular neck adaptors for worn trunnions or to change stem offset and version.
- Thin, curved osteotomes for removing uncemented hips:
  - Explant acetabular cup removal system
  - High-speed burr/cebotome
  - Flexible femoral canal reamers

Anaesthesia and positioning

This is usually the same as in primary arthroplasty, bearing in mind the procedure is likely to take considerably longer. Also initial antibiotic dose is usually delayed until after microbiological samples have been taken.

Surgical technique

Approach

Either the posterior or lateral approach can be used. Some surgeons argue that the posterior approach is best for posterior acetabular defects.

An extended trochanteric osteotomy can be beneficial particularly when needing to remove a well-fixed stem or there is a risk of trochanteric fracture during the surgical approach. The greater trochanter is osteotomised with gluteus medius and vastus lateralis attached, allowing it to be mobilised well out of the way. The length of the osteotomy required is dependent on the length of the stem and may be as long as the implant itself, which can be judged with image intensifier or from preoperative planning (**Figure 10.14**).

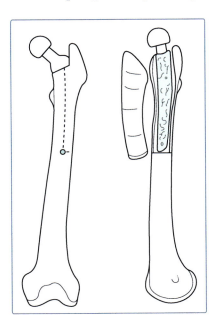

Figure 10.14 An 'extended' trochanteric osteotomy.

Identification of the sciatic nerve is important, particularly in the posterior approach. The nerve can be isolated by carefully passing a vascular sloop around it, thus ensuring that its location is known at all times.

Procedure

Following dislocation, the femoral head of a modular component is removed with a head and neck separator. Many implants have a specific extraction device and, if available, these should be used.

Removal of a cemented stem

It is sometimes possible to simply pull the implant out of the cement mantle. If this is not the case, some of the proximal cement mantle will need to be removed, particularly from the lateral margin of the implant. This is almost always necessary if removing a curved femoral stem. This can be achieved with cement osteotomes or a high-speed burr.

The rest of the cement can be left *in situ* at this time as it tamponades bleeding from the femoral canal and may reduce the chances of femoral fracture during acetabular exposure. When cement is to be removed, it can be done with cement osteotomes and an ultrasonic cement remover. The cement restrictor must also be removed.

Removal of an uncemented stem

This can be very difficult in well-fixed stems, particularly if extensively coated.

The use of specialised, flexible osteotomes, K-wires or high-speed burs is recommended. Care must be taken to avoid unnecessary breach of the proximal femoral cortex. Following removal, the femoral canal is packed with swabs to tamponade bleeding.

Assessing femoral bone loss

The two most commonly used grading systems are the Paprosky and the American Academy of Orthopedic Surgeons (AAOS) systems. *Table 10.1* shows the Paprosky system together with possible reconstructive solutions.

Removal of a cemented socket

If the acetabular component is loose, it will often come free with minimal effort, typically along with the majority of its cement attached.

In a well-fixed socket, a curved osteotome is used to develop a plane between the cup and the cement. Alternatively, a pilot hole can be drilled into the centre of the component and a slap-hammer screwed into it. Once loose, the socket is removed and the cement is then removed piecemeal with small osteotomes. This method ensures the least amount of bone loss and minimises the likelihood of acetabular fracture.

If this method also fails, the acetabular socket can be cut into quarters with a power saw and can then be removed. It is important that all cement is also removed.

Removal of an uncemented socket

If the cup is well fixed, it should be remembered that it may not need to be removed. In this case, the liner can be removed, but this must be done carefully to avoid damage to the cup-to-liner locking mechanism. If the locking mechanism is still functioning, a simple liner exchange can be performed, remembering that the replacement liner need not be of the same internal diameter or have the same augment or 'lip' size. An alternative measure,

Table 10.1 Paprosky classification of femoral defects at revision hip surgery

Paprosky grade	Diagram	Treatment options
Type I – has an intact metaphysis and isthmus		Typically treated with a primary implant
Type II – has metaphyseal damage but an intact isthmus		Long stem cemented implant; distally fixed uncemented stem
Type IIIA – distal fixation can be achieved at the isthmus, despite damage to the isthmus and the metaphysis		Long stem cemented implanted with impaction allograft; long stem distally fixed uncemented stem
Type IIIB – damage to the metaphysis and isthmus prevent distal fixation from being achieved		Long stem cemented implant with morcellized and corticocancellous strut graft; long stem distally fixed uncemented stem with corticocancellous strut graft; massive tumour prosthesis proximal femoral replacement
Type IV – extensive metaphyseal damage and an eroded isthmus		Proximal femoral replacement

in a well-fixed socket with a destroyed or obsolete locking mechanism, is cementation of a smaller liner within the shell.

If the shell is to be removed, any screws are removed first. The well-fixed cup is carefully removed by developing a plane between the bone and the implant with curved osteotomes or a suitable removal system, such as Explant (Zimmer, Warsaw, Indiana). In either case, care must be taken to minimise bone destruction and avoid excess bone loss.

Assessing acetabular bone loss

The most commonly used grading systems are the Paprosky and AAOS systems. *Table 10.2* shows the AAOS grading system together with possible reconstructive solutions.

Revision of infected implants

If the revision is for infection, this can be performed as either a single-stage or a two-stage procedure. Two-stage revision is believed to result in lower re-infection rates but may result in significant functional impairment. In appropriately selected patients, single-stage revision can be associated with similar reinfection rates when compared with two-stage revision with superior functional outcomes. For a two-stage procedure, the initial stage is removal of all implants and cement. It is vital that multiple samples (usually five) from around all implants are sent for microbiological assessment. The whole surgical field should be thoroughly debrided and then washed out with a minimum of 6 L of saline pulsatile lavage.

A polymethylmethacrylate cement spacer is then inserted. This can be preformed or can be made with moulds of varying sizes. The cement should contain heat-stable antibiotics, such as gentamicin or tobramycin. Closure is performed and the patient may mobilise, although usually only partially weightbearing.

The patient should be followed up clinically and have regular checks of inflammatory markers. Postoperative antibiotics can be given once the microbiological sensitivities have been received. These cases often require combination antibiotic therapy and should be managed together with a microbiologist. Once the inflammatory markers are normal, the second stage can be undertaken, with reconstruction depending on the extent of femoral and acetabular bone loss. Particular care must be taken with the soft tissues as multiple procedures will often have taken their toll on the surrounding musculature. Many surgeons prefer the use of a cemented stem in this situation as extra antibiotics can be added to decrease the chance of recurrence. Some surgeons may opt to perform a single-stage revision in selected patients, which involves a thorough debridement, removal of implants and re-implantation of definitive prosthesis at the same time. Whichever approach is taken it is important to manage these complex patients within a multidisciplinary team structure consisting of orthopaedic surgeons, plastic surgeons and microbiologists.

Table 10.2 American Academy of Orthopedic Surgeons (AAOS) classification of acetabular bone loss at revision hip surgery

AAOS grade	Diagram	Treatment options
Segmental		Small defects, allowing for 70% implant to bone contact, require no additional treatment; larger defects can require the use of structural allograft or asymmetric acetabular shells, e.g. the S-ROM oblong (DePuy, Warsaw, Indiana); loss of the medial wall can be managed with a malleable mesh and morcellized allograft as long as there is peripheral support.
Cavitatory		If small, these are usually reamed to provide contact in 70% or more of the bone surface. An uncemented cup with screw augmentation is a typical prosthesis used; larger defects require grafting – this can be with morcellized graft obtained from fresh frozen femoral head allograft. It can need structural graft, again usually obtained from femoral head or distal femoral allograft, fixed with *screws* or a buttress plate.
Combined		The segmental defect is first reconstructed to provide a stable rim; persisting cavitatory loss is grafted with morcellized allograft.
Pelvic discontinuity		This is a difficult problem, requiring reconstruction with plates and screws or even an entire acetabular allograft; CAD/CAM sockets can be very useful to provide fixation to the ilium, ischium and pubis.

Abbreviations: CAD/CAM, computer-aided design/computer-aided manufacturing.

Closure and postoperative care

These are broadly in line with the guidelines for primary hip arthroplasty. It may be necessary to consider additional precautions, particularly in limitation of range of motion and weightbearing. It is usual to continue antibiotics until microbiological results are available.

Recommended references

Gruen TA, McNeice GM, Amstutz AC. 'Modes of failure' of cemented stem-type components: A radiographic analysis. *Clin Orthop Relat Res*. 1979;**(141)**:17–27.

Jasty M, Harris WH. Total hip reconstruction using frozen femoral head allografts in patients with acetabular bone loss. *Orthop Clin North Am*. 1987;**18**:291–299.

Valle CJ, Paprosky WG. Classification and an algorithmic approach to the reconstruction of femoral deficiency. *J Bone Joint Surg Am*. 2003;**85(Suppl 4)**:1–6.

Hip resurfacing

Hip resurfacing can be technically more challenging than a primary THA but shares many similar principles.

Preoperative planning

Indications and contraindications

The indications and contraindications of hip resurfacing are almost the same as those for THA. In addition, there are further contraindications that reflect the need to maintain the femoral neck:

- Femoral head cysts greater than 1 cm diameter
- Osteoporosis – recommended to investigate with dual-energy X-ray absorptiometry (DEXA or DXA) in perimenopausal women/high-risk groups
- Neck length of less than 2 cm
- Significant lateral head-neck remodelling
- Head:neck ratio less than 1.2

Consent and risks

- The consent process and risk profile are equivalent to THA.
- In addition the risks of femoral neck fracture or intraoperative conversion to THA (e.g. due to notching or size mismatch) must be mentioned.

Operative planning

Performing up-to-date radiographs and preoperative templating are essential. The surgeon should have a guide available to check the compatibility of the femoral and acetabular components.

Anaesthesia and positioning

This is performed as for THR.

Surgical technique

Surface replacement is possible through any of the common approaches to the hip. The posterior approach is commonly used, and the following description describes this approach.

The dissection is exactly as described in the THA section. In order to gain visibility around the whole of the femoral neck, some further steps are applied:

- The quadratus femoris should be released prior to dislocation.
- The gluteus maximus tendon can be released off its insertion into the linea aspera, allowing more rotation and visualisation.
- The capsular incision is much more significant. This is essential in order to allow 360° visualisation of the neck to check that notching is not going to occur.
- The capsulotomy is carried out from superior to inferior around the femoral neck, carrying on down the inferior neck as far as can be visualised.
- This incision is then carefully continued with heavy 'capsulotomy' scissors, releasing the capsule inferiorly and medially. Great care is taken to stay close to the bone of the femoral neck.
- The hip is dislocated and the capsulotomy continued until the capsule is released right around the femoral neck, such that the head and proximal femur can be viewed all the way around (**Figure 10.15**).

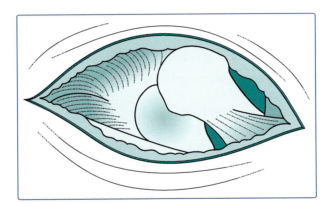

Figure 10.15 Extensive release of the hip capsule to allow full delivery of the femoral head into the wound.

Femoral head displacement

In order to adequately visualise the acetabulum, the femoral head must be displaced. If there are any particularly large osteophytes, these should be removed at this stage. A pocket is created for the femoral head, lying under the gluteus medius and upon the iliac wing above the acetabulum. This can be created by sweeping a blunt periosteal elevator or bone spike under the gluteus medius. Once a sufficient pocket is created, the leg is lowered sufficiently to place a sharp retractor over the anterior lip of the acetabulum. This is used to lever the femur anteriorly as the leg is dropped down onto the table, and the femoral head is guided into the pocket already created.

If the head is very large, it can be debulked further by the initial stages of femoral head preparation (described later) prior to displacing it into the pocket.

Acetabular preparation

This is very similar to the technique described in the section on THA for uncemented cup insertion and the position is the same. Care should be taken not to over-ream the acetabulum as the implants are press-fit and cannot be augmented with screws. In addition, selection of the femoral head size is guided by the size of the acetabular component as they must fit together.

Femoral preparation

Femoral shaping is done to create a cut surface that will fit with the femoral component. A variety of jigs are available depending upon the implant manufacturer, and reference to the individual technical guides is recommended. They all aim to place a guide wire in the centre of the neck, in both the anteroposterior and mediolateral planes. The fovea does not correspond to the midpoint of the neck so the entry point will be some way above this. This critical step can be helped by drawing a line up the centre of the posterior and lateral margins of the neck and carrying this up onto the head as a guide. The position to aim for is equal to the native anteversion and 0–10° of valgus compared with the patient's femoral neck.

Once the guide wire is passed, a jig is placed over it and swept around the entire neck to ensure that there is clearance around the whole diameter, i.e. it will not be notched. If the entry point or angle is incorrect, the guide wire is removed and replaced.

Once the guide wire is correctly positioned a post drill is used to create a central hole for the post to be inserted into the femoral head. This is then the guide for further cuts. Again, equipment varies but all have specific cutters and reamers for shaping of the proximal femur. Care should be taken to ensure the size chosen fits with the acetabular component and that notching of the neck is prevented. If a significant notch is created, the surgeon must convert to a THA. While cutting and shaping, drapes should be placed over the surrounding soft tissues to prevent bone swarf from entering tissue planes.

A profile reamer is then used to shape the head and a step drill to create around six holes in the bevelled edge, to act as cement keys. The intended final resting place of the component is marked on the femoral head-neck junction.

The head is thoroughly washed with pulsed normal saline and the appropriate head is cemented *in situ,* typically with low-viscosity cement. It is impacted up to the previously created mark to ensure that it is in place. The hip is reduced and assessed for stability.

Closure and postoperative care

At closure, the gluteus maximus tendon and quadratus femoris are closed, then closure is as for THA. Postoperative care and rehabilitation are also equivalent to THA.

Hip arthrodesis

Preoperative planning

The following is a description of one common technique although there are many described in the literature.

Indications

Hip arthrodesis is rapidly becoming a procedure of historical interest only, as improvements in THA allow implantation in younger patients. It has limited indications now but was used in younger adults in order to allow return to manual labour. Continuing indications are

- Failed arthroplasty
- Sequelae of infection, particularly tuberculosis
- Sickle cell anaemic arthropathy

Contraindications

- Contralateral hip disease
- Ipsilateral knee disease
- Pre-existing lower back pain
- Inflammatory arthropathy – relative

Consent and risks

- Lower back pain: 60%
- Leg length discrepancy: 100% (typically up to 5 cm)
- Knee pain: 45%
- Failure of fusion: 2% clinically but up to 30% radiographically
- Malpositioning (it has been shown that the rates of back pain are higher in malpositioned hips)

The patient must understand that walking will be abnormal and running impossible. There is a significant reduction in walking speed and increase in energy expenditure.

Operative planning

Planning the position of fusion is vital. The optimum position is

- Flexion of 20°–25°
- Rotation neutral to 10° of external rotation
- Adduction of 0°–5°

A variety of intra-articular or extra-articular techniques can be used to achieve fusion.

Anaesthesia and positioning

This is performed as for THA, except the patient is in a supine position with a sandbag under the ipsilateral buttock.

Surgical technique

Approach

The lateral approach to the hip is used, as described in the primary arthroplasty section. The supine position allows for more accurate assessment of leg length and, upon removal of the sandbag, the surgeon can perform a Thomas' test at the end of the fusion in order to assess the position of arthrodesis.

Procedure

The gluteus medius and minimus complex is left attached to the greater trochanter and their anterior and posterior borders defined carefully. An oscillating saw is used to create an osteotomy, separating the greater trochanter from the proximal femur. The abductors, proximally and vastus lateralis distally, remain attached to the greater trochanter. The greater trochanter and abductor complex are reflected upwards; this may require some dissection of the undersurface of the abductors away from the superior capsule.

The bony surface around the superior acetabulum is defined by blunt dissection, revealing the sciatic notch, posteriorly and the anterior inferior iliac spine, anteriorly. A blunt Hohmann retractor is inserted into the sciatic notch (this protects the sciatic nerve and the superior gluteal vessels) and another is hooked around the iliopectineal eminence anteriorly. A horizontal osteotomy is carefully created between the two retractors, running just above the superior surface of the acetabulum. This can be started with an oscillating saw but should be completed with an osteotome to reduce the danger of sciatic nerve injury.

A corresponding horizontal surface is created on the top of the femoral head by removing a small portion of the head with an oscillating saw. Curettes are used to remove any areas of persistent cartilage on the femoral head and the acetabulum. A retractor is inserted into the pelvic osteotomy and used to lever the osteotomy and displace the distal portion approximately 1 cm medially with respect to the proximal ilium. By removing the sandbag from under the buttock, the position for arthrodesis can be accurately assessed.

The cobra plate is attached over the osteotomy site; this only requires one screw into the pelvis and one into the femur at this stage. Careful palpation of the pelvis, patella and malleoli is carried out to confirm the correct position of the leg before the arthrodesis is completed. The author recommends the use of an image intensifier at this stage to further confirm positioning.

The flexion position of 20°–25° is confirmed by performing the Thomas test. The greater trochanter is then repositioned at the anatomical site. This can now be attached back onto the femur with a screw through the greater trochanter and the cobra plate (**Figure 10.16**). The remaining screw holes are drilled and further cortical screws inserted to strengthen the arthrodesis.

Closure

Similar to lateral approach for THA.

Postoperative care and instructions

Thromboembolism should be prevented by early mobilisation and the addition of chemical and mechanical measures in patients at increased risk. Two further doses of the antibiotic given at induction should be given at 8 hours and 16 hours after surgery.

Excision hip arthroplasty (Girdlestone procedure)

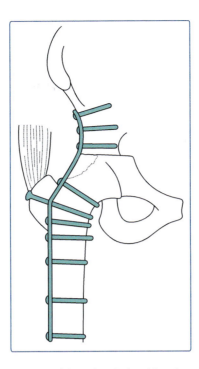

Figure 10.16 A hip arthrodesis with cobra plate.

Early mobilisation is non-weightbearing, with the aid of crutches. Radiographic signs of union are sought before a return to weightbearing is allowed. This often takes around 3 months. If the patient has significant shortening, i.e. greater than 15 mm, a shoe raise can be provided and used as the patient deems necessary.

Recommended references

Murrell GA, Fitch RD. Hip fusion in young adults. Using a medial displacement osteotomy and cobra plate. *Clin Orthop Relat Res.* 1994;**(300)**:147–154.

Sponseller PD, McBeath AA, Perpich M. Hip arthrodesis in young patients: A long term follow up study. *J Bone Joint Surg Am.* 1984;**66**:853–859.

Excision hip arthroplasty (Girdlestone procedure)

Preoperative planning

Indications

- It is a last resort operation and used as a salvage procedure, generally in patients with resistant infections or co-morbidities which necessitate a quick operation.
- Sepsis of either THA or the native hip.
- Aseptic loosening of THA.
- Painful hip conditions in a patient otherwise immobile, particularly in degenerative neuromuscular conditions.

> **Consent and risks**
> - Nerve injury
> - Limb length discrepancy: it is usually 3–12 cm, depending on resection
> - Recurrence of infection (if a septic indication): 10%
> - Nearly all will be reliant on walking aids after surgery; many have poor function but most have good pain relief

Anaesthesia and positioning
This is performed as for THA.

Surgical technique
One of the approaches for THA is selected. If the hip is septic, a thorough washout and debridement of infected tissue is essential.

The excision is carried out as in THA femoral head resection. All non-viable bone should be resected; however, the best functional results are achieved with a greater amount of retained proximal femur. A considered excision of bone should be performed.

Postoperative care and instructions
This is similar to THA in many respects. Traction is often used for the first 2 weeks after surgery. Almost all patients will require walking aids and shoe raises.

Femoroacetabular impingement surgery
Preoperative planning
Indications
Pain and/or restricted range of motion associated with a recognised anatomical deformity.

This can be of two types: cam or pincer; these can also co-exist (**Figure 10.17**). The cam deformity of the femur is also referred to as a 'pistol grip' deformity. The most typical presentation is groin pain worse on prolonged flexion, e.g. sitting. The impingement test of the hip is usually positive. This is performed with the hip held in 90° flexion and passively internally rotated and adducted.

Contraindications
- Active infection
- Moderate or severe existing arthritis on radiographs

Femoroacetabular impingement surgery

Consent and risks (as applicable to open femoroacetabular impingement surgery)
- DVT: Less than 1%
- Infection: Less than 1%
- Femoral neck fracture: Incidence related to amount of femoral 'bump' removed
- Avascular necrosis of the femoral head: Unknown incidence (many studies of open surgery show 0%)
- Heterotopic ossification: 3%
- Progression to frank osteoarthritis: Up to 100%

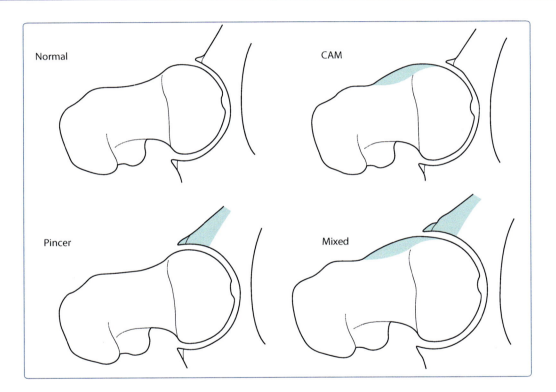

Figure 10.17 The common variants of femoroacetabular impingement.

Operative planning

Recent radiographs must be available – anteroposterior (AP) views of the hip and a shoot-through lateral with the leg in maximal internal rotation best demonstrates the anatomy. Hip and impingement morphology is best demonstrated with computer tomography (CT) scan. Magnetic resonance imaging (MRI), MR arthrography or arthroscopy are often used to examine for labral pathology. Conventional arthrography and local anaesthetic injection are frequently used to provide evidence that the pain is originating in the hip.

The surgeon must decide the approach to be taken. There are three common options:

- The arthroscopic approach (see 'Hip arthroscopy', next section).
- The lateral open approach, using a trochanteric flip osteotomy, as popularised by Ganz. The hip is then surgically dislocated to reveal the impingement.
- A more recent approach has been a 'mini-open' modified Smith-Peterson approach. This has the advantage of visualisation without dislocation of the hip. This approach is described here.

Anaesthesia and positioning

Anaesthesia is general with supine positioning. The use of an intraoperative image intensifier is optional.

Surgical technique

Landmarks

The anterior superior iliac spine is palpated. Slight external rotation of the hip aids location of the interval between the tensor fascia lata and sartorius.

Incision

A 7–10 cm incision is created, running from just below the anterior superior iliac spine, along the border between the tensor fascia lata and sartorius. This incision should not stray medially into the area overlying sartorius and it is preferable to create the incision a few millimetres lateral to the border of sartorius to ensure that this does not occur. The direction of the incision is towards the lateral border of the patella.

Superficial dissection

> **Structure at risk**
> - Lateral femoral cutaneous nerve

Dissection is continued through fat and superficial fascia. The lateral femoral cutaneous nerve is identified, running over the fascia between the tensor fascia lata and sartorius. The nerve is retracted medially and the fascia incised between the two muscle bellies. This provides an interval with the muscle belly of tensor fascia lata laterally and that of sartorius medially.

The dissection is continued down between the tensor fascia lata and sartorius, until the direct and reflected heads of the rectus femoris are identified.

Deep dissection

Structures at risk

- *Femoral nerve and artery*: These lie medial to the sartorius, anterior to the pectineus muscle. They will not be damaged if dissection is lateral and deep to the sartorius.
- *Medial femoral circumflex artery*: 1 cm proximal to the lesser trochanter, underlying the iliopsoas tendon. If not identified and accidentally damaged, profuse bleeding can be expected.

The reflected head of the rectus femoris is identified and dissected off its origin on the superior acetabular margin. Its fibres also blend with the anterior hip capsule, and these fibres are dissected free from the capsule. The direct head is retracted medially to reveal the iliopsoas tendon. This also requires dissecting free from the capsule as it is attached by the iliocapsularis tendon. Subsequently, the iliopsoas too can be retracted medially.

The underlying capsule is exposed and can be incised in line with the femoral head-neck junction. This is most easily identified at the anteromedial portion of the femoral head as the impingement bump in a cam-impinging hip will prevent palpation of the head-neck junction laterally. Thus, it is advisable to begin the incision medially and proceed laterally.

Procedure

The osteoplasty of the head-neck junction is carried out with a small (10–15 mm) osteotome or a high speed burr. An assistant internally and externally rotates the hip to allow complete excision of the cam lesion. The resection is directed distally to produce a bevelled resection, restoring the offset between the femoral head and neck. This creates a 'V'-shaped valley over the anterior head-neck junction. The depth of the valley can be assessed by bringing the hip back into the position of the impingement test. The aim is a gain in both internal rotation and flexion of the hip by over 10°. If the valley is not deep enough, it can be further deepened in a similar manner. The aim is complete excision of the protuberant bump, until the remaining femoral head is spherical and no longer impinging on the anterior acetabular rim. Similarly, if there is evidence of pincer impingement, the acetabular osteophytes or calcified labral tissue can be removed with an osteotome and excised.

Bleeding from exposed bone can be reduced by application of bone wax. The wound is thoroughly irrigated and any loose bone and cartilage carefully removed.

Closure

- The capsulotomy, reflected head of rectus and tensor fascia lata-sartorius interval are all closed in a layered manner with heavy absorbable suture. Skin closure is performed as per surgeon preference.

Postoperative care and instructions

The patient may begin mobilisation as soon as comfortable – this should be toe-touch weightbearing, with crutches, for 6 weeks. Active flexion is avoided for 6 weeks to allow healing of the reflected head of rectus femoris. Active abduction is begun straight away. Mobilisation without crutches is slowly begun after 6 weeks. High-impact sports, including running, are not permitted for 6 months.

Hip arthroscopy
Preoperative planning
Indications

Hip arthroscopy is indicated in a variety of painful conditions of the hip. The most frequent are

- Femeroacetabular impingement
- Septic arthritis of the hip joint
- Osteoarthritis
- Labral pathology
- Osteochondral defect
- Removal of loose bodies
- Synovectomy or synovial biopsy

Contraindications

- Infection of overlying skin.
- Hip ankylosis or significant protrusion of the hip.
- Lack of proper instrumentation. The instruments are specific to hip arthroscopy and surgery should not be attempted without fluoroscopy, appropriate portal instruments, a long arthroscope (30° or 70° angle) and distraction equipment.
- Gross osteoarthritis is a relative contraindication.

Consent and risks

- *Nerve injury*: Less than 1%. The lateral femoral cutaneous nerve (anterolateral portal) or the femoral nerve (anterior portal) are at risk.
- *Vascular injury*: Less than 1%.
- *Infection*: Less than 1%. As risk is very low routinely, prophylactic antibiotics are not recommended.
- *Trochanteric bursitis*: 1%.
- *Iatrogenic injury/failure*: 2%. Injury to articular cartilage or labrum is possible. A small number of patients cannot be sufficiently distracted for arthroscopy to be performed.
- Deep vein thrombosis.
- *Traction-related nerve injury*: Pudendal or peroneal nerves.

Operative planning

Recent radiographs, CT scans, MR images and MR arthrograms, where indicated, should be available. The equipment must be available and should be checked by the surgeon.

Anaesthesia and positioning

Anaesthesia is general, and the supine or lateral position can be used. In the supine position, a peroneal post is well padded and used to provide counter-traction. The hip and knee are extended and the hip slightly externally rotated. The foot is placed in a foot holder on a traction table. This should have a simple mechanism for internal or external rotation as it is useful for an assistant to be able to move the hip during arthroscopy.

Under fluoroscopic control the hip joint is distracted, aiming for 10 mm of opening. The surgical field is prepared with a germicidal solution and draped.

Surgical technique

Landmarks

The greater trochanter is palpated and outlined with a cutaneous marker. Lines should be marked to indicate the anterior, middle and posterior thirds of the greater trochanter. The anterior superior iliac spine is also palpated and marked.

Approach

A variety of portals have been described. The details of most are beyond the scope of this book.

The 'workhorse' portals are two lateral portals (described later), although anterior portals can be added in specific situations. The anterior portal is created at the intersection of a line descending vertically from the anterior superior iliac spine and a line passing horizontally from the pubic symphysis.

The lateral portals are created just above the superior surface of the greater trochanter; hence they are sometimes known as superolateral portals. Using a long, 14G spinal needle, an approach is made lying just above the anterior third of the greater trochanter (**Figure 10.18**). Fluoroscopy can be used at this stage to confirm entry into the joint.

The approach must be relatively flat (i.e. parallel to the floor) to avoid the superior acetabular labrum. Normal saline is injected through the needle, both to confirm entry and to further distend the joint. Another 14G spinal needle is passed over the superior edge of the greater trochanter, this time in line with the posterior third. It should be passed at the same angle. A guide wire is placed through each spinal needle and the needles removed. Dilators are then used sequentially to enlarge the portal in a controlled manner, e.g. a 5 mm, 7 mm, then 10 mm dilators.

The final dilator is removed and an arthroscopic cannula is inserted into the anterior and slightly more posterior portals. These two portals are generally referred to as the anterolateral and the lateral portals, to avoid confusion with true anterior portals and the rarely used and more dangerous posterior portals. Initially, the anterolateral portal will be used for introduction of instrumentation, and the lateral portal will house the arthroscope.

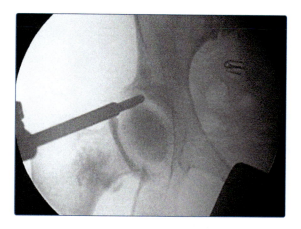

Figure 10.18 Entry to the hip joint.

Either a 30° or 70° arthroscope can be used. Some authors advocate a 70° scope as it can overcome some of the limitations in the viewing field with hip arthroscopy. The fluid irrigation should be controlled with an inflow pump and an outflow integrated within the portals.

Procedure

A systematic approach is essential if pathology is not to be missed. The authors recommend beginning posteriorly, following the posterior labrum and acetabulum. The arthroscope is then drawn superiorly, again specifically viewing the acetabulum and its labrum, then anteriorly.

Throughout the process the femoral head can also be viewed centrally, as the acetabular labrum is seen in the periphery of the view. A hooked probe is introduced and used to assess the soft tissues, particularly the labrum and the articular cartilage.

Specific instruments can be used for removal of loose bodies or debridement of labral tissues (**Figure 10.19**).

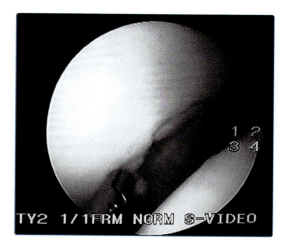

Figure 10.19 Arthroscopic debridement.

Closure

Non-absorbable suture is used to close the skin incisions.

Postoperative care and instructions

The patient is fully weightbearing as tolerated. Specific precautions are rarely required. Hip strengthening exercises are commenced once a full range of movement has been achieved.

Recommended references

Mason JB, McCarthy JC, O'Donnell J et al. Hip arthroscopy: Surgical approach, positioning, and distraction. *Clin Orthop Relat Res.* 2003;**(406)**:29–37.

McCarthy JC, Lee JA. Hip arthroscopy: Indications, outcomes, and complications. *J Bone Joint Surg Am.* 2005;**87**:1137–1145.

McCarthy JC, Lee JA. Hip arthroscopy: Indications, outcomes, and complications. *Instr Course Lect.* 2006;**55**:301–308.

Hip arthrography

Preoperative planning

Indications

- Osteoarthritis/rheumatoid arthritis – to assess the degree of cartilage loss
- Sequelae of paediatric disorders, particularly developmental dysplasia of the hip and Perthes disease
- Impingement syndrome
- Assessment of loose total hip implants, including aspiration in suspected prosthetic joint infection

Contraindications

- Contrast allergy
- Uncontrolled bleeding dyscrasias

Operative planning

Preoperative AP and lateral views of the pelvis and hip should be available. Appropriate equipment including a fluoroscope and contrast medium need to be available.

Anaesthesia and positioning

Hip arthrography is uncomfortable. It is recommended that it is performed under at least sedation but a short general anaesthetic is preferred. The supine position is used. The hip is placed in the position of maximum joint volume to aid injection:

- 10° abduction
- 10° flexion
- 10° internal rotation

The fluoroscope is positioned over the hip.

Surgical technique

Landmarks and approach

Useful landmarks include the anterior superior iliac spine, the greater trochanter and palpable femoral artery. Approaches include anterior, lateral or medial.

Procedure

Using the surgeon's preferred approach, a long 22G needle is guided towards the hip joint under fluoroscopic guidance. A 'pop' is felt as the needle penetrates the capsule. The correct position is checked by injecting a small amount of contrast and checking that it is intra-articular with fluoroscopy. Once the position is confirmed, further contrast is injected and the needle removed. The hip is gently manipulated to distribute the contrast throughout the joint.

Imaging is performed; a typical series includes

- AP view of the hip in neutral
- AP view with the hip in internal and external rotation both in flexion and extension
- Shoot-through lateral

If impingement is suspected, an image in flexion and internal rotation is particularly useful.

If the arthrogram is being performed for planning an osteotomy, live screening can be used to locate a position of best fit of the femoral head in the acetabulum. This is particularly useful in cases of Perthes disease.

If imaging a total hip implant, digital subtraction can be used by taking a plain AP view prior to injection of contrast and superimposing it on the contrast view. This will show areas of contrast intrusion around the implant while subtracting the image of the implant and cement.

Postoperative care and instructions

The patient may fully weightbear immediately. Risks are very low, with infection and an adverse reaction to contrast medium occurring at less than 1%.

Recommended reference

O'Neill DA, Harris WH. Failed total hip replacement: Assessment by plain radiographs, arthrograms, and aspiration of the hip joint. *J Bone Joint Surg Am.* 1984;**66**:540–546.

Viva questions

1. How does revision surgery differ when infection is suspected?
2. What are the indications, benefits and drawbacks for hip arthrodesis?
3. What are the surgical options for a 50-year-old man with symptomatic osteoarthritis of the hips?
4. Describe the anatomy of the sciatic nerve around the hip.
5. How do you classify bone loss around a femoral/acetabular component of a hip replacement?
6. What complications do you warn the patient about prior to hip replacement? What are their incidences?
7. What are the indications for Girdlestone's procedure?
8. When would allograft be used in hip replacement? What types of allograft are used and why?
9. Which approach do you use for total hip replacement and why?
10. What factors influence your choice of hip implant for total hip replacement?
11. What are the contraindications to total hip replacement?
12. What factors affect the quality of the cement mantle in cemented hip replacement?
13. Which nerves can be injured in hip surgery?
14. What factors contribute to dislocation in total hip replacement?
15. Describe the portals used in hip arthroscopy.
16. How do you perform a hip arthrogram?
17. What are the potential advantages of hip resurfacing over total hip replacement?
18. What imaging would you consider before revising a total hip replacement?
19. What are the options for reconstruction of cavitary bone loss in acetabular revision surgery?
20. How can femoroacetabular impingement be treated surgically?

11 Surgery of the Knee

Alexander D Liddle, Lee A David and Timothy WR Briggs

Primary total knee replacement	279	Distal femoral osteotomy	309
Revision total knee replacement	293	Proximal tibial osteotomy	313
Patellofemoral replacement	302	Knee arthrodesis	317
Unicompartmental knee replacement	305	Viva questions	320

	Range of motion	Position of arthrodesis
Flexion	150°	10°–15°
Extension	0 to −5°	
Internal/External rotation	10°	10°

Primary total knee replacement
Preoperative planning
Indications
Total knee replacement (TKR) is indicated in the treatment of pain and deformity from the following conditions, when non-operative management has failed or is futile:

- Osteoarthritis
- Post-traumatic osteoarthritis
- Rheumatoid arthritis and other inflammatory arthropathies
- Spontaneous osteonecrosis of the knee (SONK)

Contraindications
- Active or recent local or generalised infection
- Critical arterial ischaemia
- Non-functioning extensor mechanism
- Severe neurological disorders (relative)
- Age (relative): Very young or very old patients should be carefully selected depending on severity of arthritis, level of symptoms and quality of life

Severe deformity or instability may be a contraindication to the use of an unconstrained, condylar implant and may require the use of a semi-constrained and stabilised or a constrained, hinged prosthesis (see section 'Revision total knee replacement', p. 293).

Consent and risks

- *Infection*: 1%–2% in the general population. Increased in diabetics, smokers, those with a high body mass index (BMI) and those with a history of infection.
- *Bleeding*: Haematoma formation increases the risk of wound problems, arthrofibrosis and infection. Hypovolaemia and anaemia may cause cardiovascular, cerebral or renal complications.
- *Venous thromboembolism*: Below-knee deep vein thrombosis (DVT) occurs in approximately two-thirds of patients following TKR. The risk of fatal pulmonary embolism (PE) is approximately 0.1%. The prevention of DVT and PE remains a controversial topic, but it is almost universally accepted that mechanical and some form of chemical thromboprophylaxis should be used.
- *Neurovascular injury*: Damage to the infrapatellar branch of the saphenous nerve during the incision is often unavoidable and leads to sensory change on the anterolateral shin; this occurs in upwards of 70% of patients but generally improves over time. Damage to important nerves and blood vessels is rarer, and can be caused by direct transection, traction or pressure. Discrete arterial damage is rare (approximately 0.05%) but must be recognised and dealt with immediately. Distal arterial thromboembolism must be promptly recognised, pressure dressings released and a vascular surgical opinion sought. Common peroneal nerve (CPN) injury has an incidence of approximately 0.5% and should initially be managed by release of pressure dressings with exploration indicated if caused by haematoma. Traction injury to the CPN is most common if a severe valgus deformity is corrected, particularly if combined with a fixed flexion deformity. In these cases, a foot drop splint should be used to prevent equinus contracture and nerve conduction studies may be performed at a later date.
- *Fractures*: The risk of fracture is increased in osteoporosis and rheumatoid arthritis. Significant notching of the anterior distal femoral cortex is thought to increase the risk of postoperative periprosthetic fracture, but the evidence is weak. Excessive patella resection during resurfacing increases the risk of patella fracture. Intraoperative fractures usually require immediate fixation and the use of stemmed implants.
- *Extensor mechanism injury*: Avulsion of the patellar tendon is a disastrous complication and must be avoided as it severely compromises the outcome following TKR. In the event of this occurring, the tendon must be reattached to the tibial tuberosity and protected, although the result is usually poor.
- Stiffness may be caused by true arthrofibrosis, but other causes must be ruled out. These include infection and mechanical problems, such as oversizing the femoral component, errors of rotation leading to patellar maltracking, reversing the tibial slope or making an inadequate bone resection. Treatment depends on the underlying problem.
- Instability may be caused by unequal flexion/extension gaps, soft tissue imbalance, ligamentous insufficiency, insufficient insert thickness, polyethylene wear or patellofemoral maltracking. Treatment depends on cause.
- *Revision surgery*: 4% at 10 years according to worldwide national joint registries. A recent meta-analysis suggested that over 80% of TKRs survive to at least 25 years. The majority of patients undergoing knee replacement will never undergo revision.

Operative planning

Clinical examination should pay careful attention to alignment, deformity, instability, range of movement and extensor mechanism function. Scars should be carefully noted, and a distal neurovascular assessment must be performed.

Recent weightbearing anteroposterior, lateral and skyline radiographs must be available and long-leg alignment views are helpful to establish the mechanical axis of the leg (**Figure 11.1**). It is imperative that the patient's symptoms should correlate with the radiographic findings. Templating of preoperative radiographs should be performed if possible, and it is the responsibility of the surgeon to ensure that the required implants are available.

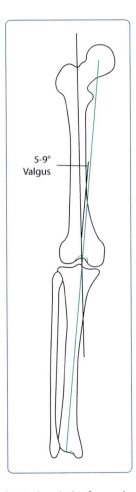

Figure 11.1 The mechanical and tibiofemoral axes of the lower limb.

Choice of implant

Most implants in current use are evolutions of the condylar knee designs popularised in the late 1960s and early 1970s; the great majority are cemented. In most cases, the femoral component is polyradial in the sagittal plane to recreate the 'J-curve' of the native condyles. The tibial component is usually modular with a metal baseplate and an ultra-high molecular weight polyethylene insert, although monoblock (metal-backed or all-polyethylene) tibial components have good published results and are generally cheaper. The tibiofemoral articulation is minimally constrained, but the tibial component is dished to mitigate for the loss of the anterior cruciate ligament. In cruciate retaining (CR) implants the posterior cruciate ligament (PCL) is retained; in posterior stabilised (PS) designs, the PCL is resected and a cam-post mechanism is used to maintain stability; in most studies the outcomes are similar. As designs have evolved, the femoral components have gone from being symmetrical in the coronal plane to being sided (with the asymmetry either restricted to the trochlear flange or involving different radii of the medial and lateral condyles as in the native knee); newer designs are generally more conforming to prevent subtle but symptomatic instability. Variations include rotating platform tibial components, medial rotation knees where the medial side represents a ball and socket joint and the lateral side is unconstrained, and femoral components with a single radius of curvature (which is designed to maintain collateral ligament tension through the range of flexion). There is little published evidence to suggest the superiority of one philosophy over any other.

In the end, the choice of implant remains at the discretion of the surgeon or, increasingly, the purchasing agreements of the trust. It is the surgeon's responsibility to ensure that he or she is familiar with the implants used, that all necessary equipment is available and that the appropriate range of sizes are readily to hand.

Anaesthesia and positioning

Anaesthesia is usually general, regional or combined, depending on the preferences of the anaesthetist and surgeon and the patient's co-morbidities.

The patient is positioned supine on the operating table with a lateral thigh support and foot bolster, allowing free flexion and extension of the knee. Pressure areas should be protected with gel pads. Most, but not all, surgeons use a tourniquet for all or part of the procedure unless contraindications exist (such as arterial insufficiency). The tourniquet should be well padded and placed high on the thigh. Tourniquet time should be clearly documented and should not exceed 2 hours. A dose of an appropriate antibiotic is administered intravenously prior to the inflation of the tourniquet. The skin in the area of the incision should be shaved immediately prior to surgery. The surgical field is prepared with an antiseptic solution. The foot should either be thoroughly prepared or wrapped with an impervious 'shut-off' drape. Appropriate waterproof drapes should be carefully applied. An antibacterial, transparent adhesive drape is usually applied to the surgical field.

Surgical technique

By far the most common approach to the knee joint in TKR is the medial parapatellar approach, which is discussed later. The subvastus, midvastus and direct lateral approaches are used much less frequently. Other extensile approaches are discussed in the section 'Revision total knee replacement'.

Landmarks and incision

The position of the patella, patellar tendon and tibial tubercle should all be noted. An anterior midline longitudinal incision is made, usually with the knee in flexion. The incision needs to be long enough to allow adequate exposure and avoid excessive skin stretching; this runs proximally from the level of the tibial tubercle for approximately 20 cm, although the length is heavily dependent on the patient's build.

Dissection

> ### Structures at risk
>
> The medial collateral ligament (MCL) may be damaged during medial release. The risk of this can be minimised by careful subperiosteal release using either a periosteal elevator or coagulating diathermy.
>
> The patellar tendon may be damaged during excision of the fat pad, which can be prevented by always cutting away from the tendon itself. The patellar tendon may be avulsed at its insertion to the tibial tubercle during eversion of the patella and flexion of the knee. This is a disastrous complication and can be prevented by extending the deep dissection proximally, dividing any lateral plicae and performing a lateral parapatellar release to allow eversion of the patella. External rotation of the tibia also relaxes the extensor mechanism.

Dissection continues in the midline, until the quadriceps tendon is identified. The medial and lateral skin, subcutaneous fat and deep fascia should be reflected in matching thick flaps to allow exposure of the quadriceps tendon, medial patellar retinaculum and patellar tendon.

The medial parapatellar incision is extended from the quadriceps tendon proximally, through the medial parapatellar retinaculum and along the medial border of the patellar tendon distally (**Figure 11.2**). There should be at least a 3 mm cuff of quadriceps tendon left attached to vastus medialis and a cuff of medial retinaculum attached to the patella to allow closure.

The medial capsule is released subperiosteally off the proximal tibia to gain exposure to the medial compartment. In a varus knee, this dissection should include the deep medial collateral ligament and, depending on the degree and correctability of the varus deformity, may extend as far as the posteromedial corner. In a valgus knee, this medial release should be kept to the minimum required to allow exposure.

With the knee in extension, the patella is everted and the knee flexed. The retropatellar fat pad may be partially or fully excised if necessary. The visible remnants of the medial and lateral menisci may be resected at this stage and the anterior cruciate ligament (ACL) must be divided and resected. If a PS implant is to be used the PCL can be resected now by dissecting it from its femoral attachment with diathermy. Osteophytes may be debrided at this stage.

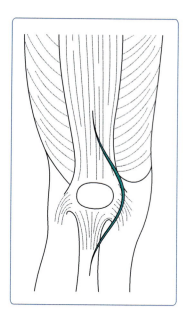

Figure 11.2 The medial parapatellar approach to the knee.

Procedure

The primary goals of surgery are relief of pain, restoration of function and longevity of the prosthesis. The immediate technical aims of the operation are to restore alignment, allow a good range of motion, good stability and ligamentous balance throughout the range of motion with good patellar tracking.

The primary requirement to allow a TKR to function is for the gaps between the femur and the tibia to be symmetrical and equal in flexion and extension. This can be achieved by one of two main routes, 'measured resection' and 'gap balancing'. Measured resection is the more common approach and involves performing anatomically consistent bone cuts on the femur and tibia and restoring symmetry and equality of gaps by performing sequential soft tissue releases. In gap balancing, the femoral and tibial cuts are made in order to maintain the tension of the medial and lateral collateral ligaments without significant releases. Some surgeons will perform a measured resection of the distal femur and proximal tibia with flexion gap and femoral rotation achieved using a gap balancing technique. Either way, the surgeon must appreciate that a TKR is as much a soft tissue operation as a bony procedure.

Bone cuts

In most cases, the bony cuts are made using a measured resection technique using standard instrumentation. Whether the femoral or tibial cut is made first depends on the surgeon's preference and type of prosthesis used; however, it is advisable to perform the distal femoral and proximal tibial cuts before final femoral preparation. This ensures that the extension gap is adequate and symmetrical, and allows the flexion gap (dictated by the anteroposterior size and position of the femoral component) to be fine-tuned to match the extension gap.

Structures at risk

- The MCL must be carefully protected during saw cuts.
- Patellar tendon.
- Common peroneal nerve may be injured by injudicious placement of the lateral retractor or by stretch in large corrections.
- Popliteus tendon can be damaged during posterior femoral saw cut or resection of meniscus.
- Popliteal vessels and tibial nerve can be injured during removal of posterior osteophytes, posterior capsular release, PCL resection and when cutting the posterior tibial cortex with the saw, if not protected. The anatomy of the popliteal artery in relation to the knee joint is extremely variable.

Femoral cuts

The femur should be prepared with the use of an intramedullary alignment jig if possible. The tibial cut can be made by using intra- or extramedullary alignment jigs, depending on the surgeon's preferred method and the degree of extra-articular deformity of the tibia. There is evidence to show that intramedullary referencing of the tibial cuts is more accurate, but it has also been shown to increase the risk of fat embolism.

Femoral preparation is undertaken with the knee flexed and the patella everted. A large drill bit is used to create an entry point in the distal femoral canal at a point approximately 1 cm anterior to the insertion of the PCL within the trochlear notch. The intramedullary rod should be inserted into the canal with care, especially if a previous total hip replacement has been performed. The distal femoral cutting jig is positioned over the rod and adjusted so that the distal cut is set at a 5°–9° valgus angle to the appropriate side of the knee to be replaced (**Figure 11.3**). Ideally, this should be chosen to match the anatomical axis of the contralateral limb, if normal.

The distal cutting jig is secured with two or three pins that should be fully inserted to ensure that the saw is not hampered and to allow the saw blade to make ample excursion to complete the cut. The amount of distal femoral resection performed depends upon the thickness of the implant (usually around 9 mm) and any fixed flexion deformity present (see later). It is imperative that the medial and lateral soft tissues are retracted and protected with either Hohmann or Trethowan retractors. The cut bone surface should be of sufficient surface area and quality to allow adequate fixation and must expose trabecular bone. If the distal femur is particularly sclerotic in parts, a 'second pass' with the saw blade may be required to achieve a flat surface, but one must bear in mind that repeated passes with a power saw generates heat, necrosis and metal debris from the jig.

The distal femur must then be sized to enable placement of the appropriate cutting block. Sizing jigs generally work on an anterior or posterior referencing system, using either the anterior distal femoral cortex or the posterior femoral condyles as the baseline, measuring the amount of anteroposterior resection required accordingly. If the sizing is perfect, the size and position of the implant will be the same whether anterior or posterior referencing is used. If there is over- or under-sizing, then the use of a posterior referencing system will

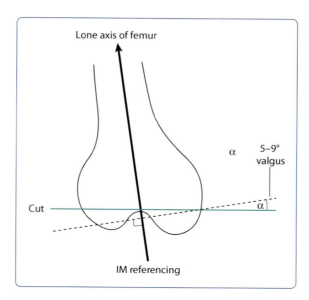

Figure 11.3 Distal femoral resection.

lead either to notching of the anterior femur or 'overstuffing' of the patellofemoral joint. If an anterior referencing system is used, then a gap mismatch will occur, with the flexion gap being either tight, resulting in stiffness, or loose, resulting in instability in flexion. If the knee is found to be between sizes of implant, generally the smaller implant is chosen. The typical sizing jig has an anterior stylus that must be seated down onto the anterior cortex, and it may be necessary to remove the overlying synovium to ensure accurate sizing. When the desired size is estimated, marker holes are made on the distal femur through the appropriate holes on the jig, to enable positioning of the femoral cutting block. Attention must be paid to femoral rotation as mistakes (usually too little external rotation) will result in flexion gap asymmetry and patellar maltracking. Rotation should be set parallel to the interepicondylar axis, which is perpendicular to Whiteside's line. The transepicondylar axis is usually around 3° externally rotated to the posterior femoral condyles and in most systems, the holes made by the femoral sizing jig are set in 3° of external rotation to the posterior condylar axis to match this. In the valgus knee the lateral condyle may be hypoplastic, and relying on the jigs may result in internal rotation of the femoral component. In such cases, additional external rotation should be introduced, guided by the transepicondylar axis.

The cutting block corresponding to the measured size is placed onto the cut surface of the distal femur, with pegs sitting into the previously drilled marker holes. Cuts (particularly the anterior cut) can be estimated using an 'angel wing'. The cutting block is firmly impacted until seated flat onto the cut surface of the distal femur and secured with obliquely placed pins. Again, the soft tissues must be carefully retracted during the placement of instrumentation. If there is any difficulty in seating either the sizing jig or cutting block, the surgeon must check that all osteophytes are removed, that there is adequate meniscal resection, that the bone cuts are complete and that the soft tissues are retracted sufficiently. Anterior and posterior cuts should be made prior to the chamfer cuts to prevent destabilising the cutting block. If it is apparent that there will be significant notching of the distal femur, the cutting block should be removed and the sizing reassessed (**Figure 11.4**). If there is a possibility of minor notching occurring, this should be controlled and any sharp edge of anterior cortex should be smoothed off with the saw or a bone file. The cut bone fragments can then be removed with knife and forceps and the posterior condylar cuts can be removed with a broad osteotome. The distal femur is then examined to ensure that the cuts are complete. Large posterior osteophytes apparent on the preoperative lateral radiograph or evident after bone cuts can be removed by lifting up the femur and carefully using a broad osteotome under direct vision.

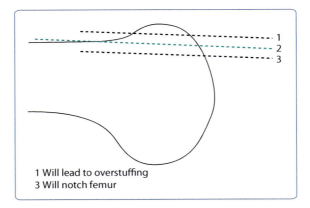

Figure 11.4 The anterior femoral cut.

Tibial cut

The tibial cut should be made perpendicular to the axis of the tibia in the coronal plane ensuring a sufficient anterior to posterior slope (**Figure 11.5**). If intramedullary referencing is used, the entry point should be made with a drill at the centre point of the tibia. The intramedullary rod should be inserted comfortably into the tibial canal. With intramedullary referencing, the slope is generated using an appropriately angled cutting block. If extramedullary referencing is used, the rod should be in line with the tibial tubercle, and the distal tip of the rod should lie just medial to the centre of the ankle joint (as this is where the mechanical axis of the limb passes). Use of anatomical landmarks in the foot, such as the second metatarsal, is less reliable as rotation can occur within the hindfoot and midfoot. With extramedullary referencing, the anteroposterior slope of the tibial cut can be introduced either by use of an angled cutting block (as with the intramedullary technique) or by adjustment of the extramedullary jig itself. Depth of resection is estimated using a stylus. Generally, either the depth of the implant (usually 8–10 mm) is taken from the preserved tibial plateau (the lateral plateau in varus arthritis) or 2 mm is taken from the depth of the wear scar to ensure an adequate resection has been made. In valgus disease, the preserved tibial plateau is the medial, which is concave, and it may be appropriate to take a smaller resection than would be appropriate in varus disease.

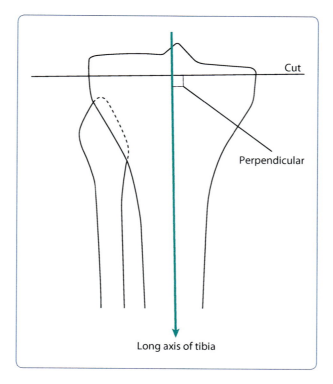

Figure 11.5 The tibial cut.

After the tibial resection is complete, the remaining meniscal remnants can be excised and the tibial component is sized. Following a trial of the components, the tibia can be prepared to accept the stem or keel of the prosthesis. Sizing the tibial component is a balance between achieving adequate coverage of the cut surface to provide support to the implant and avoiding overhang which may cause symptoms. The midpoint of the tibial component should be in line with the medial third of the tibial tubercle, but the surgeon should err on the side of external rotation. Often, particularly with symmetrical tibial components, an oversized tibial component may fit the cut surface but only with the introduction of excessive internal rotation. In this situation, a smaller size should be chosen and care taken to position the implant accurately.

Balancing the knee
Balancing flexion/extension gaps
As stated previously, prior to implantation the flexion and extension gaps should be equal and symmetrical in full extension and 90° of flexion (**Figure 11.6**). Inequality or asymmetry can be addressed using bony or soft tissue adjustment. Adjustment of the bone resection on the tibia will affect the flexion and extension gaps equally. Adjustment of the bone resection on the femur will affect either the extension gap (adjustment of the distal cut) or the flexion gap (adjustment of the posterior femoral cut) individually.

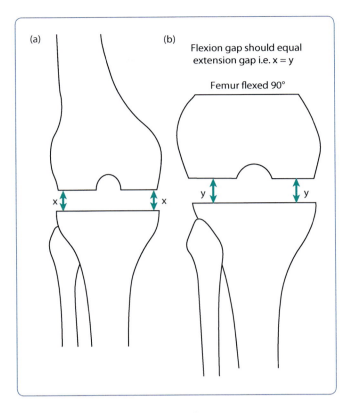

Figure 11.6 Flexion and extension gaps.

Unequal but symmetrical gaps

If the flexion gap and extension gap are different, but the medial and lateral tensions are similar, the following steps can be taken:

- Tight in extension, flexion satisfactory
  - *Solution*: Increase distal femoral resection. Recess the PCL or convert to PS design. Beware of raising the joint line with excessive distal femoral resection.
- Tight in flexion, extension satisfactory
  - *Solution*: Resect more posterior femur by downsizing the femur (in anterior referencing implant) or translating the femur more anteriorly. Check that the tibial slope is adequate and increase it if necessary.
- Tight in flexion and extension
  - *Solution*: Increase tibial resection. This may necessitate a smaller size of tibial component due to the tapering morphology of the proximal tibial metaphysis.
- Loose in flexion and extension
  - *Solution*: Increase thickness of insert. Ensure that laxity has a firm endpoint and no ligamentous injury has occurred. If there is ligamentous injury, a more constrained implant may be necessary (see the section 'Revision total knee replacement').

Soft tissue balancing
When a measured resection technique is used, soft tissue balancing is used to ensure symmetry of flexion and extension gaps. The extent and sequence of soft tissue releases depends upon the pre-intervention deformity. Often, only minimal releases are necessary – it is better to start with a small release and increase them later than to perform large releases initially which turn out to be excessive.

- *Varus deformity*: This is the most common deformity seen in osteoarthritis and generally leads to a tight medial collateral ligament in extension. The flexion gap may be equal or tight in flexion. The sequence of releases is
    - Resection of osteophytes and subperiosteal release of capsule and deep MCL.
    - Distal extension of release to involve superficial MCL and pes anserinus.
    - Recession or resection of PCL.
    - Release of posteromedial capsule or semimembranosus.
- *Valgus deformity*: This is the most common deformity in rheumatoid arthritis and can be seen in osteoarthritis and post-traumatic or post-meniscectomy arthritis. The lateral side is tight in extension (commonly), flexion (less commonly) or both. In all cases, a minimal medial release is performed. A PS implant may be chosen. The sequence of releases is
    - Removal of osteophytes.
    - If tight in extension, 'pie-crusting' of the iliotibial band or release from Gerdy's tubercle.
    - If tight in flexion, popliteus release.
    - If tight in both flexion and extension, the lateral collateral ligament may need to be 'pie-crusted' or released from the femur.
    - Finally, in a severe combined valgus and fixed flexion deformity, posterolateral capsule and lateral head of gastrocnemius may be released.
- *Fixed flexion deformity*: This can be the result of posterior osteophytes and contracture of the posterior capsule in severe disease. Either bony or soft tissue releases may be performed:
    - Taking care not to excessively elevate the joint line, extra bone may be removed from the distal femur (1 mm for every 2°–3° of fixed flexion).
    - Osteophytes should be removed from the posterior femur with osteotomes and Kocher's forceps under direct vision.
    - Posterior capsule may be released using a curved osteotome.
    - PCL may be recessed or resected.

The patella

Whether the patella should be resurfaced is still a controversial issue. Some surgeons always resurface, some never resurface and some do only if there are patellofemoral symptoms or if the retropatellar surface is severely affected. The evidence on patellar resurfacing is mixed. The Knee Arthroplasty Trial, the largest randomised trial of TKR in osteoarthritis, suggests that patellar resurfacing results in no difference in patient-reported outcome but reduces the rate of revision by eliminating secondary patellar resurfacing. Inflammatory arthropathy is considered to be a disease of the whole joint and patellar resurfacing is mandatory in rheumatoid and other inflammatory arthropathies (unless the patellar bone stock precludes it).

The majority of patella buttons used are monoblock and all-polyethylene. There are two types of patella button – onlay and inlay. As the respective names suggest, these designs utilise a prosthesis that is implanted either onto or into the resected retropatellar surface. To resurface the patella, the knee should be extended and the patella fully everted. Peripheral osteophytes can be removed with a bone nibbler to demarcate the actual articular surface. The thickness of the patella should be measured and the amount of bone/cartilage removed should approximately correspond to the thickness of the implant, although if there is severe damage it may be less. Resecting too little bone runs the risk of overstuffing the knee and if a sclerotic surface is left behind, fixation is compromised, whereas resecting too much increases the risk of fracture. Many implants now have calibrated clamps and jigs that help indicate the correct resection level.

To avoid an increase in the 'Q'-angle and therefore reduce the likelihood of maltracking, the patella button should be slightly medialised and both the femoral and tibial components should be lateralised and externally rotated. Patellar tracking should be adequate even before the patellar retinaculum is closed. Maltracking of the patella is usually related to problems with rotation of the femoral or tibial components; rarely, if the patella maltracks with well-positioned implants then a lateral retinacular release may be necessary. This should be performed with a diathermy (as it may lead to significant bleeding and bruising postoperatively) and should be carried out from distal to proximal and from deep to superficial. There are often palpable fibrous bands, and release of these is sometimes enough. To enable the release to be performed, the patella is lifted anterolaterally with the knee in extension. If possible, the superior lateral geniculate artery should be preserved to avoid devascularisation of the patella. Superficial releasing with a resultant subcutaneous flap and undermining of the lateral skin should be avoided. Where TKR is performed following a previous patellectomy, a PCL substituting implant should be used in order to avoid excessive anterior subluxation of the femur on the tibia due to an already relatively attenuated extensor mechanism.

Implantation of prostheses

While cementless and hybrid designs are available, most TKRs are implanted using cement. In cemented knee replacement, two mixes of antibiotic-impregnated polymethylmethacrylate (PMMA) bone cement should be used. The surgeon should be familiar with the biomechanical properties of the cement and its mixing technique. Following satisfactory trials, the selected components are checked by the surgeon and opened. The knee is flexed and the patella everted allowing the tibia to be subluxed anteriorly, with a Hohmann retractor or similar, and the prepared surface of the tibia exposed medially and laterally with spiked retractors. The knee is washed out thoroughly with normal saline pulsed lavage in order to expose the bone trabeculae and maximise the mechanical fixation of the cement. If sclerotic bone surfaces are present, a small drill can be used to make multiple small 'key holes'. The knee should be thoroughly dried with suction and swabs. The cement can then be mixed and the whole surgical team should change the outer layer of gloves. In most situations, cementing of both components can be performed simultaneously, but on occasions it may be desirable to perform cementing of the components separately with different mixes of cement.

To ensure a satisfactory and efficient cementation process, everything should be prepared and ordered in a logical fashion. The tibial component is usually implanted first. Cement can be applied onto the surface of the tibia, or the implant, or both, using a gun with short nozzle or a spatula. The tibial component is positioned in the correct orientation and firmly seated with a soft impactor and hammer. Excess cement is removed. Cement is applied to the cut surface of the femur and the posterior surface of the implant taking care not to apply too much cement to the posterior condyles as removal of excess cement can be difficult from the posterior part of the femur. The femoral component must be positioned carefully in relation to the distal femur; in particular flexion of the femoral component should be avoided. The femoral component must be firmly impacted and any excess cement should be removed. Either a trial or definitive insert is attached to the tibial baseplate, the knee is extended and axial compression applied. (Note: Hyperextension leads to uneven cement pressurisation and may cause posterior 'lift-off' of the tibial baseplate.) If the patella is resurfaced the orientation should be checked; once positioned, the patella is compressed and held with a clamp. The knee can then be flexed again and any further cement extruded can be removed quickly. The knee is then extended and further axial compression applied.

Closure

Once the cement has set, the knee can be washed out again with pulsed lavage. Some surgeons prefer to deflate the tourniquet and gain haemostasis prior to closure. Intravenous or topical tranexamic acid may be given at this stage. Alternatively, the knee can be closed and a pressure dressing applied prior to deflation of the tourniquet. The use of drains has declined over recent years and the evidence for their use is weak.

The actual closure technique varies with surgical preference, but it is important that the repair is watertight and that range of motion is maintained with no patella maltracking. Closure of the knee in flexion ensures that the correct tension is achieved. The deep layer is closed with a heavy suture (e.g. number 1 Vicryl), by means of a continuous repair of the quadriceps tendon, interrupted repair of the parapatellar retinaculum and continuous repair of the medial capsule to patellar tendon. The deep fascia can be closed as a separate layer if desired or the subcutaneous fat can be opposed with deep interrupted sutures. The deep dermal layer is closed with a continuous absorbable suture to allow tension-free closure of the skin with surgical staples or a continuous absorbable subcuticular suture. A sterile occlusive dressing and a padded compression bandage are applied.

Postoperative care and instructions

Regular neurovascular, cardiovascular and respiratory observations are mandatory. Urine output, temperature and drainage (if a drain is used) should also be monitored. Adequate analgesia should be administered. Mechanical and chemical thromboprophylaxis should be given according to local and national protocols. Haemoglobin levels should be checked 24–48 hours after the procedure. Any drains, urinary catheters, epidural lines and intravenous cannulae should be removed as soon as appropriate to avoid unnecessary portals of infection. Pressure dressings should be reduced and ice applied. Full weightbearing and active range-of-motion exercises should be commenced as soon as possible. The wound should be inspected and radiographs performed prior to discharge should be checked. The patient must be declared safe for discharge and for routine cases should be able to straight leg raise and flex the knee from 0° to 90°.

Skin clips should be removed 10–14 days after surgery, and an outpatient appointment should be arranged approximately 6 weeks postoperatively. Ideally, patients undergoing TKR should be followed up for life with serial radiographs, but in reality this is rarely possible.

Recommended references

Bayliss LE, Culliford D, Monk AP et al. The effect of patient age at intervention on risk of implant revision after total replacement of the hip or knee: A population-based cohort study. *Lancet*. 2017;**389**: 1424–1430.

Evans JT, Walker RW, Evans JP, Blom AW, Sayers A, Whitehouse MR. How long does a knee replacement last? A systematic review and meta-analysis of case series and national registry reports with more than 15 years of follow-up. *Lancet*. 2019;**393**:655–663.

Murray DW, MacLennan GS, Breeman S et al. A randomised controlled trial of the clinical effectiveness and cost-effectiveness of different knee prostheses: The Knee Arthroplasty Trial (KAT). *Health Technol Assess*. 2014;**18**;1–235.

Shetty AA, Tindall A, Ting P, Heatley FW. The evolution of total knee arthroplasty. Part III: Surface replacement. *Curr Orthop*. 2003;**17**:478–481.

Whiteside LA. *Ligament Balancing in Total Knee Arthroplasty: An Instructional Manual*. Berlin, Germany: Springer, 2004.

Revision total knee replacement

This section is not intended as a comprehensive guide to revision knee replacement but rather covers the principles of the procedure. This section refers extensively to the section 'Primary total knee replacement' (p. 279).

Preoperative planning

Indications

Revision TKR is indicated in the treatment of pain, stiffness or instability from a failed TKR. The cause of failure must be diagnosed prior to embarking on revision surgery: revision for unexplained pain has poor outcomes. Knees may fail for a single reason or several in combination. The most common indications for revision are

- Infection
- Aseptic loosening/osteolysis
- Polyethylene wear
- Instability
- Stiffness
- Patellofemoral dysfunction
- Periprosthetic fracture

Contraindications

- Medically unfit for surgery or anaesthetic
- Critical arterial ischaemia
- Non-functioning extensor mechanism
- Unexplained pain
- Insufficient skin coverage (relative)
- Severe neurological disorders (relative)
- Age (relative): Very elderly patients should be carefully selected depending on severity of symptoms, quality of life and options available

Consent and risks

All of the risks and complications of primary TKR occur at increased rates following revision. The overall complication rate for revision knee replacement is approximately 25%, while the outcome of a successful revision is significantly inferior to the results of a successful primary. In revision for infection, the best centres report rates of clearance of infection at up to 95%.

- Infection (or failure to eradicate)
- Bleeding
- Venous thromboembolism
- Wound problems
- Neurovascular injury
- Fractures
- Extensor mechanism injury
- Stiffness
- Instability
- Wear
- Loosening
- Pain

Operative planning

A thorough history and examination is essential to rule out pain referred to the knee from elsewhere and to assess the level of pain and functional disability. Special consideration should be given to potential risk factors, and realistic goals should be identified. The examination should pay careful attention to ligamentous instability, range of movement and extensor mechanism function. In cases of apparent aseptic loosening, stiffness or pain, infection must be excluded: inflammatory markers should be performed, and there should be a low threshold for performing an aspiration or biopsy. Scars should be carefully noted, and a distal neurovascular assessment must be performed. If the skin over the knee is of poor quality, it may be necessary to consult a plastic surgeon.

Recent weightbearing anteroposterior, lateral and skyline radiographs must be available, and long-leg alignment views are helpful in diagnosing malalignment. Computed tomography is helpful to assess the degree of bone loss in cases of osteolysis and can be useful in diagnosing rotational malalignment. It is absolutely essential that a cause for the failure is found. Templating of preoperative radiographs should be performed if possible; it is the responsibility of the surgeon to ensure that the required implants are available.

Choice of implant

When selecting an implant for revision TKR, the aim is to confer sufficient constraint at the joint to address any ligamentous deficiency, to provide sufficient fixation to support the more constrained implant in compromised bone stock, and to fill any bony defects that may be present.

The native knee joint is effectively unconstrained at its bony surfaces. The femur and tibia are connected by the cruciate and collateral ligaments, capsule, extensor mechanism, hamstrings and gastrocnemius. Unicompartmental knee replacement is similarly unconstrained as all of these structures are preserved. Primary TKR is minimally constrained, introducing a dish to substitute for the ACL and, in PS designs, a cam and post. As more capsular and ligamentous structures are lost, more constraint is necessary – this is the 'ladder of constraint' (see box). Generally, except in exceptional circumstances (such as revision of unicompartmental or patellofemoral replacement), a condylar constrained design is the minimum acceptable degree of constraint.

The more constraint that is present at the knee joint, the more forces are transferred to the bone-implant interface. As a result, increasing constraint necessitates more secure fixation within bone. A useful concept for fixation of revision knee prostheses is that of zonal fixation. Fixation can be achieved in three zones – the epiphysis/joint surface (zone 1), the metaphysis (zone 2) and the diaphysis (zone 3); fixation in two of the three is considered to be adequate. Traditionally, revision implants achieve fixation in zones 1 and 3: sufficient epiphyseal bone is identified by re-cutting, and may be supplemented using wedges or augments (augments are very frequently used on the femoral side to avoid raising the joint line). Zone 3 fixation is achieved using stems, which may be broad to allow a cementless press-fit, or may be narrower and cemented. Fixation in zone 2 can be achieved using metaphyseal sleeves or cones. Sleeves attach to the component via a morse taper to form a monolithic structure. They are wedge shaped and are designed to provide metaphyseal fixation in a similar way to a cementless total hip replacement. If a stem and a sleeve is present, secure fixation in zone 1 is unnecessary. Cones are separate from the implant and come in a variety of shapes – cones are designed to fill defects and provide supplementary fixation in the metaphysis.

Bone loss can be addressed using bone graft (for contained defects in the metaphysis, for example) or by the use of augments, cones and sleeves. Massive bone loss may necessitate the use of a distal femoral or, rarely, a proximal tibial replacement.

> ### Ladder of constraint (from least to most constrained)
>
> - Unicompartmental knee replacement
>   - Round on flat or mobile bearing design results in a completely unconstrained joint surface
>   - Requires functionally intact ACL, PCL, collateral ligaments
> - Cruciate retaining TKR
>   - Minimal constraint through dishing at joint surface to substitute for absent ACL
>   - Requires functionally intact PCL and collaterals
> - Posterior stabilised TKR
>   - Additional constraint through cam-post mechanism to substitute for absent PCL
>   - Provides no mediolateral constraint so requires functionally intact collaterals
> - Condylar constrained revision knee replacement ('high post posterior stabilised')
>   - Large central cam-post substitutes for PCL and provides a degree of mediolateral constraint
>   - Will allow for a degree of ligamentous laxity but not for a completely absent MCL
> - Rotating hinge
>   - Direct connection of femur to tibia removes the need for any functional collateral ligaments
>   - Rotating hinge design reduces the degree of torsion transmitted to interface
>   - Requires an intact extensor mechanism
> - Fixed hinge
>   - Rarely necessary; has significantly inferior survival compared to rotating hinge
>   - Useful in those with neuromuscular disorders
>   - Can be used to treat patellofemoral dysfunction following rotating hinge
>   - Requires an intact extensor mechanism

Anaesthesia and positioning

See 'Primary total knee replacement' (p. 279). The operation is likely to last longer than a primary knee replacement, leading to more physiological disturbance. It can be helpful to exsanguinate the leg after preparation and draping to save tourniquet time.

Surgical technique

Although many revision procedures can be performed via the medial parapatellar approach, as described in primary TKR, other extensile approaches may be required to gain adequate exposure.

Landmarks and incision

All scars should be marked with a sterile pen. If possible, a generous midline incision is used. If there are multiple longitudinal incisions in front of the knee, the most lateral scar should be used to avoid necrosis of the intervening strip of skin due to the fact that the blood supply passes from medial to lateral. The incision needs to be long enough to allow adequate exposure and avoid excessive skin stretching.

Superficial dissection

Skin flaps should be kept as thick as possible and should not be undermined. The quadriceps and patellar tendons should be defined. Identification of the correct tissue plane is easier if the incision is extended to an area previously untouched.

Deep dissection

Structures at risk

- The medial collateral ligament is at risk from aggressive synovectomy and medial release.
- The patellar tendon is usually thickened, tight and at risk of avulsion. The patellar tendon and quadriceps tendon should be thinned down by excision of any thickened fibrous tissue and the articulating surface of the patella should be exposed. If the patella does not evert or subluxate easily, one or more of the following measures needs to be performed.
- All other important structures around the knee are at greater risk of injury during revision surgery than in the primary procedure due to scar tissue, difficulty in exposure and stiffness or laxity.

The standard medial parapatellar approach is usually performed initially. It is usually necessary to perform an extensive synovectomy in order to improve exposure and to recreate the suprapatellar pouch and medial and lateral gutters. The fat pad is excised. Medial release should be performed to allow exposure of the tibia. There is usually a plane visible between the pseudocapsule and normal tissue, and this can be developed with knife or diathermy and the pseudocapsule carefully pulled away under tension. The PCL is usually sacrificed, this can be performed following implant removal.

Lateral parapatellar release

It is almost always necessary to perform some degree of lateral parapatellar release to allow eversion of the patella. It is usually beneficial to perform the lateral release early on. The release should be performed from deep to superficial and from distal to proximal, alongside the lateral border of the patellar tendon and lateral retinaculum. To reduce subsequent blood loss, it can be performed using diathermy. Full-thickness lateral release should be avoided if possible, but if this is necessary to gain exposure the superior lateral geniculate artery should be left intact and the lateral parapatellar retinaculum should be closed later.

Quadriceps snip

This involves a lateral incision into the quadriceps tendon from the proximal extent of the standard medial parapatellar approach (**Figure 11.7a**). A quadriceps snip can be performed in combination with a more distal lateral release, provided that the superior lateral geniculate artery is preserved.

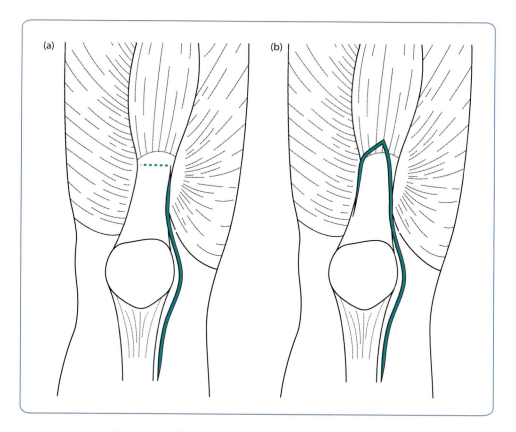

Figure 11.7 (a) Quadriceps snip; (b) quadriceps turndown.

Quadriceps turndown
This consists of an incision passing distally and laterally from the proximal extent of the standard medial parapatellar approach (**Figure 11.7b**). The superior lateral geniculate artery should be preserved. The inverted V thus formed can be closed as a Y, thereby advancing the quadriceps tendon and patella distally.

Tibial tubercle osteotomy
This requires an osteotomy of approximately 6 cm of the tibial tuberosity, hinging on the lateral soft tissues in order to maintain vascularity (**Figure 11.8**). The tuberosity can be proximalised in cases of patella baja. The osteotomy may be performed with a saw or sharp osteotome from the medial side and should be wide enough to include the patellar tendon insertion, tapering distally along with the anatomy of the tibial tubercle. It needs to be fixed with screws or wires at the end of the procedure.

Procedure
The ultimate goals of revision knee replacement are pain relief, functional stability and eradication of infection, if present. In order to achieve these goals, the important factors

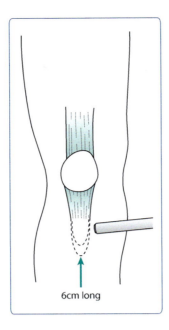

Figure 11.8 Tibial tubercle osteotomy (leaving the lateral soft tissues undisturbed).

are preservation of bone stock, reconstruction of defects, adequate fixation of implants, ligamentous balancing and restoration of the joint line.

Implant removal

Safe and careful implant and cement removal should involve preservation of as much bone stock as possible. It is necessary to use fine, sharp osteotomes (e.g. Lambotte osteotomes), and it may be helpful to have cement-splitting osteotomes, a thin saw blade, Gigli saw and burr available. If a modular polyethylene insert is present it can be removed prior to the cemented components. It is usually preferable to remove the femoral component first as this facilitates easier extraction of the tibial component. With adequate retraction, the bone-cement interface should be carefully disrupted with osteotomes of appropriate width. If the implant is well fixed it may be safer to disrupt the implant-cement interface and remove the cement separately. Only when fully loosened should the implant be removed with the appropriate extraction device using a longitudinal distraction force. The tibial component can be removed in a similar manner. The tibial component should never be 'levered' out of bone. It is usually necessary to remove the cement from around the tibial keel and stem with cement-splitting osteotomes or gouges. If a polyethylene patella button has been used it should only be removed if significantly worn, in cases of infection, or if there is a patellofemoral problem. Metal-backed patella components can be very difficult to remove and are often best left if possible.

Reconstruction

Following successful removal of implants and cement, any fibrous membrane on the distal femur and proximal tibia is carefully removed with a small, sharp curette and bone nibblers. Even in cases where infection is not suspected, multiple samples should be sent

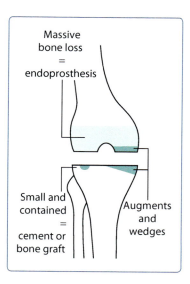

Figure 11.9 Reconstructive options for bone loss in revision knee surgery.

for microbiology using clean instruments. Ideally, the remaining bone surfaces should consist of trabecular bone to allow optimum cementation. Any small, contained, cavitatory defects can be filled with morsellised bone graft or cement but larger, uncontained, segmental defects need to be reconstructed with augments, wedges (**Figure 11.9**) or rarely, endoprosthetic replacement.

The tibia should be prepared first with the knee flexed, the proximal tibia exposed and subluxated anteriorly and the patella everted if possible. The canal is opened with a drill. Sequential reamers are used to the desired stem length until there is good endosteal engagement of the reamer. Using stable intramedullary referencing, which may be in the form of an intramedullary rod and sleeve, the proximal tibia is then resected to the correct level. If a tibial cutting jig is used with an inbuilt anteroposterior slope, the rotation should be referenced from the medial third of the tibial tubercle. Tibial resection should usually be conservative, but depends on the previous resection level and bone stock. If a flat, level cut cannot be achieved a wedge or augment may be used.

Attention is then turned to the femur. The canal is prepared as earlier. Distal femoral cuts are made with intramedullary referencing and a cutting jig. Distal femoral augments are used to prevent elevation of the joint line; if the condyles are resected at different levels, the additional resection must be compensated for by using a larger augment on that side. The femoral anterior, posterior and chamfer cuts are then performed with the cutting block positioned in the correct rotational orientation. This can be estimated from the transepicondylar axis. This is essential to ensuring a symmetrical flexion gap. Again, augments can be used to make up differences in resection levels of the posterior condyles. Thought must constantly be given to achieving equal flexion and extension gaps (see 'Primary total knee replacement', p. 279) and to restoration of the joint line. If the knee is looser in flexion than extension, the femoral component is upsized with posterior augmentation. If the knee is loose in extension compared with flexion, the distal femur is augmented. This is preferred to using a thicker insert and elevating the joint line. The level of the joint line should be approximately one finger breadth below the inferior pole of the patella or at the level of the meniscal scar. Femoral and tibial coverage and rotation are optimised; most systems allow the introduction of an offset between the stem and the component to facilitate this. Final trials should be performed with all trial stems, augments and wedges in place and the thickness of insert can be determined and final ligamentous releases performed. If the patella is to be revised, care must be taken with further resection. The femoral and tibial components are assembled – it can be useful to compare the completed implants to the trials to ensure no errors have been made prior to implantation. Usually, the tibia is implanted first and a separate batch of cement is used for the femur.

Two-stage revision for infection
Revising a TKR for infection is even more challenging. Two-stage revision is the current gold standard but single-stage revision is being used increasingly in cases where the soft tissues and microbiological profile allow it. Single-stage revision has better functional outcomes and exposes the patient to less surgical and anaesthetic risk. Single-stage revision should be approached in the same way as two-stage revision, with a full re-drape and change of gowns and instruments after the debridement.

At the first stage, all implants and cement are removed. Aggressive debridement is performed with excision of all infected-looking tissue, and multiple fluid and tissue samples are sent to microbiology and histopathology. The knee is thoroughly washed out. It may be helpful to perform preliminary bone cuts at this stage. A pre-moulded antibiotic-impregnated cement spacer is inserted and lightly cemented in place to avoid displacement. Appropriate antibiotics are continued and inflammatory markers checked on a regular basis. The knee should be mobilised to preserve range of motion if possible. When confident that infection has been eradicated, the second-stage revision can be performed with implantation of the definitive prosthesis. Occasionally, if not settling, the first stage may need to be repeated.

Closure
Routine cases can be closed in a similar fashion to primary knee replacements. Occasionally, especially after repeated revision cases or following infection, closure can be difficult and it may even be necessary to consider gastrocnemius muscle flap coverage and skin grafting, where the assistance of a plastic surgeon may be required.

Postoperative care and instructions
If a standard approach has been used, in aseptic cases, the postoperative regimen is similar to that following primary knee replacement. The results of microbiology samples must be obtained.

If a quadriceps turndown or tibial tubercle osteotomy has been performed, flexion should be limited for approximately 6 weeks to allow the tendon or osteotomy to heal and active quadriceps extension should be avoided.

Recommended references

Morgan-Jones R, Oussedik SIS, Graichen H, Haddad FS. Zonal fixation in revision knee arthroplasty. *Bone Joint J.* 2015;**97–B**:147–149.

Saleh KJ, Rand JA, Ries MD et al. Revision total knee arthroplasty. *J Bone Joint Surg Am.* 2003;**85**(**Suppl 1**).

Younger AS, Duncan CP, Masri BA. Surgical exposures in revision total knee arthroplasty. *J Am Acad Orthop Surg.* 1998;**6**:55–64.

Patellofemoral replacement

Preoperative planning

Indications

Patellofemoral replacement is indicated in the treatment of pain from isolated patellofemoral osteoarthritis when non-operative or more conservative operative management has failed.

The lateral facet of the patella and trochlea are most commonly involved, and there is commonly some degree of dysplasia, malalignment or laxity present as a predisposing factor.

Contraindications

General contraindications to knee replacement (see 'Primary total knee replacement', p. 279) include

- Tibiofemoral osteoarthritis
- Inflammatory arthritis

Consent and risks

- See 'Primary total knee replacement' (p. 279).
- Significantly higher rate of revision at 10 years compared to primary TKR (the National Joint Registry for England and Wales reports a 10-year revision rate of 18.7%).
- Specific problems with the patellofemoral articulation include patella fracture, lateral subluxation, impingement, anterior knee pain.

Operative planning

Recent weightbearing anteroposterior, lateral and skyline radiographs must be available, and Schuss or Rosenberg views may be helpful. The Rosenberg view is a posteroanterior weightbearing view with the knee in 45° of flexion (the Schuss view is the same with the knee at 30°). Both views are more sensitive in detecting subtle tibiofemoral osteoarthritis, particularly on the lateral side. It is essential that the symptoms and signs should be consistent with patellofemoral osteoarthritis. Some surgeons consider it necessary to perform magnetic resonance imaging (MRI) or arthroscopy to assess the rest of the joint surfaces, although in most cases the decision can be made from the history, examination and plain radiographs. Occasionally, however, the final decision is made at the time of operation.

Choice of implants

Current designs of patellofemoral replacement are 'onlay' designs, and their geometry is based on existing designs of TKR. The most popular design in use in the United Kingdom, the Avon (Stryker, Newbury, United Kingdom) is based on the geometry of the Kinemax TKR and has a symmetrical trochlear groove. Others are based on more modern TKR designs and are sided. Aside from that, systems vary in their workflows, methods of femoral preparation and instrumentation. Ultimately, the decision on which implant to use rests with the surgeon and the unit.

Anaesthesia and positioning

Anaesthesia, positioning, preparation and draping are similar to that for primary TKR.

Surgical technique

Patellofemoral replacement is usually performed using a medial parapatellar approach.

Landmarks and incision

The position of the patella, patellar tendon and tibial tubercle should all be noted. An anterior midline longitudinal incision is made with the knee in flexion. It is not usually necessary to extend the excision as far distally as in TKR, but it needs to be long enough to allow eversion of the patella and adequate exposure of the distal femur.

Superficial dissection

The medial and lateral skin, subcutaneous fat and deep fascia should be reflected in a thick flap to allow exposure of the quadriceps tendon, medial patellar retinaculum and patellar tendon and to allow mobilisation of the patella.

Deep dissection

Structures at risk

- The anterior horns of the medial and lateral menisci should be carefully preserved, unlike with TKR where they are sacrificed. The incision at the level of the joint line must be done with great care not to extend into meniscal tissue.
- The medial femoral condyle can be damaged during the medial parapatellar approach.
- If the patellar tendon is contracted, there may be a risk of patellar tendon avulsion from the tibial tubercle during eversion of the patella. This can be prevented by extending the deep dissection proximally, dividing any lateral plicae and performing a lateral parapatellar release to allow eversion of the patella.

The medial parapatellar incision is extended from the quadriceps tendon proximally, through the medial parapatellar retinaculum and along the medial border of the patellar tendon distally. There should be an adequate cuff to ensure a good soft tissue repair. The retropatellar fat pad can be incised or partially excised to facilitate eversion of the patella, and it may be necessary to perform a lateral parapatellar release. Osteophytes may be debrided at this stage.

Procedure

The aims of the operation are pain relief, good patella tracking and patellofemoral stability. This is achieved by accurate bone resection, correct alignment of implants and parapatellar soft tissue balancing.

Patella

To resurface the patella, the knee should be extended with the patella fully everted and held with a clamp. Peripheral osteophytes can be removed with a bone nibbler to demarcate the articular surface. It is often difficult to accurately assess the amount of patella to be resected, as the articular cartilage wear is usually not uniform. If the median ridge is of normal height, the thickness of the patella should be measured, and the amount of bone and cartilage removed should correspond to the thickness of the implant. If there is severe damage, a measured resection technique is unreliable. In this situation, the insertions of the quadriceps tendon and the lateral border of the patellar tendon can be exposed carefully with a diathermy and used as reliable landmarks. Resection 2 mm above this plane results in two-thirds of the original patella thickness being left behind. Resecting too little bone runs the risk of overstuffing the knee and if a sclerotic surface is left behind, fixation is compromised, whereas resecting too much increases the risk of fracture. A clamp is then applied and used as a cutting guide. The amount of resection should be carefully inspected and adjusted if necessary. There will usually be more bone resected from the medial than lateral facet, and the remaining cut surface may be sclerotic. This can be roughened with a saw or burr and small drill holes made to improve cement fixation; a partial lateral facetectomy may be performed if there is significant overhang. The patella is then subluxated or everted and the knee flexed to allow the femur to be prepared. Care must be taken to avoid fracture of the patella during flexion if the remaining patella is thin.

Femur

To expose the distal femur, two Hohmann retractors are placed medially and laterally. The anterior surface of the distal femur is exposed by excising the overlying synovium with coagulating diathermy. The femoral component should sit flush with the anterior distal femur without notching, with the correct degree of rotation to ensure restoration of the lateral ridge and good tracking. The implant should not be situated too far distal within the notch, as this can cause impingement and catching of the patella in full flexion. Intra- or extramedullary referencing may be used to determine the position of the implant in the coronal plane; rotation may be based on femoral landmarks (such as the transepicondylar axis or Whiteside's line) or the long axis of the tibia, depending on the system used.

Trials are then performed and tracking assessed. Final adjustments and preparations can then be made including lateral parapatellar release if necessary. Components are cemented in place.

Closure
The knee should be closed in flexion in a similar manner to a primary TKR. Again, the use or not of drains is a surgical decision, but drain use is more frequently indicated if a lateral release has been performed.

Postoperative instructions
These are the same as for primary TKR.

Recommended references
Odgaard A, Madsen F, Kristensen PW et al. The Mark Coventry Award: Patellofemoral Arthroplasty Results in Better Range of Movement and Early Patient-reported Outcomes Than TKA. *Clin Orthop Relat Res.* 2018;**476(1)**:87–100.

Metcalfe AJ, Ahern N, Hassaballa MA et al. The Avon patellofemoral arthroplasty. *Bone Joint J.* 2018; **100–B**:1162–1167.

Unicompartmental knee replacement
Preoperative planning
Indications
Unicompartmental knee replacement (UKR) is indicated in the treatment of painful end-stage osteoarthritis when non-operative management has failed. The following criteria must be met:

- Bone-on-bone osteoarthritis or osteonecrosis in a single compartment
- Presence of full-thickness cartilage in the remaining compartment
- Varus or valgus deformity must be correctable to normal
- Fixed flexion deformity less than 10°
- Functionally intact knee ligaments

Contraindications
- General contraindications to knee replacement (see 'Primary total knee replacement', p. 279).
- Inflammatory arthritis.
- Relative contraindications are controversial. Some authors (most notably the Oxford group) recommend offering UKR to all patients in whom the pathoanatomy is suitable, with no restrictions based on patient factors. Others have suggested contraindications including obesity, youth, high activity levels, the presence of chondrocalcinosis, the presence of generalised knee pain or the presence of a lateral osteophyte (in medial UKR). A number of clinical studies from various centres have been performed which suggest that these factors are unimportant in determining outcome following UKR.
- Patellofemoral osteoarthritis is particularly controversial, and some surgeons suggest strongly that UKR should not be performed in patients with PFJ disease. Again, there are several studies demonstrating no effect of clinical or radiological evidence of patellofemoral osteoarthritis (aside from severe lateral wear) on outcome.

Consent and risks

- Most risks and complications of primary TKR can occur in UKR.
- Medial knee pain may occur and usually resolves with time. Persistent anteromedial knee pain may be associated with changes in loading of the medial bone or damage to the MCL intraoperatively.
- The rate of revision of UKR is two to three times that of TKR. This is partly due to additional mechanisms of failure (including progression of osteoarthritis) and partly due to a lower threshold for revision of UKR. High-volume centres report revision rates similar to those of TKR.
- In common with TKR, most patients undergoing UKR never undergo revision surgery. Outcomes of revision of UKR to TKR are closer to the outcomes of a revision TKR than to those of a primary TKR. For these reasons UKR should be performed in those with end-stage disease and should not be considered as a temporising measure for TKR.
- Dislocation of the insert can occur with mobile bearings, especially if ACL laxity is present.
- Revision of UKR usually results in a 'primary' knee replacement but bone loss around the tibial baseplate may necessitate stems and wedges.

Operative planning

Recent weightbearing anteroposterior, lateral and skyline radiographs must be available, and Rosenberg views can be helpful in identifying subtle disease in the preserved compartment. Some surgeons advocate the use of valgus and varus stress views to determine suitability for UKR. *Anteromedial arthritis* is the most common indication; the presence of an anterior wear scar on the lateral radiograph implies the presence of an intact ACL (**Figure 11.10**). Some surgeons advocate the use of MRI or arthroscopy to determine eligibility for UKR, but in most cases the decision can be made by the history, examination and plain radiographs. However, the final decision is made at the time of operation.

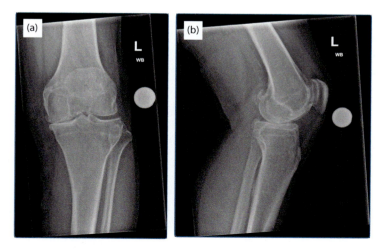

Figure 11.10 Anteromedial arthritis. Note the anterior wear scar on the lateral radiograph.

Choice of implant

All implants in UKR have the same aim, which is to restore the affected joint surface and recreate native kinematics by reconstructing the joint with the minimum of constraint. To do this there are two main design rationales. Most designs of UKR have a fixed bearing, flat tibial component, which may be all-polyethylene or metal-backed, and a polyradial femoral component. The most commonly used UKR, the Oxford Knee (Zimmer Biomet, Bridgend, United Kingdom) uses a different rationale, with a spherical femoral component and a mobile polyethylene bearing, which has a highly conforming articulation with the femur on the superior surface and a flat-on-flat articulation with the metal tibial base plate on the underside. Proposed advantages of the mobile bearing include improved wear properties and kinematics, but this comes with a risk of dislocation of the bearing, which occurs in just under 1% of cases in large series. Most designs of UKR are cemented but cementless fixation is becoming increasingly popular and has excellent published results.

Anaesthesia and positioning

This is essentially similar to that described for TKR. However, as UKR is usually performed via a less invasive approach, the use of regional anaesthesia can be avoided, if desired, by the administration of local anaesthetic into the wound and deep tissues. Some surgeons prefer to use a leg holder with the knee flexed, the hip abducted and the leg over the side of the operating table or the foot of the table removed. This allows the knee to be stressed and can improve exposure.

Surgical technique
Medial unicompartmental knee replacement
Landmarks and incision
With the knee flexed, a longitudinal incision is made along the medial border of the patellar tendon from patella to tibial tubercle and can be extended proximally or distally as required.

Dissection
The incision is deepened along the same line and the medial border of the patella and tendon identified. It is continued along the medial border of the patellar tendon and proximally up to the medial parapatellar retinaculum. The medial capsule is dissected subperiosteally off the proximal tibia to gain exposure to the medial compartment. The dissection should not extend beyond the anteromedial corner and should not involve any release of the MCL. The medial portion of the fat pad can be excised. The anterior two-thirds of the medial meniscus can be excised at this point, with the posterior horn removed later following bone cuts. This should give adequate exposure of the medial compartment, and it should be possible to inspect the ACL, patellofemoral joint and lateral compartment.

This operation can usually be performed through a relatively minimally invasive approach, with the skin incision being used as a 'mobile window' to gain access to the femur or tibia with varying degrees of knee flexion. However, if exposure is difficult, the skin incision and deep dissection should be extended to allow the patella to be subluxated laterally, although it should not usually be necessary to involve the quadriceps tendon or vastus medialis.

Procedure

> ### Structures at risk
> - The MCL must be protected throughout.
> - The ACL is at risk during the sagittal tibial cut with the reciprocating saw and should be retracted.
> - The patellar tendon can be damaged during reaming of the femoral condyle.

Osteophytes on the medial tibial plateau and femoral condyle are excised. The exact nature and sequence of bone preparation are dependent on the implant used and manufacturer's recommendations but the aims are restoration (or slight undercorrection) of pre-disease alignment, equal flexion/extension gaps, optimum range-of-motion and good fixation of implants.

The tibial cut is usually made first, with extramedullary referencing and a tibial cutting guide. The vertical cut is performed, with a reciprocating saw, just medial to the ACL insertion. The horizontal cut is made with an oscillating saw, perpendicular to the long axis of the tibia. The wedge of tibia can then be removed with a Kocher forceps.

The femoral preparation uses femoral intramedullary alignment and the tibial cut as a combined reference (**Figure 11.11**). The flexion gap is usually set by making the posterior condylar cut first. The mechanism of setting the extension gap varies by implant and can involve saw cuts or reaming.

Final trials and preparations can then be made and the definitive implants inserted. If there is impingement of the bearing anteriorly on the femoral condyle in full extension, trimming of the condyle can be performed to allow clearance.

Closure
Closure is in layers, with continuous absorbable sutures and a continuous subcuticular suture or staples to the skin. It is not usually necessary to use a drain.

Lateral unicompartmental knee replacement

This is much less commonly performed than medial UKR. It can be performed via either a midline approach with the patella everted, or a direct lateral parapatellar approach. The procedure itself is analogous to that of medial unicompartmental surgery, although some surgeons use a window in the patellar tendon to perform the vertical saw cut. Due to the increased excursion of the lateral compartment during knee movement, and the relative laxity of the lateral compartment in flexion the rate of bearing dislocation is significantly higher in mobile bearing UKR, and fixed bearings are often used.

Postoperative care and instructions

Patients should be encouraged to mobilise the knee and bear weight as quickly as possible. Recovery is significantly faster than after TKR and patients leave hospital on average a day earlier. The use of day-case UKR is increasing around the world.

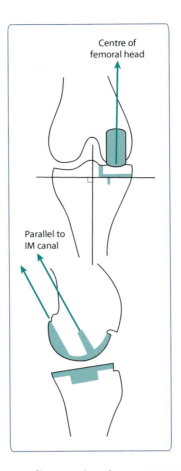

Figure 11.11 Component alignment in unicompartmental knee replacement.

Recommended references

Argenson JN, Blanc G, Aubianiac JM, Paratte S. Modern unicompartmental knee arthroplasty with cement: A concise follow-up, at a mean of twenty years, of a previous report. *J Bone Joint Surg Am.* 2013;**95**:905–909.

Liddle AD, Judge A, Pandit H, Murray DW. Adverse outcomes after total and unicompartmental knee replacement: A study of 101,330 matched patients from the National Joint Registry for England and Wales. *Lancet.* 2014;**384**:1437–1445.

Pandit H, Jenkins C, Gill HS et al. Unnecessary contraindications for mobile-bearing unicompartmental knee replacement. *J Bone Joint Surg Br.* 2011;**93**:622–628.

Distal femoral osteotomy
Preoperative planning

Distal femoral osteotomy is used to correct valgus deformity of the knee and consists of a varus osteotomy which may either be a medial closing wedge or a lateral opening wedge. The authors' preference is the lateral opening wedge varus osteotomy and this is described next.

Indications

Distal femoral osteotomy is indicated in the treatment of pain and deformity caused by valgus osteoarthritis in relatively young patients when non-operative management has failed.

It can also be used to correct malunion following supracondylar fractures of the femur.

Contraindications

- Distal lower limb ischaemia
- Significant medial or patellofemoral osteoarthritis
- Flexion limited to less than 90°
- Fixed flexion deformity greater than 15°
- Inflammatory arthritis
- Osteoporosis
- Inability to comply with the rehabilitation protocol

Consent and risks

- Delayed/non-union
- Inadequate/loss of correction
- Failure of fixation
- Stiffness
- Iliotibial band irritation
- Progression of arthritis may require revision to TKR. Although this can be relatively straightforward, it may be advisable to remove the metalwork at a separate operation prior to performing TKR
- There may be difficulty in achieving the desired valgus intramedullary alignment of the distal femoral bone cut following distal femoral osteotomy
- Infection
- Bleeding
- Venous thromboembolism
- Neurovascular injury

Operative planning

Recent weightbearing anteroposterior, lateral and skyline radiographs must be available. Long-leg alignment films must be performed and stress views may be helpful. It is essential that the symptoms and signs should correlate with radiographic findings. It is sometimes necessary to perform MRI or arthroscopy to assess the integrity of the ligaments and the state of the joint surfaces. Although instability has historically been thought of as a contraindication to osteotomy, it may be performed as a precursor to or in association with ligament reconstruction in malaligned ligament deficient knees. Accuracy of correction is of paramount importance and the osteotomy must be planned using templating software; there may be a role for patient-specific instrumentation. The rule of thumb is that each millimetre of opening in the coronal plane corresponds to 1° of correction.

Anaesthesia and positioning

General anaesthesia is used. Regional anaesthesia can be avoided, if desired, by the administration of local anaesthetic into the wound and deep tissues. The patient is positioned supine on the operating table. Provided that there are no contraindications, a tourniquet is applied as proximally as possible. An image intensifier is needed throughout the operation.

Prior to preparation and draping, in order to reference the mechanical axis of the limb, the centre of the femoral head can be screened with the image intensifier and a radio-opaque electrocardiogram (ECG) sticker is placed on the skin directly overlying the centre of the femoral head. If a tri-cortical wedge of iliac crest bone graft is to be used, the iliac crest must be prepared, draped and exposed to allow bone graft harvesting.

Surgical technique

The aim of a varus osteotomy is to correct valgus malalignment, shift the mechanical axis to the medial compartment and offload the diseased lateral compartment (**Figure 11.12**). The goal is to overcorrect to a tibiofemoral angle of 0°. Traditionally, a distal femoral osteotomy is preferred for varus osteotomy as this more reliably achieves a horizontal joint line.

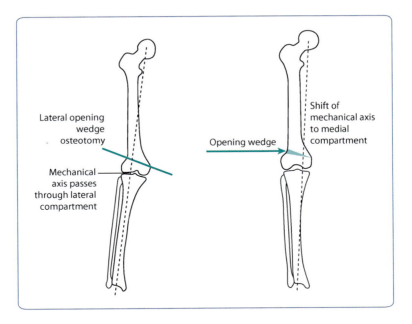

Figure 11.12 Lateral opening wedge distal femoral osteotomy in a valgus knee.

Landmarks and incision

An opening wedge osteotomy is performed via a lateral approach to the distal femur. A longitudinal incision is made over the lateral aspect of the thigh in the supracondylar region. Correct placement of the incision site is ensured by screening with the image intensifier.

Dissection

The incision is deepened along the same line until the fascia lata is exposed. The fascia lata is split and the vastus lateralis can either be divided or incised and lifted off the femur at its posterior border. Any blood vessels encountered should be coagulated and subperiosteal dissection is continued anteriorly and posteriorly around the femur. Insertion of the appropriate retractors anteriorly and posteriorly gives good exposure of the distal femur.

Procedure

Structures at risk

- The popliteal artery must be protected by the subperiosteal retractor throughout the procedure. The risk of major arterial injury may be reduced by performing the osteotomy with the knee in flexion as this moves the artery away from the posterior femur.
- The medial distal femoral cortex should be left intact. If breached, a staple can be inserted to maintain stability.

The ECG sticker placed over the femoral head is palpated through the drapes and an alignment rod can be placed to lie between this point and the centre of the articular surface of the ankle joint. When the osteotomy is opened by the correct amount, the mechanical axis is shifted to the desired point, i.e. the centre of the medial tibial plateau. This improves the efficiency of the use of fluoroscopy, minimises X-ray exposure and helps to minimise operation time.

A first guide wire is inserted with the power driver from the lateral cortex in a medial and slightly caudal direction. The wire should emerge in the metaphyseal region of the distal femur at the junction of the medial femoral condyle and the supracondylar ridge. A second wire is then introduced to lie exactly superimposed on the first true anteroposterior fluoroscopic image, indicating that the wires are exactly parallel to the joint surface. This second wire can be introduced through a parallel guide.

The osteotomy can then be performed with an oscillating saw, using either the guide wires or cutting jig to help control the saw. The saw is placed on the proximal side of the wires and advanced approximately two-thirds of the distance across the femur under fluoroscopic control. Care must be taken not to penetrate the medial cortex. The osteotome is then used to complete the osteotomy through the anterior and posterior cortices but should stop approximately 1 cm short of the medial cortex. The blade of the osteotome can be marked at a level where penetration of the far cortex will not occur, and this marking can be observed carefully as the osteotome advances.

The osteotomy is then opened with distraction osteotomes using a screwdriver under fluoroscopic control. When the osteotomy is opened, metal wedges can be gently inserted into the osteotomy to the desired level. The amount of correction can be checked with the image intensifier using the alignment rod as previously described. A locking plate with interposition wedge of the desired size is then inserted into the osteotomy in the correct position and screws inserted and checked with fluoroscopy. The opening wedge can be filled with bone graft or calcium triphosphate wedges.

Closure

Closure is performed in layers with continuous absorbable sutures and a continuous subcuticular suture or staples to the skin. It is not usually necessary to use a drain.

Postoperative care and instructions

Regular neurovascular observations should be performed and the patient carefully monitored for signs of compartment syndrome. Adequate analgesia is administered. Mechanical and chemical thromboprophylaxis is recommended. Two further doses of prophylactic antibiotics are administered at 8 hours and 16 hours postoperatively. The wound should be inspected and radiographs performed prior to discharge should be checked. If the fixation is stable, range-of-motion exercises are encouraged from the first postoperative day. Patients should remain non-weightbearing in a hinged knee brace for 2 weeks. Repeat radiographs are taken and clips removed at this stage. Touch weightbearing only is commenced in a hinged knee brace for a further 4 weeks. If radiographs are satisfactory at 6 weeks, partial weightbearing can be commenced and if the osteotomy has united at 12 weeks the patient can build up to full weightbearing.

Recommended references

Brouwer RW, Raaij van TM, Bierma-Zeinstra SM et al. Osteotomy for treating knee osteoarthritis. *Cochrane Database Syst Rev.* 2007;(18):CD004019.

Cameron JI, McCauley JC, Kermanshahi AY, Bugbee WD. Lateral opening-wedge distal femoral osteotomy: Pain relief, functional improvement, and survivorship at 5 years. *Clin Orthop Relat Res.* 2015;**473**:2009–2015.

Wylie JD, Scheiderer B, Obopilwe E et al. The effect of lateral opening wedge distal femoral varus osteotomy on tibiofemoral contact mechanics through knee flexion. *Am J Sports Med.* 2018;**46**:3237–3244.

Proximal tibial osteotomy

Preoperative planning

Proximal tibial osteotomy is used to correct varus deformity of the knee and consists of a valgus osteotomy which may either be a lateral closing wedge or a medial opening wedge. The authors' preference is the medial opening wedge valgus osteotomy; this is described later.

Indications

Proximal tibial osteotomy is indicated in the treatment of pain and deformity caused by varus osteoarthritis in relatively young patients when non-operative management has failed.

Contraindications

- Distal lower limb ischaemia
- Significant lateral or patellofemoral osteoarthritis
- Significant bone loss from the medial tibial plateau
- Flexion limited to less than 90°
- Fixed flexion deformity greater than 15°
- Inflammatory arthritis
- Osteoporosis
- Inability to comply with rehabilitation protocol

Consent and risks

Progression of arthritis may require revision to TKR. Although this can be relatively straightforward, it may be advisable to remove the metalwork prior to performing TKR. There may be problems caused by patella baja. Other specific complications include

- Infection
- Bleeding
- Venous thromboembolism
- Common peroneal nerve injury (usually associated with fibular osteotomy in closing wedge proximal tibial osteotomy)
- Major arterial injury
- Compartment syndrome
- Lateral tibial plateau fracture
- Delayed/non-union
- Inadequate/loss of correction
- Overcorrection
- Failure of fixation
- Stiffness

Operative planning

This is the same as for distal femoral osteotomy.

Anaesthesia and positioning

This is the same as for distal femoral osteotomy.

Surgical technique

The aim of a valgus osteotomy is to correct malalignment, shift the mechanical axis to the lateral compartment and offload the diseased medial compartment (**Figure 11.13**). The goal is to correct to a tibiofemoral angle of 5°–9°. The advantages of an opening wedge valgus osteotomy include the fact that there is no need for a fibular osteotomy, there is more control over the correction and it may correct instability in anterior or posterior cruciate ligament deficiency by adjustment of the tibial slope. It has the disadvantage of creating a degree of patella baja.

Landmarks and incision

A medial opening wedge valgus osteotomy is performed via an anteromedial approach to the proximal tibia. A longitudinal or oblique incision is made over the anteromedial aspect of the proximal lower leg in the region of the insertion of the pes anserinus and 3 cm medial to the lower border of the tibial tubercle.

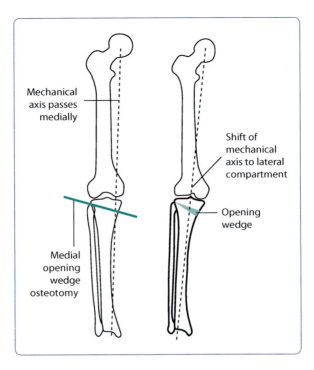

Figure 11.13 Medial opening wedge proximal tibial osteotomy in a varus knee.

Dissection

The incision is deepened until the fascia overlying the pes is exposed. The fascia is incised and the pes anserinus is reflected posteriorly, with the superficial medial collateral ligament. Any blood vessels encountered should be coagulated and subperiosteal dissection is continued anteriorly and posteriorly around the tibia. Insertion of the appropriate retractors anteriorly and posteriorly gives good exposure of the proximal tibia and protects the patellar tendon anteriorly with the popliteal artery and tibial nerve posteriorly.

Procedure

Structures at risk

- Popliteal artery: The risk of major arterial injury may be reduced by performing the osteotomy with the knee in flexion.
- Patellar tendon.
- Superficial MCL.
- The lateral tibial cortex should be left intact. If breached, a staple should be inserted laterally to maintain stability.
- The lateral tibial plateau can be fractured if the anterior cortex has not been fully osteotomised prior to distraction of the osteotomy. If this occurs, the osteotomy should be advanced and the fracture stabilised with one or more interfragmentary screws from the lateral side.

The ECG sticker placed over the femoral head is palpated through the drapes and an alignment rod can be placed to lie between this point and the centre of the articular surface of the ankle joint. When the osteotomy is opened by the correct amount, the mechanical axis is shifted to the desired point, i.e. at the junction of the medial two-thirds and lateral third of the articular surface of the tibia. Using an alignment rod to show the mechanical axis improves the efficiency of the use of fluoroscopy, minimises X-ray exposure and helps to minimise operation time. It is imperative that a 'true' anteroposterior radiograph of the knee be obtained in order to gauge the anteroposterior slope of the tibia.

A first guide wire is inserted, with the power driver, from the medial cortex in a lateral and slightly cephalad direction. The wire should emerge in the metaphyseal region of the proximal tibia at the level of the tip of the fibula head. A second wire is then introduced to lie exactly superimposed on the first on a true anteroposterior fluoroscopic image, indicating that the wires are exactly parallel to the joint surface. This second wire can be introduced through a parallel guide.

The osteotomy can then be performed with an oscillating saw, using either the guide wires or a cutting jig to help control the saw. The saw is placed on the distal side of the wires and advanced approximately two-thirds of the distance across the tibia under fluoroscopic control. Care must be taken not to penetrate the lateral cortex. The osteotome is then used to complete the osteotomy through the anterior and posterior cortices but should stop approximately 1 cm short of the lateral cortex. The blade of the osteotome can be marked at a level where penetration of the far cortex will not occur, and this marking can be observed carefully as the osteotome advances.

The osteotomy may pass above the insertion of the patellar tendon, but if it crosses the anterior tibial cortex at the level of the tibial tuberosity it may be necessary to make a step cut beneath the tuberosity from the transverse osteotomy proximally to ensure that the tuberosity and patellar tendon insertion remain intact (**Figure 11.14**).

The osteotomy is then opened with distraction osteotomes using a screwdriver under fluoroscopic control. When the osteotomy is opened, metal wedges can be gently inserted into the osteotomy to the desired level. The amount of correction can be checked with the image intensifier using the alignment rod as previously described. A locking plate with interposition wedge of the desired size is then inserted into the osteotomy in the correct position and screws inserted and checked with fluoroscopy. The opening wedge can be filled with bone graft or calcium triphosphate wedges. Autograft is still advocated for larger corrections or revision procedures.

Closure

Closure is undertaken in layers with continuous absorbable sutures and a continuous subcuticular suture or staples to the skin. It is not usually necessary to use a drain.

Postoperative care and instructions

These are the same as for distal femoral osteotomy.

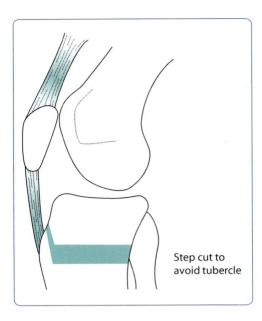

Figure 11.14 A step cut to avoid tibial tuberosity.

Recommended references

Brinkman JM, Lobenhoffer P, Agneskirchner JD et al. Osteotomies around the knee: Patient selection, stability of fixation and bone healing in high tibial osteotomies. *J Bone Joint Surg Br.* 2008;**90**:1548–1557.

Coventry MB, Ilstrup DM, Wallrichs SL. Proximal tibial osteotomy. A critical long-term study of eighty-seven cases. *J Bone Joint Surg Am.* 1993;**75**:196–201.

Niinimäki TT, Eskelinen A, Mann BS, Junnila M, Ohtonen P, Leppilahti J. Survivorship of high tibial osteotomy in the treatment of osteoarthritis of the knee: Finnish registry-based study of 3195 knees. *J Bone Joint Surg Br.* 2012;**94**:1517–1521.

Knee arthrodesis
Preoperative planning
Indications

The most common indication for knee arthrodesis is as a salvage procedure in failed revision knee replacement either where infection has been resistant to eradication or when there is a non-functioning extensor mechanism.

In the past and currently still in some parts of the world, knee arthrodesis is more commonly performed in patients with postinfective arthritis, tuberculosis, poliomyelitis and severe trauma.

Contraindications

- Critical arterial ischaemia
- Extensive bone loss (relative)
- Ipsilateral hip arthrodesis (relative)

> **Consent and risks**
>
> - Infection (or failure to eradicate existing infection)
> - Bleeding
> - Venous thromboembolism
> - Wound problems
> - Neurovascular injury
> - Fractures
> - Delayed or non-union
> - Pain
> - Immobility
> - Risk of subsequent amputation
> - Increased risk of osteoarthritis in other joints of the lower limbs

Operative planning

The indication for arthrodesis, severity of bone loss and adequacy of soft tissue coverage all need to be taken into account prior to deciding on whether the arthrodesis should be a single or staged procedure or an intramedullary or extramedullary fixation and whether it is necessary to enlist the help of a plastic surgeon. The patient should be thoroughly counselled before the operation.

Anaesthesia and positioning

See 'Revision total knee replacement' (p. 293).

Surgical technique

This depends on indication, type of fixation and need for bone grafting.

Landmarks and incision

A longitudinal, anterior midline incision is used, usually through a previous TKR scar.

Dissection

The quadriceps tendon and patellar tendon are split and a patellectomy performed. A synovectomy can be carried out and ligaments released or divided to gain exposure.

Procedure

The goals of arthrodesis are pain relief, eradication of infection and sound bony fusion in the correct alignment. In order to achieve these goals the important factors are good apposition of healthy bone surfaces, preservation of bone stock and stable fixation with compression.

Implants are removed as described in the section 'Revision total knee replacement' (p. 293). It is important to preserve as much bone as possible. Bone surfaces must be viable. In the presence of infection, it is usually desirable to perform a two-stage procedure with the first stage involving thorough debridement, insertion of an antibiotic-impregnated cement spacer and temporary fixation. The second stage involves the definitive arthrodesis. This is commonly achieved in one of two ways.

External fixation
The tibia is cut perpendicular to the long axis. The femur is cut to enable apposition at approximately 15° of flexion, 7° valgus and 10° external rotation. Bone graft may be used if desired. Compression must be achieved with the external fixator. Any form of external fixator can be used, from simple monoaxial fixators to fine wire frames.

Intramedullary fixation
Bone cuts are made as described earlier. The femoral and tibial intramedullary canals are reamed. The distal femur/proximal tibia can be reamed in a concave/convex fashion to increase contact surface area. Fixation can be achieved either with a long nail or with a two-part nail with a locking device between the femur and tibia which can also provide compression, correct alignment and restore length in cases with significant bone loss. The nail can be locked proximally and distally.

Closure
In some cases closure can be difficult. Occasionally, especially after repeated revision cases or following infection, closure can be such a challenge that it may even be necessary to consider gastrocnemius muscle flap coverage and skin grafting, where the assistance of a plastic surgeon may be required.

Postoperative care and instructions
The amount of weightbearing allowed depends on the stability of fixation, but generally touch weightbearing should be commenced immediately, gradually built up to partial weightbearing over approximately 6 weeks and to full weightbearing over the next 6 weeks.

Recommended references
Conway JD, Mont MA, Bezwada HP. Arthrodesis of the knee. *J Bone Joint Surg Am.* 2004;**86**:835–848.
White CJ, Palmer AJR, Rodriguez-Merchan EC. External fixation vs intramedullary nailing for knee arthrodesis after failed infected total knee arthroplasty: A systematic review and meta-analysis. *J Arthroplasty.* 2018;**33**:1288–1295.
Wiedel JD. Salvage of infected total knee fusion: The last option. *Clin Orthop Relat Res* 2002;**(404)**:139–142.

Viva questions

1. What are the risks and complications of TKR?
2. What are the contraindications to TKR?
3. Which TKR would you choose and why?
4. Discuss the advantages and disadvantages of posterior cruciate ligament retaining and sacrificing TKR.
5. Describe how you would address an imbalance in flexion/extension gaps.
6. What releases would you perform to correct alignment in a valgus knee?
7. How do you deal with a fixed flexion deformity during TKR?
8. What measures do you take to ensure correct patella tracking in primary TKR?
9. How would you manage a patient with a painful knee replacement?
10. Describe the modes of failure of TKR.
11. What extensile approaches are available in revision knee replacement?
12. What is your rationale for choosing an implant in revision knee replacement?
13. What are the treatment options for a 50-year-old man with medial compartment osteoarthritis?
14. What criteria need to be met for a medial UKR?
15. How would you select the ideal patient for a patellofemoral replacement?
16. How would you ensure adequate realignment in proximal tibial osteotomy?
17. Why is a distal femoral osteotomy preferred to proximal tibial osteotomy in a valgus knee?
18. Discuss the pros and cons of opening versus closing wedge proximal tibial osteotomy.
19. What are the indications for knee arthrodesis?
20. Describe the general principles and fixation options in arthrodesis.

12 Soft Tissue Surgery of the Knee

Stephen Key, Jonathan Miles and Richard Carrington

Knee arthroscopy	321	Posterolateral corner reconstruction	353
Arthroscopic meniscal knee surgery	328	Posterior cruciate ligament reconstruction	356
Lateral patellar retinaculum release	332	Medial collateral ligament reconstruction	360
Patellofemoral instability	334	Viva questions	365
Cartilage reconstruction surgery	339		
Anterior cruciate ligament reconstruction	342		

	Range of motion	Position of arthrodesis
Flexion	140°	0°–20°
Extension	0°	(10° external rotation and 5°–8° valgus)

Knee arthroscopy

Preoperative planning

Indications

Knee arthroscopy is used as a diagnostic and interventional tool in a wide variety of conditions. Because of advances in other imaging modalities, particularly magnetic resonance imaging (MRI), it is becoming less common for arthroscopy to be used for diagnosis alone. The frequent indications include:

- Meniscal tears
- Cruciate ligament injury
- Chondral defects
- Removal of loose bodies
- Washout of sepsis
- Synovectomy, including cases of pigmented villonodular synovitis
- Patella realignment procedures
- Intra-articular knee fracture assessment and reduction

Contraindications
- Infection – particularly cellulitis over the potential portal sites
- Ankylosis of the knee
- Rupture of the joint capsule (allows extravasation of the irrigation fluid)

Consent and risks
- *Venous thromboembolism*: Less than 1%
- *Septic arthritis*: Less than 1%
- *Superficial wound infection*: Less than 1%
- *Neurapraxia (secondary to tourniquet use)*: Less than 1%
- *Effusion*: Virtually universal and can last for several months

Operative planning
Any preoperative imaging should be available. Appropriate instrumentation should be available and checked by the surgeon, including the arthroscope, camera, light lead, arthroscopic instruments, irrigation fluid pump and the 'stack', which must include a functioning light source and monitor. The arthroscope used for knee arthroscopy has a 4 mm diameter and 30° viewing angle.

Anaesthesia and positioning
Anaesthesia is usually general, though regional anaesthesia is acceptable. The position is supine. A side support can be used, at the level of the upper- to mid-thigh, to provide a lever when opening up the medial compartment.

Tilting the patient toward the operative side, either by tilting the table or placing a sandbag under the contralateral buttock, reduces internal rotation when applying a valgus stress and allows better opening of the medial compartment in more extended positions when visualising the posterior part of the meniscus.

An appropriately padded tourniquet is applied and inflated at the level of the upper thigh. If the patient is hirsute, the anterior knee is shaved. The surgical field is prepared with a germicidal solution. Waterproof drapes are used with adhesive edges to provide a seal to the skin. Specific arthroscopy drapes with fluid collection pouches and suction ports can help to reduce flooding the operating theatre floor. The foot and lower leg are covered with a stockinette. The arthroscope is connected to the camera and light source. With the arthroscope applied against a clean white swab, the white balance button is pushed to prevent colour casts (unwanted colour tints affecting the picture) during the arthroscopy.

Surgical technique
Examination under anaesthesia
The first stage of any arthroscopy is vital and occurs before any incision is made. The knee is assessed for its full range of movement (which includes any hyperextension) and stability of its ligaments. The patella height and tracking are noted.

Landmarks

The patella, patellar tendon, medial and lateral joint lines are palpated carefully with the knee in around 70° of flexion.

Portals

All arthroscopy requires at least two portals with by far the most common two being the anterolateral and anteromedial portals (**Figure 12.1**). The anterolateral portal is almost always created first and other portals can be created under direct vision. The following is a general description of portal placement for diagnostic arthroscopy, but the precise location may be adapted to reach specific pathology or perform specific procedures anticipated from the clinical features and imaging. Similarly, it may be necessary to switch viewing and working portals to perform specific tasks.

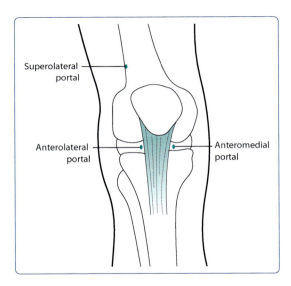

Figure 12.1 The three common knee arthroscopy portals.

The *anterolateral portal* is created 1 cm above the lateral joint line and 1 cm lateral to the lateral border of the patellar tendon. This corresponds to a level just below the inferior pole of the patella. It can be palpated by pushing a thumb against the angle between the lateral border of the patella and the anterolateral border of the upper tibia. If the thumb is left on the upper tibial border, the incision can be made just above the thumb to guide the surgeon to the correct position. It is best done with a pointed, rather than curved, blade, with the blade facing away from the patella tendon. A vertical incision or horizontal incision is acceptable. If using a horizontal incision, once the skin is breached the blade is turned to face vertically upwards to perform the capsulotomy. This reduces the risk of damaging the lateral meniscus.

The *anteromedial portal* is created under direct vision with the arthroscope viewing the medial compartment. It lies 1 cm above the medial joint line and 1 cm medial to the medial border of the patellar tendon. A 16G needle is inserted at this point, facing slightly downwards towards the tibia. This can be visualised directly to ensure that it exits just above the medial meniscus and is directed appropriately to perform any subsequent procedures. If not, it can be withdrawn and replaced correctly. Once the correct entry point has been identified, the needle is withdrawn and the scalpel used to enlarge the portal in the same fashion as the anterolateral portal.

The superior portals are made with the knee in extension. The *superomedial portal* is 2 cm above the superior pole of the patella, in line with the medial border of the patella. It was historically used for an outflow cannula. These are rarely used now, as modern pumps obviate their use.

The *superolateral portal* is 2 cm above the superior pole of the patella, in line with the lateral border of the patella. It can be used in suprapatellar synovectomy, for visualisation of the patellofemoral joint such as in surgery for patellar maltracking, or to visualise the patellar tendon and infrapatellar fat pad.

The *posteromedial portal* is 1 cm above the posteromedial joint line, in line with the medial border of the medial femoral condyle. This represents the 'soft spot' between the tendon of semimembranosus, the medial head of gastrocnemius and the medial collateral ligament (MCL). The portal is created under direct vision with the knee in 90° flexion, allowing the saphenous nerve to fall out of the surgical field. It can be used to visualise the posterior cruciate ligament (PCL) or posterior horn of the medial meniscus, in total synovectomy of the knee, or for removal of loose bodies. It utilises a longitudinal skin incision to avoid neurovascular damage. Following skin incision, an artery clip is used to dissect down to and through the capsule.

Structures at risk

- Sartorial branch of the saphenous nerve
- *Long saphenous vein*: Can be transilluminated by the arthroscope to help its identification

These structures pass together, approximately 1 cm behind the portal incision.

The *posterolateral portal* is placed in a soft point between the lateral head of gastrocnemius, the lateral collateral ligament (LCL) and the posterolateral tibial plateau. It is very infrequently used, but it can be used to visualise the posterior horn of the lateral meniscus or to retrieve a loose body from the posterior compartment of the knee. Again, a longitudinal incision is used. The portal is placed under direct vision in a similar fashion to the posteromedial portal. Remaining anterior to the biceps femoris tendon helps to reduce the risk to the common peroneal nerve, which lies posteriorly.

Structures at risk

- Common peroneal nerve, running lateral to the lateral head of gastrocnemius, 15 mm below the portal
- Lateral superior and inferior geniculate arteries, passing just below and above the incision site, respectively

A transpatellar tendon portal can be placed to access centrally or for passing additional grasping instruments into the knee. A longitudinal incision is made in line with the fibres of the patellar tendon approximately 1 cm below the inferior pole of the patella.

Insertion of the arthroscope

> **Structures at risk**
> - Articular cartilage
> - Anterior horn of lateral meniscus

This is the only step of arthroscopy which must be carried out blind: it must be done with great care to prevent gouging of the articular surfaces. The anterolateral portal is created as described earlier. The trochar and sleeve are inserted at 70° of knee flexion. Firm, gradual pressure is applied until there is a reduction in resistance, indicating that the trochar has passed through the joint capsule. At this point the knee is extended to around 20° of flexion and the trochar advanced, passing through the patellofemoral joint. Its intra-articular position can be confirmed by sweeping the arthroscope gently from side to side – it can be felt to be beneath the patella. If it is outside the knee joint, it will not sweep from side to side. The position of the arthroscope should be confirmed before removing the trochar, introducing the camera and turning on the saline inflow.

Arthroscopic inspection of the knee

It is good practice to follow the same 'route' around the knee as this helps to prevent any omissions. It is the authors' practice to address any pathology as it is located, rather than to proceed with a full inspection before beginning intervention. *Table 12.1* gives a suggested route, which many surgeons find the most effective one.

Closure

The portals are closed with either single sutures or adhesive paper stitches. Adhesive dressings, then wool and crepe, are applied before the tourniquet is deflated.

Postoperative care

The specific rehabilitation will depend on procedures performed, but for a simple diagnostic arthroscopy or meniscectomy weightbearing mobilisation is begun early, together with range-of-motion exercises. Anti-thromboembolism stockings are recommended for 6 weeks. The wool and crepe are removed 24 hours after surgery, to increase mobility. Sutures are removed at 10–14 days after surgery.

Recommended references

Jaureguito JW, Greenwald AE, Wilcox JF et al. The incidence of deep venous thrombosis after arthroscopic knee surgery. *Am J Sports Med.* 1999;**27**:707–710.

Kim SJ, Kim HJ. High portal: Practical philosophy for positioning portals in knee arthroscopy. *Arthroscopy.* 2001;**17**:333–337.

Kramer DE, Bahk MS, Cascio BM et al. Posterior knee arthroscopy: Anatomy, technique, application. *J Bone Joint Surg Am.* 2006;**88**:110–121.

Moseley JB, O'Malley K, Petersen NJ et al. A controlled trial of arthroscopic surgery for osteoarthritis of the knee. *N Engl J Med.* 2002;**347**:81–88.

Table 12.1 Arthroscopic inspection of the knee

Step	Area of inspection	Position of knee	Position of arthroscope	Structures to inspect	Technical notes
1	Suprapatellar pouch	20° flexion	Upright/upside down	Synovium; loose bodies	Turning the arthroscope through all angles allows visualisation of the synovium throughout the whole cavity.
2	Lateral gutter	20° flexion	Upright	Loose bodies	Best inspected at this stage so that it is not forgotten after tibiofemoral joint inspection.
3	Patellofemoral joint	20° flexion	Upright/upside down	Medial + lateral patella facets; synovial plica; trochlea; patellar tracking	The arthroscope is turned upside down to inspect the patellar cartilage and kept upright to view the trochlea. It must be withdrawn to just inferior to the patella to view tracking.
4	Medial gutter	20° flexion	Upright	Loose bodies	
5	Medial compartment	90° flexion initially 30° flexion to view the posterior horn	Normal/viewing laterally to improve visualisation of the posterior horn	Medial femoral condyle; medial tibial plateau; medial meniscus; loose bodies; creation of medial portal	Viewing the posterior horn is easier with the knee straighter and with the arthroscope swung to look laterally.

(Continued)

Table 12.1 (Continued) Arthroscopic inspection of the knee

Step	Area of inspection	Position of knee	Position of arthroscope	Structures to inspect	Technical notes
6	Intercondylar notch	90° flexion	Upright	Anterior cruciate ligament (ACL); posterior cruciate ligament; loose bodies; both posterior horns	In ACL surgery, the portals are created a little closer to the patella tendon to improve access to the notch. The posteromedial and posterolateral compartments can be visualised by driving the arthroscope through the notch between the cruciate ligament and respective femoral condyle. The posteromedial compartment is best accessed with the arthroscope in the anterolateral portal, then switching to the anteromedial portal to access posterolaterally.
7	Lateral compartment	Figure-four position	Upright/viewing medially	Lateral femoral condyle; lateral tibial plateau; lateral meniscus; loose bodies; popliteus tendon	Move the knee into the figure-four position with the arthroscope in the notch (**Figure 12.2**). Drive into the lateral compartment as it opens and comes into view.

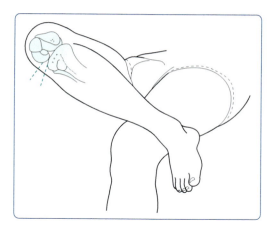

Figure 12.2 The figure-four position for lateral compartment viewing.

Arthroscopic meniscal knee surgery
Preoperative planning
See 'Knee arthroscopy' (p. 321) for further details of consent and operative planning, as well as postoperative care.

Indications
- *Acute tears of the meniscus*: Radial, longitudinal, complex and bucket-handle forms (**Figure 12.3**)
- *Degenerative tears of the meniscus* (commonly posterior horn of medial meniscus): If fails conservative management or there are clear mechanical symptoms
- *Meniscal repair*: In non-degenerative, longitudinal tears within 3 mm of the periphery (i.e. within the vascular zone of the meniscus)

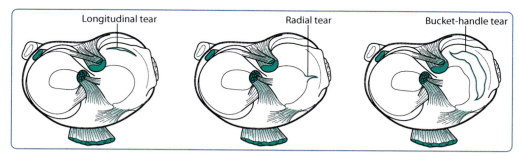

Figure 12.3 The common forms of acute meniscal tear.

Surgical technique
Partial meniscectomy
Partial meniscectomy is the most common procedure performed by trainees throughout the developed world and is considered a required skill by trainers and programme directors. It must be part of a full diagnostic arthroscopy, as described in the previous section.

Initial inspection of the meniscus can often reveal the presence, though not extent, of a tear. The smooth outline of the meniscus will be lost. The first stage is to probe the meniscus with an arthroscopic probe. The probe is inserted under the meniscus and the hook turned to point upwards, into the meniscus; the probe is withdrawn and will catch any inferior tear that was not previously visible.

Large posterior horn tears and even displaced bucket-handle tears can flip into the intercondylar notch and will not be seen unless specifically looked for in the posterior part of the notch. Using the probe, the surgeon can determine the extent of the tear and decide on the boundary between unstable, torn meniscal remnants and well-fixed, stable meniscal rim (**Figure 12.4**).

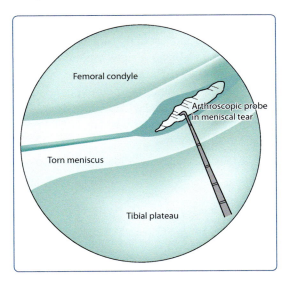

Figure 12.4 Use of an arthroscopic probe to show a meniscal tear.

The meniscus can be resected using a number of instruments. The author prefers to use simple punches for the majority of the resection and an arthroscopic shaver to smooth over the final remnant. An 'upbiter' is very useful during resection of very posterior tears, particularly of the medial meniscus (**Figure 12.5**).

The resection should be careful and methodical, leaving all stable meniscus behind. After resection, the meniscus must be probed again to ascertain that all remaining meniscus is stable.

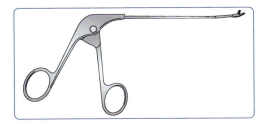

Figure 12.5 An 'upbiter' is useful in posterior horn resection.

Bucket-handle tear surgery

A bucket-handle tear is a large, longitudinal tear in which the internal portion is mobile and can flip over and become stuck in the intercondylar notch. It is three times as common in the medial as the lateral meniscus. The following discussion uses the medial meniscus as an example, though the principles are transferrable to the lateral meniscus.

Entry of the arthroscope into the medial compartment can be difficult. Careful creation of an anteromedial portal, as described, is recommended, followed by use of a probe through this portal to gently push the displaced fragment medially. This will usually afford a good view. Assessment can be made as to whether the tear is repairable (see the following section).

A probe is used to define the attachments of the tear, both posteriorly and anteriorly (**Figure 12.6**). If the fragment is found to be irreparable then a punch is used to detach 90% of the tear at its posterior origin. It is easiest to do this with an upbiter curved to the left for a left medial meniscus and to the right for a right medial meniscus. A straight punch or side-biter is used to resect completely through the anterior attachment. A strong, locking arthroscopic grasper is introduced through the medial portal and locked onto the middle of the torn remnant. The remnant is removed with a 'crocodile roll' – the graspers are rolled over several times while carefully watching with the arthroscope.

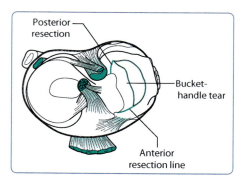

Figure 12.6 Resection points of a bucket-handle medial meniscal tear.

Once the meniscal remnant has been freed, it is removed through the medial portal. In large tears, this portal often requires enlargement. Careful inspection of the meniscal remnant is carried out, with debridement of any further unstable tissue.

Meniscal repair

Repair is possible if the tear is within 5 mm of the periphery, but more commonly undertaken if the tear is within 3 mm of the periphery, i.e. within the vascular zone. In order to be worthy of repair, the tear should be between 8 and 30 mm long.

The results of meniscal repair are better in patients with a concurrent anterior cruciate ligament (ACL) reconstruction than in repair alone. Repair should not be undertaken in a knee with ligament injury that has not been addressed. A variety of methods are described including outside-in, inside-out and all-inside suturing (**Figure 12.7**). In addition, meniscal darts can be used. The details of this surgery are beyond the scope of this book. Sutures are placed, usually vertically, about 3–4 mm apart from each other.

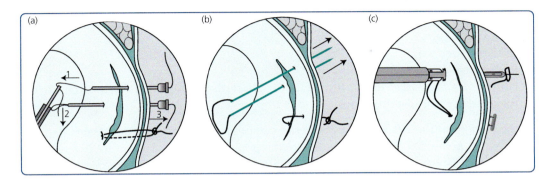

Figure 12.7 Meniscal repair: (a) outside-in, (b) inside-out and (c) all-inside technique.

Most surgeons recommend avoidance of weightbearing for around 4 weeks after surgery, particularly avoiding weightbearing in flexion.

Discoid meniscus surgery

Discoid malformation more frequently affects the lateral meniscus and is bilateral in one-fifth of cases. The majority are stable (i.e. have peripheral attachments to the rim). These are treated by partial meniscectomy, if symptomatic, to create a more normal meniscus.

If a discoid meniscus becomes suddenly painful, it is likely that it is torn and should be examined and treated as such. The rarer unstable, or Wrisberg variant, discoid meniscus is hypermobile due to absent peripheral attachments. These are usually treated by complete excision as there is no stable rim to leave *in situ*.

Postoperative care

See 'Knee arthroscopy' (p. 321).

Meniscal repair has a more controversial rehabilitation regimen. The author uses a brace, limited to 0°–60° range for 1 month then full range of motion within the brace for a further 2 months. Return to sports is gradual following the initial 3 months in the knee brace.

Recommended references

Fabricant PD, Jokl P. Surgical outcomes after arthroscopic partial meniscectomy. *J Am Acad Orthop Surg.* 2007;**15**:647–653.

Min S, Kim J, Kim LM et al. Correlation between type of discoid lateral menisci and tear pattern. *Knee Surg Sports Traumatol Arthrose.* 2004;**10**:218–222.

Rankin CC, Lintner DM, Noble PC et al. A biomechanical analysis of meniscal repair techniques. *Am J Sports Med.* 2002;**30**:492–497.

Lateral patellar retinaculum release

Preoperative planning

Indications

Lateral release of the patella is indicated in patients with a tight lateral patellar retinaculum who meet the following criteria:

- Anterior knee pain
- Positive patella tilt test, less than 5°
- Failure of conservative measures, including physiotherapy specifically, to strengthen the quadriceps and hamstrings

Associated conditions that may worsen the symptoms include chondromalacia patellae, patella alta, abnormal Q angle and trochlear hypoplasia, but these alone are not sufficient to perform a lateral release. In cases of malalignment, it may need to be combined with more advanced procedures, including osteotomy or tibial tubercle transfer. It can also be performed in conjunction with medial patellofemoral ligament reconstruction and vastus medialis advancement.

Contraindications

Lateral release is not indicated in patients with generalised hypermobility or patellar hypermobility – it will worsen the symptoms.

Operative planning

Very careful history and examination are required to elucidate the features. Plain radiography, including patella views, is essential. If malalignment is suspected, reconstruction in computed tomography is useful.

Anaesthesia and positioning

See 'Knee arthroscopy' (p. 321).

Consent and risks

- The complications are essentially those of any knee surgery: bleeding, infection, thrombosis and numbness, whether carried out open or arthroscopically
- Mention of haemarthrosis should be made in particular as it is very common and can be major
- Medial subluxation is a rare, late complication

Surgical technique

Open lateral release

Landmarks
- Lateral border of the patella
- Gerdy's tubercle (insertion of the iliotibial band on the lateral tibia)

Incision
A straight incision is created 1 cm from the lateral border of the patella, running from the level of the superior pole of the patella to 1 cm above Gerdy's tubercle. The incision is carried down to the lateral retinaculum.

Technique
The superficial lateral retinaculum is incised in line with the skin incision. The deeper fibres and synovium are not incised. The surgeon now assesses whether the release has been sufficient. If the patella is now able to be tilted 45° or more laterally, it is sufficient.

If the release is insufficient, the superficial retinaculum is dissected off the deep retinaculum for 2 cm on the lateral side of the incision. The deep retinaculum can now be incised parallel to the superficial retinacular incision but 2 cm further lateral. If this is required, the lateral portion of the superficial retinaculum is sutured to the medial edge of the deep retinaculum – this helps to lessen haemarthrosis.

Closure
The subcutaneous fat is opposed with interrupted sutures and the skin closed with the surgeon's chosen method. Occlusive dressing and heavy wool and crepe bandages are applied.

Arthroscopic lateral release

Technique
A complete arthroscopy is carried out first – the lateral release is done last as it causes bleeding. A tourniquet is not used as it interferes with patellar tracking and causes more bleeding postoperatively.

A horizontal line is drawn laterally from the superior pole of the patella and another line 1 cm away from the lateral border of the patella. A needle is inserted into the knee joint at the level where these lines cross.

Structures at risk

- The superior geniculate artery

The needle serves as a proximal limit of the release to prevent damage to the artery and subsequent bleeding that cannot be controlled arthroscopically.

Release is carried out, with cautery, running from the needle to the anterolateral portal; it is continued until subcutaneous fat is seen from within the knee.

Closure
The portals are closed with either single nylon sutures or adhesive paper stitches. Adhesive dressings, then wool and crepe, are applied.

Postoperative care and instructions

Weightbearing is begun immediately. The wool and crepe are removed after 24–36 hours and range-of-motion exercises are begun early (to prevent lateral adhesions within the knee). The patient is referred to physiotherapy to reinstate medial quadriceps exercises.

Recommended references

Kolowich PA, Paulos LE, Rosenberg TD et al. Lateral release of the patella: Indications and contraindications. *Am J Sports Med.* 1990;**18**:359–365.

Mulford JS, Wakeley CJ, Eldridge JD. Assessment and management of chronic patellofemoral instability. *J Bone Joint Surg Br.* 2007;**89**:709–716.

Patellofemoral instability

A careful assessment of patients with recurrent patellar instability is required to identify the underlying pathoanatomy and confirm the surgical target. The mainstays of surgical treatment, which are discussed here, are medial patellofemoral ligament (MPFL) reconstruction and tibial tubercle transfer, but other abnormalities that should be sought and may require surgical correction include trochlear dysplasia, coronal malalignment and torsional malalignment. Combined procedures may be warranted. The problem may be compounded by generalised hypermobility disorders. Additionally, poor strength of the quadriceps, glutei and core muscles leads to dynamic alignment problems, particularly evident on attempted single-leg squatting, that should be targeted with intensive physiotherapy. Isolated lateral release is not indicated for patellar instability and may even exacerbate the problem.

Medial patellofemoral ligament reconstruction

Preoperative planning

Indications

Recurrent patellar instability with MPFL deficiency. May require combined procedures if other pathoanatomical features are identified. The MPFL is the primary restraint to lateral patella displacement from full extension to 20°–30° of flexion, at which point the patella should engage in the trochlea. Apprehension in extension is typical of MPFL deficiency, whereas apprehension beyond 30° of flexion is suggestive of additional abnormalities.

Consent and risks

- Increased contact pressures, pain and degeneration
- Patella fracture
- Stiffness
- Rerupture, recurrent or persistent instability

Operative planning

Various graft options and reconstruction techniques have been described. Regardless of the technique chosen, accurate graft positioning and avoidance of over-tensioning are important in optimising outcome. Intraoperative fluoroscopy may be used to confirm the femoral attachment site.

The need for additional procedures will be dictated by the presence and severity of other risk factors for instability. This may include tibial tubercle transfer for lateralisation or patella alta, trochleoplasty for dysplasia or osteotomies to correct torsional or coronal abnormalities.

Anaesthesia and positioning

The patient is positioned supine under general or regional anaesthesia. Antibiotic prophylaxis is administered on induction of anaesthesia according to local protocols. A thigh tourniquet is used, the skin is shaved as required and standard skin antisepsis with adhesive sterile drapes are used to create a sterile surgical field.

Surgical technique

Landmarks

- Superior and medial patellar borders
- Medial epicondyle
- Adductor tubercle

Incision and approach

Arthroscopy can be performed to identify and address any additional lesions. Visualisation through the superolateral portal provides a good assessment of patellar tracking, which can be compared before and after the procedure.

Three incisions are made for the MPFL reconstruction. The reconstruction is performed with an autologous gracilis graft, harvested through an incision over the medial proximal tibia and whip-stitched with number 1 suture for 10 mm at each end (see section 'Hamstring graft', p. 348). An 18 cm length of graft is required.

A 2 cm longitudinal incision is made in line with the proximal half of the medial border of the patella. Access is required from the superomedial corner to the centre of the medial edge of the patella. Dissection is continued through layer 1 of the medial tissues; soft tissue is cleared from the upper half of the medial patella while remaining extra-articular.

The third incision is a 1–2 cm longitudinal incision placed between the medial epicondyle and adductor tubercle. Fluoroscopy can be used to help identify the correct position for femoral tunnel placement. The radiographic landmark (Schoettle point) is 1 mm anterior to a line extending distally from the posterior femoral cortex, 2.5 mm distal to the superior margin of the posterior articular border of the medial femoral condyle, and proximal to the posterior end of Blumensaat's line (**Figure 12.8**). Dissection is continued down to the bone where the femoral tunnel will be placed.

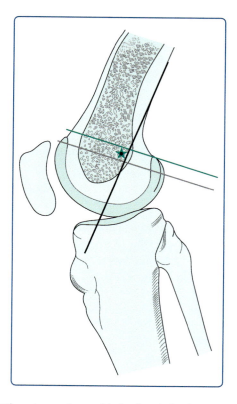

Figure 12.8 Schoettle point: radiographic landmark for femoral tunnel placement in MPFL reconstruction.

Procedure

Two parallel 2.4 mm guide wires are placed transversely across the patella. They are positioned so that both are in the upper half of the patella and separated by approximately 15 mm. The two guide pins are over-drilled with a 4.5 mm cannulated drill to a depth of 25 mm. The two whip-stitched ends of the gracilis graft are secured in the patella with 4.75 mm knotless anchors to leave a central loop of graft that will be secured to the femur.

The femoral insertion point is identified between the medial epicondyle and adductor tubercle (confirmed radiographically if desired). A Beath pin guide wire is inserted and directed to exit the lateral femoral cortex and advanced out through the skin of the lateral thigh. The femoral tunnel is created by over-drilling the Beath pin to a diameter of 6–7 mm. The Beath pin is left in place for passage of the graft.

Blunt dissection is performed deep to the fascia of layer 1, remaining extra-articular, to connect the two incisions at the medial patella and medial epicondyle. A loop of heavy suture is passed around the central loop of the graft and passed through the track created from the incision at the medial patella to the medial epicondyle. The loop of graft is pulled down through the same channel and out through the incision at the medial epicondyle. The free ends of the suture looped around the graft are then passed through the eye of the Beath pin and pulled into the femoral tunnel and out through the skin of the lateral thigh. The loop of graft can then be pulled into the femoral tunnel with the suture, ensuring equal tension on both limbs of the graft. It is tensioned to align the lateral patella facet with the lateral femoral condyle in 30° of flexion. Over-tensioning must be avoided; approximately 1 cm of lateral displacement should be possible in full extension. The graft is secured in the femoral tunnel with an interference screw.

Closure

The suture used to pull the graft into the femoral tunnel can be pulled out through the lateral thigh, and the free ends of the whip-stitches are cut short. The skin is closed with the surgeon's preferred method.

Postoperative care and instructions

A hinged knee brace allowing motion between 0° and 90° is worn for the first 6 weeks. Weightbearing is protected with crutches for the first 2 weeks, which are then weaned off as tolerated. Full range-of-motion and light exercise are allowed after 6 weeks, aiming for return to full activity after 12 weeks.

Tibial tubercle transfer

Preoperative planning

Indications

In the context of patellar instability, tibial tubercle osteotomy is indicated in the presence of patella alta or a laterally placed tibial tubercle, represented by high tibial tubercle–trochlear groove (TT-TG) distance. The precise thresholds used for these parameters are variable in the literature, but TT-TG greater than 20 mm and Caton-Deschamps ratio greater than 1:1.4 are definitely abnormal. Tibial tubercle transfer is often combined with MPFL reconstruction. Apprehension present at 30°–60° of knee flexion is typical of tibial tubercle abnormalities, while apprehension persisting in deeper flexion typically represents more significant coronal or torsional malalignment issues.

Consent and risks

- Over-medialisation, increased contact pressures, pain and degeneration
- *Non-union*: Approximately 1%
- *Tubercle fracture*: More common with shallow cuts of insufficient length
- *Tibial fracture*: Approximately 1% – more common with deeper and more oblique cuts
- *Recurrent instability*: Approximately 10%
- *Hardware irritation*: May require later removal

Operative planning

A number of different tibial tubercle transfers are described. Medialisation alone (Elmslie-Trillat) may increase contact pressures, pain and degeneration, particularly in the presence of pre-existing patellofemoral degeneration. In such cases an anteromedialisation (Fulkerson) is preferred. The extent of the transfer is dependent on the preoperative abnormality and aims to correct TT-TG to 12 mm and Caton-Deschamps ratio to 1:1.1. If anteromedialisation is performed then the length of transfer in the plane of the osteotomy (which will be measured intraoperatively) can be calculated from the required medialisation in the coronal plane and the planned angle of the osteotomy using trigonometry (**Figure 12.9**).

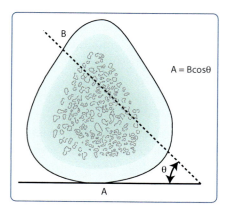

Figure 12.9 Tibial tubercle anteromedialisation. The length of medialisation is related to the measured length of displacement in the plane of the osteotomy by $A = B\cos\theta$.

Anaesthesia and positioning

This is the same as for MPFL reconstruction.

Surgical technique

Landmarks

- Patella tendon
- Tibial tubercle

Incision and approach

A 6 cm longitudinal incision is made over the tibial tubercle. Full-thickness flaps are elevated to expose the medial and lateral attachments of the patella tendon to the tubercle and continued for a distance 5 cm distal to the attachment for full exposure of the planned osteotomy site. The anterior compartment muscles are elevated off the anterolateral tibial cortex.

Procedure

The line of the planned osteotomy cut is marked on the periosteum with diathermy. A minimum thickness of 5 mm at the point of tendon attachment is required, tapered distally to produce a 5–6 cm osteotomy length. Larger transfers require thicker cuts. Medialisation alone is achieved with a medial-to-lateral cut in the coronal plane. For anteromedialisation the cut is from anteromedial to posterolateral. Parallel guide wires can be placed in the plane of the cut and used as a saw guide. The longitudinal cut is made in the required plane with an oscillating saw. A distal hinge is left intact if possible. The proximal transverse cut is made with an osteotome, proximal to the tendon attachment. The tubercle is freed with an osteotome and rotated on the distal hinge to medialise it by the planned distance, measured with a ruler at the level of the tendon attachment.

If distalisation is also required then the distal hinge is cut to free the fragment fully. The length of bone equivalent to the planned distalisation distance is removed from the distal end of the osteotomised tubercle fragment, which is then pulled distally to align flush with the distal osteotomy cut.

When the desired transfer has been achieved the fragment is provisionally held in place with two 1.2 mm K-wires. Patella tracking through the range of movement is confirmed, and the fragment can then be definitively fixed with two or three countersunk 3.5 mm cortical screws using a lag technique.

Closure
Debris is washed out of the surgical field and layered closure is performed using the surgeon's preferred technique.

Postoperative care and instructions
Mobilisation is non-weightbearing with a hinged knee brace locked in extension for the first 6 weeks. Passive range-of-motion exercises are allowed initially from 0° to 30°, increasing by 30° every 2 weeks. Provided radiographs at 6 weeks are satisfactory, weightbearing and range of motion can be progressed from 6 to 12 weeks, with resumption of full range of motion and full weightbearing thereafter. Strengthening and light exercise can resume after full range and weightbearing are achieved, with return to full sport after 6 months.

Recommended references
Grimm NL, Lazarides AL, Amendola A. Tibial tubercle osteotomies: A review of a treatment for recurrent patellar instability. *Curr Rev Musculoskelet Med.* 2018;**11**:266–271.

Koh JL, Stewart C. Patellar instability. *Orthop Clin N Am.* 2015;**46**:147–157.

Rhee S-J, Pavlou G, Oakley J et al. Modern management of patellar instability. *International Orthopaedics (SICOT).* 2012;**36**:2447–2456.

Cartilage reconstruction surgery
Preoperative planning
Indications
- Articular cartilage injury (most common on the medial femoral condyle).
- Osteochondritis dissecans (most common on the lateral part of the medial femoral condyle).
- Atraumatic osteonecrosis of the knee.
- The National Institute for Health and Care Excellence (NICE) supports the use of autologous chondrocyte implantation for symptomatic defects greater than 2 cm² failing conservative management provided it is the primary surgical procedure, there is minimal osteoarthritis and it is performed in a tertiary centre.

Contraindications
- *Degenerative knee changes*: None of the techniques developed to date are successful on osteoarthritic lesions.

- *Age over 55 years*: Poor cartilage regeneration and may be more suitable for arthroplasty techniques.
- Active infection.

> ### Consent and risks
> - Same as for 'Knee arthroscopy' (p. 321)
> - Unpredictable outcome (worse if long-standing injury or high body mass index)
> - Donor site morbidity (mosaicplasty and autologous chondrocytes transplants [autologous chondrocyte implantation, ACI])
> - Need for second procedure (ACI)

Operative planning

Details of previous imaging and surgery should be available. Suitable equipment for the chosen technique of chondroplasty consists of:

- Microfracture picks/K-wire (microfracture)
- Plug harvest and implant equipment (mosaicplasty)
- Chondrocytes (ACI)

Anaesthesia and positioning

See 'Knee arthroscopy' (p. 321).

Surgical technique

Debridement

- Simple removal of loose chondral material and smoothing of the damaged edges.
- 'Roughening' of the underlying, subchondral bone may allow clot formation and encourage fibrocartilage formation.
- May be suitable for small lesions.

Microfracture

Following debridement, an awl is inserted into the ipsilateral arthroscope portal and used to create microfractures in the subchondral bone at the defect (**Figure 12.10**). The microfractures are 5 mm apart and approximately 5 mm deep. This allows penetration of the tidemark and the release of pluripotential cells from the cancellous bone. This produces a more pronounced and longer-lasting healing response than abrasion alone and increases the prospect of fibrocartilage formation at the defect.

Mosaicplasty

Small plug grafts are taken from a non-weightbearing area of the knee, typically the peripheral areas of the superior trochlea, and grafted into the defect until it is filled. Grafts are taken with a core drill and are 4–8 mm in diameter and 20 mm deep. Matching cores are removed from the defect and the graft plugs impacted in a mosaic pattern (**Figure 12.11**).

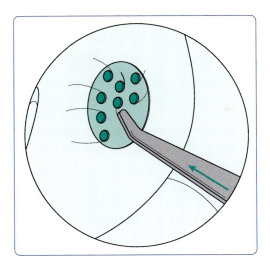

Figure 12.10 Microfracture of a chondral injury of the medial femoral condyle.

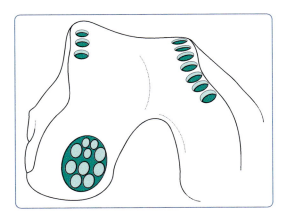

Figure 12.11 Femoral condylar defect treated with mosaicplasty medial femoral condyle.

Care must be taken to leave the graft plugs flush with the surrounding cartilage. The defects between the plugs fill in with fibrocartilage. Results are variable and highly dependent on the skill of the surgeon. There are questions over their use in defects over 4 cm^2.

Autologous chondrocyte implantation

Autologous chondrocyte implantation is performed as a two-stage procedure. The first stage is arthroscopic and includes a diagnostic arthroscopy and debridement of any chondral flaps around the area of chondral damage. This should be done to provide a rim of stable or healthy cartilage all around the lesion and is essential for attachment of the graft. At the end of the first-stage arthroscopy, small segments of healthy cartilage are harvested from the outer border of the anterosuperior femur, usually on the medial side of the trochlea. This is performed with a small gouge to loosen the segment and rongeurs to retrieve it. A venous blood sample is taken to screen for infectious diseases.

The chondrocytes can be prepared in a number of ways and can be provided suspended in solution or can be implanted onto a membranous matrix. This usually takes 3–6 weeks. The steps of preparation are similar in each technique: collagenases dissolve the matrix to leave the chondrocytes, then the cells are washed and put in a culture medium derived from the patient's serum. The cells adhere to a culture surface and proliferate to provide a large number of healthy chondrocytes.

The second procedure is carried out once the chondrocytes have been grown and returned. This is a larger procedure and is performed open. The incision is dependent on the site: for example, a medial femoral condyle defect requires an 8 cm medial parapatellar incision. The defect is exposed and any further loose material is debrided. The defect is then covered with an appropriately shaped membrane that is stitched or glued in place. If the cells are embedded on the membrane, this is the final stage; if the cells are in suspension, the liquid is injected under the membrane. The wound is closed in layers.

Postoperative care and instructions

Movement encourages chondrocyte growth, so after ACI or mosaicplasty, the patient is rested for up to 2 weeks, in either a bulky dressing or a cylinder plaster, then passive mobilisation is begun. In all cases, the patient is allowed to toe touch weightbear for 6–8 weeks, to reduce the force on the grafts. Running is not allowed for 6 months and contact sports for 12 months after ACI or mosaicplasty.

Recommended references

Briggs TWR, Mahroof S, David LA et al. Histological evaluation of chondral defects after autologous chondrocyte implantation of the knee. *J Bone Joint Surg Br.* 2003;**85**:1077–1083.
Hangody L, Kish G, Karpati Z et al. Mosaicplasty for the treatment of articular cartilage defects: Application in clinical practice. *Orthopaedics.* 1998;**21**:751–756.
Steadman JR, Briggs KK, Rodrigo JJ et al. Outcomes of microfracture for traumatic chondral defects of the knee: Average 11-year follow-up. *Arthroscopy.* 2003;**19**:477–484.

Anterior cruciate ligament reconstruction
Preoperative planning
Indications

ACL reconstruction is indicated in patients with symptomatic instability of the knee with a proven ACL rupture. Specific indications include:

- High-level athlete (consider early reconstruction, without rehabilitation phase)
- Inability to return to sports, particularly those which involve twisting on a planted foot (e.g. rugby, football, racquet sports)
- Ongoing instability, giving way and pain resistant to a dedicated ACL rehabilitation physiotherapy programme

Consent and risks

- Knee stiffness (due to arthrofibrosis, inaccurate tunnel placement or insufficient notchplasty)
- *Arthrofibrosis*: More common if early reconstruction used rather than delayed
- Knee pain
- Kneeling difficulty (higher risk if bone–patellar tendon–bone (B-T-B) technique is used)
- Ongoing instability (11%–25% symptomatic, 60%–89% asymptomatic)
- Failure to return to previous level of sport (up to 30%)
- *Graft failure*: Impingement or enlargement of the tunnel with time (typically 2 years)
- *Degeneration*: Found in 75% of patients beyond 10 years after surgery

Operative planning

Careful examination and judicious use of investigations are essential, both to confirm the presence of ACL rupture and to search for associated injuries, particularly associated ligament injury.

The operation notes from prior surgery should be available, along with results of previous MRIs or other imaging. If there is an associated meniscal tear, consideration should be given to concurrent repair, as the results are improved in conjunction with ACL reconstruction.

Anaesthesia and positioning

General or regional anaesthesia is used. Prophylactic antibiotics are given. The patient is positioned supine with a side support or leg holder to hold the knee in supported flexion.

Surgical technique

There are multiple options and a number of controversies surrounding the technique of ACL reconstruction. Graft choice will fall into autograft, allograft or synthetic categories. There are a number of autograft options but those available may depend on previous surgery or injuries. Synthetic grafts are generally not preferred for ACL reconstruction due to historically high failure rates, recurrent or persistent instability, debris generation leading to synovitis and chronic effusions, accelerated osteoarthritis development and possible distant effects of particulate debris. Double-bundle grafts, separately reconstructing both the anteromedial and posterolateral bundles of the native ACL, have shown mixed results when compared with single-bundle reconstruction and are not in widespread use.

Tunnel positions within the femur and tibia have been the subject of much debate. There has been a move toward more anatomical reconstruction, with tunnels being placed within the footprints of the native ACL, aiming to restore improved stability and more normal biomechanics. Fibres of the anteromedial bundle have been shown to be dominant in controlling both anterior translation and rotation, as well as remaining closer to isometric through the range of movement. Transtibial positioning of the femoral tunnel (i.e. through the tibial tunnel) risks compromising the positions of both tunnels: a non-anatomical high femoral tunnel that tends to be placed too anteriorly and risks impingement of the graft on the notch in full extension, mitigated by placing the tibial tunnel too posteriorly, resulting in a vertically oriented graft that is unable to control rotational instability. Placing the tunnels independently helps to avoid these problems. There are many devices and techniques for fixation of the graft either within the tunnel aperture itself or distant from it, again with much surrounding debate about their relative advantages and disadvantages. Here we describe two widely used techniques but accept that many variations are in clinical use.

The two common methods of reconstruction are with a B-T-B graft or a hamstring tendon graft. The harvesting of both grafts is described, along with the method of reconstruction via an arthroscopic technique. Open techniques are now uncommonly performed.

As always, careful examination under anaesthesia is essential. The technique of the arthroscopy is in common with that described in the previous sections. The anterolateral portal is placed slightly more centrally (adjacent to the patellar tendon) and higher to facilitate access to the notch. Depending on the technique used, the anteromedial portal may also need to be moved, and/or an accessory anteromedial portal created, to facilitate tunnel placement. It is wise to carefully inspect the PCL and popliteus tendon in case of associated PCL or posterolateral corner injury. Failure to address a concomitant posterolateral corner injury is associated with higher rates of ACL graft failure.

Bone–patellar tendon–bone graft
Landmarks
- Midline: Superior pole of the patella, tibial tuberosity

Incision and dissection
A midline incision is created from the superior pole of the patella to just below the tibial tuberosity. Dissection is continued to reveal the paratenon, which is then incised to expose the whole of the patella tendon. The central portion (usually 10 mm unless it is a narrow tendon, in which case use one-third of its width) of the tendon is dissected free for its entire length between the patella and the tibial tuberosity.

This dissection is continued across the patella for 30 mm proximally and the tibial tuberosity 30 mm distally. These incisions mark the sites of bone cuts for harvesting of proximal and distal blocks (**Figure 12.12**).

Structures at risk
- Anterior horns of the medial and lateral menisci, just posterior to the fat pad
- Medial femoral chondral surface: At risk as the femoral tunnel drill is passed

Procedure
With a 2 mm drill, drill two holes around 10 mm deep, in the centre of each area of bone between the dissected margins – these will be used to pass sutures for control of the graft at insertion. Using a narrow oscillating saw and then an osteotome (8–10 mm wide), dissect a block from the patella of 25 mm length. The osteotomes are directed 45° towards the

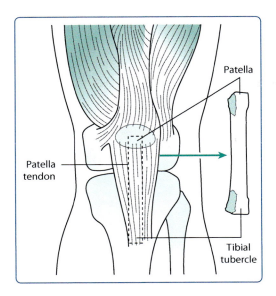

Figure 12.12 Bone–patellar tendon–bone graft harvest.

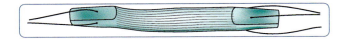

Figure 12.13 The harvested bone–patellar tendon–bone graft.

midline when performing the cuts, in order to create a trapezoidal graft shape. Care must be taken to avoid a graft which is too deep, risking subsequent patella fracture, or too thin, risking failure of fixation of the graft. The aim is creation of a block 25 mm long, 8 mm wide and 5–8 mm deep. The bone block is trimmed to a uniform size and two heavy sutures are passed through the previously drilled holes.

The same technique is used to create two holes in and harvest the tuberosity bone block, which should be of a similar size and shape. It is again trimmed and one heavy suture is passed through one of the drilled holes (**Figure 12.13**).

The graft is sized with a tunnel sizer, aiming for a snug but not too tight fit. If the grafts are of significantly different sizes, different tunnel widths can be used for the reconstruction; if this is done the tibial tunnel must be the larger one. The length of the entire graft and width of the two bone blocks should be written down and the graft wrapped in gauze presoaked in 5 mg/mL vancomycin solution for 10–15 minutes.

The ACL remnant, if present, is excised. It may be adherent to the PCL and care must be taken to avoid damage to the PCL when it is dissected free. The lateral wall is cleared of any further soft tissues and the back of the lateral wall indentified with a hook.

The femoral footprint of the ACL is identified on the lateral wall. The entire footprint is below and posterior to the lateral intercondylar (resident's) ridge; the anteromedial (AM) bundle attaches above and behind the bifurcate ridge (**Figure 12.14a**). A Beath pin guide

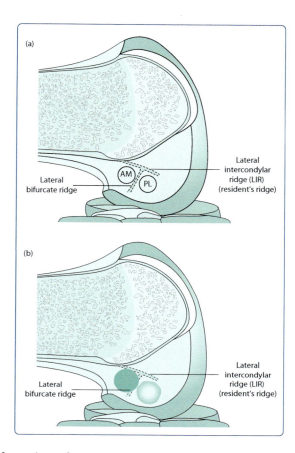

Figure 12.14 Native femoral ACL footprint position on the lateral wall of the notch (a) and position of femoral tunnel placement (b). AM, anteromedial bundle; PL, posterolateral bundle.

wire is placed through the anteromedial portal and, with the knee hyperflexed, positioned toward the AM bundle position but so the full tunnel diameter remains within the native footprint (**Figure 12.14b**). If desired, a better view of the lateral wall to confirm the tunnel position may be obtained by visualising with the scope through the anteromedial portal; an accessory anteromedial portal may be used to place the Beath pin. The Beath pin is advanced so the tip emerges through the skin of the anterolateral thigh.

The femoral tunnel is drilled with the appropriate-sized tunnel drill passing over the guide wire. The length of the tunnel should be just over the length of the bone plug to be used in the tunnel – this is usually 35 mm. The reamings are saved to graft the patellar defect from the graft harvest at the end of the procedure. A tunnel rasp is used to smooth any sharp bone edges. A heavy looped suture is passed through the eye of the Beath pin, which is pulled up through the femoral tunnel so the free ends are retrieved through the anterolateral thigh and the loop remains out of the anteromedial portal. The free suture ends can be passed through the loop and clipped to the drapes to prevent accidental displacement during tibial tunnel preparation.

To prepare the proximal tibia for tunnel creation, the area of tibia medial to the patella tendon is exposed. Using subperiosteal dissection, good bone exposure is obtained so that the tunnel jig will not slip. The ACL tibial tunnel jig is set at 50° and the aiming device

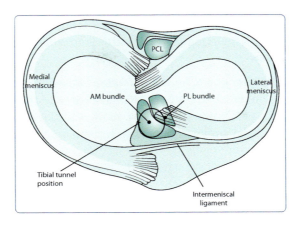

Figure 12.15 Site of the tibial tunnel for anterior cruciate ligament reconstruction. PCL, posterior cruciate ligament; AM, anteromedial; PL, posterolateral.

placed toward the anteromedial part of the tibial footprint, while allowing the full tunnel diameter to remain within the native footprint (**Figure 12.15**). Small adjustments can be made to the angle of the jig to change the tibial tunnel length, depending on the measured length of the graft, allowing the bone block at the tibial end of the graft to be pulled fully into the tunnel when the graft is in place.

An ACL guide wire is drilled, through the jig, entering the knee just in front of the medial tibial spine. The guide wire is over-drilled with the tunnel drill of appropriate size for the graft. Again, any reamings are saved and any sharp edges present at the joint surface are

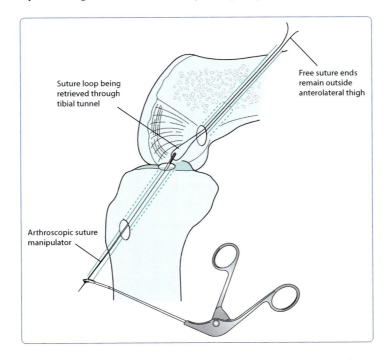

Figure 12.16 Suture loop being retrieved through tibial tunnel.

smoothed with a tunnel rasp. The previously placed suture loop is retrieved through the tibial tunnel so the loop now passes through both tunnels and the free ends remain outside the skin of the anterolateral thigh (**Figure 12.16**). This loop will be used to shuttle the graft sutures through the tunnels.

Returning to the graft, the junction of bone and tendon of the femoral block is marked with a surgical pen – the femoral block should be the smaller of the two. The two strong sutures in the femoral block are passed through the loop of the shuttle suture within the tunnels, which is then pulled up so the graft suture passes through both tibial and femoral tunnels and is retrieved through the anterolateral thigh. A second suture is passed through the tibial bone block – this should be either a strong, braided non-absorbable suture or a steel wire.

The graft is firmly, but smoothly, pulled through into position. Inspection within the knee will reveal when the marking on the femoral plug has reached the margin of the femoral tunnel. An interference screw guide wire is passed anterior to the graft within the femoral tunnel to a depth of at least 25 mm. An interference screw of appropriate size is then passed over the guide wire to secure the graft within the femur. The position and security are checked by cycling the knee through flexion and extension several times.

While the graft is tensioned, a further interference screw is inserted to secure the graft in the tibia. Securing the graft in or near full extension will reduce the risk of developing postoperative fixed flexion. The abolition of the pivot shift phenomenon can be checked at this stage. The graft saved from the tunnels is packed into the defect in the patella. Additional cancellous bone can be obtained from the harvest site of the tibial tubercle bone block to fill the patellar defect if required.

Closure

The paratenon is closed with interrupted, absorbable sutures over the tendon. The tendon itself is not closed as this would shorten the patella tendon. Adhesive dressings, then a wool and crepe dressing, are applied.

Hamstring graft

Landmarks

- Tibial tuberosity
- Patellar tendon

Incision and dissection

Structure at risk

The infrapatellar branch of the saphenous nerve can often be seen traversing the wound at the site of graft harvesting – it should be preserved if possible. Oblique incisions at the level of the pes anserinus may reduce this risk but need to be positioned carefully to allow access to both the tendons and tibial tunnel.

A diagnostic arthroscopy is carried out to identify and treat associated injuries. The anteromedial portal is kept anterior, close to the patella tendon, in order to allow good visualisation of the notch. The lateral wall is cleared with an arthroscopic shaver or a small curette. An arthroscopy hook is used to carefully identify the posterior wall.

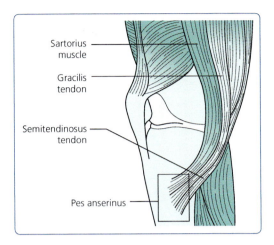

Figure 12.17 Anatomy of the pes anserinus.

A 50 mm incision, parallel with the patellar tendon, is created 20 mm medial to the tibial tuberosity. It should begin 60 mm below the joint line. Fat and deep fascia are dissected to reveal the tendons of the pes anserinus (**Figure 12.17**).

An incision is created over the upper border of the tendons, taking care not to damage the tendons themselves. The tendons are adherent to the deep surface of the sartorial fascia. Dissecting scissors are used to develop the planes between the gracilis and semitendinosus tendons, the underlying MCL and the overlying sartorial fascia.

Procedure

The tendons are then pulled forward with the scissors and a tendon hook is passed over them in turn. It is recommended that a length of surgical tape be passed over semitendinosus, which is then released but freely rediscovered via pulling on the tape.

The tendons of gracilis and semitendinosus are dissected free of soft tissue attachments in turn. The tendons are harvested in turn with a tendon stripper. The gracilis tendon is held taught and the stripper carefully pushed over it, keeping the stripper parallel to the tendon. It is advanced until the tendon is released from its muscle belly, and then the same method is used to release the tendon of semitendinosus.

The tendons can then be dissected free of the pes medially, carefully preserving as much graft length as possible. This will give a graft of two tendons, which are joined at one end and free at the other. Alternatively, the graft can be prepared *in situ*. Muscle tissue is scraped off the tendons. Each tendon is sutured, using a whip-stitch, for 30 mm at either end. The two tendons are then passed through the loop of a cortical suspensory button device and folded in half to create a four-strand single bundle graft (**Figure 12.18**). The graft is then tensioned, in order to prevent stretching *in situ*. If a tensiometer is available, it is usually tensioned to 80 N (20 lb) for 10 minutes. Next, the graft is measured: most are 8–10 mm, with 7 mm being a minimum acceptable diameter.

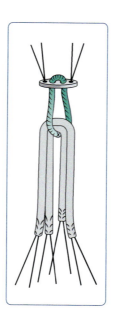

Figure 12.18 Four-strand hamstring graft prepared over a cortical suspensory button.

The femoral tunnel position is identified as for B-T-B grafts, and the guide wire is inserted through the (accessory) anteromedial portal with the knee hyperflexed in a similar fashion. The tunnel is first drilled with a 4.5 mm drill through the anterolateral femoral cortex to allow passage of the femoral cortical suspensory button. The tunnel length is noted and the femoral socket then drilled to the appropriate diameter for the graft up to, but not through, the femoral cortex. The length of graft within the femoral tunnel will be the difference between the tunnel length (total length to the outer surface of the femoral cortex) and the loop length of the suspension device, plus the thickness of the graft looped through the device (**Figure 12.19a**). A socket that ends sufficiently close to the cortex to allow the button to clear the femur and flip is required; the minimum required depth of the socket to allow this 'turning circle' will depend on the size of the button, length of the loop and thickness of the graft through the loop (**Figure 12.19b**), but drilling the socket as close as possible up to the femoral cortex will usually be sufficient. A shuttle suture loop is passed through the femoral tunnel as for B-T-B grafts.

The knee is positioned in 90° of flexion. The tibial jig is passed through the medial portal and positioned as for B-T-B reconstruction, with its aiming device passing through the previously created graft harvest incision. With the arthroscope in the anterolateral portal, the tibial tunnel guide wire is inserted and its entry point into the knee confirmed to be within the anteromedial portion of the tibial stump on the tibial surface. The tibial tunnel is then drilled and any debris at its entrance into the knee cleared with an arthroscopic shaver. Any sharp bone edges are smoothed with a tunnel rasp. The shuttle suture loop is retrieved through the tibial tunnel. The lead and flipping sutures of the suspension device are passed through the shuttle loop and pulled up through both tibial and femoral tunnels to be retrieved through the skin of the anterolateral thigh. The suspensory button and attached graft are firmly pulled through into position, the button is flipped and the graft is tensioned by pulling on the whip-stitches at the tibial end.

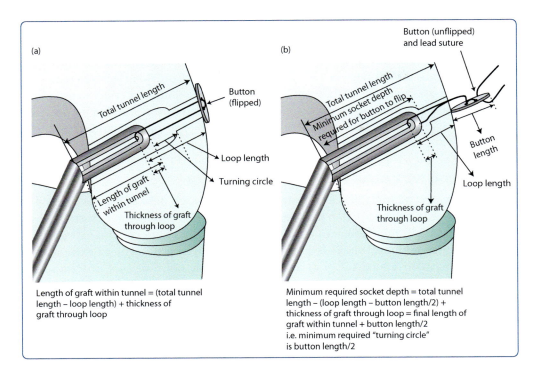

Figure 12.19 Relationship between femoral tunnel length, suspensory loop length and graft length within femoral tunnel (a) and minimum socket depth required to allow button to flip (b).

The position of the graft is checked arthroscopically and the graft fixed with a screw in the tibial tunnel as described in the section 'Bone–patellar tendon–bone graft' (p. 344).

Closure

Closure of wounds is with a combination of interrupted, absorbable deep sutures and the surgeon's chosen skin closure. The arthroscopy portals and exit wounds of guide wires can be closed with adhesive paper closure sutures alone. Adhesive dressings and a wool and crepe dressing are applied.

Postoperative care and instructions

ACL reconstruction is often performed as a day-case procedure. Full weightbearing is allowed with crutches until quadriceps function returns. The patient is not put into a brace; rather, early supervised range-of-motion exercises are begun. After 24 hours the bulky dressing is removed, leaving adhesive dressings over the wounds. With the aid of a physiotherapist, range-of-motion exercises are begun; the focus in the initial 1–2 weeks is restoration of range of motion, particularly extension, swelling control by icing and gentle quadriceps activation with leg extension activity. The wounds are inspected and sutures removed at 2 weeks after surgery.

A goal-based rehabilitation regime, with progression determined by meeting specific clinical and functional targets, is preferred over one with activities allowed at specific times. Regaining single-leg balance and muscle strength is started with simple body-weight exercises such as lunges and squats, progressing to a gym-based regime. Running, jumping, hopping and agility activities can commence when strength and balance goals are achieved, followed by a return to sport-specific exercises and training tailored to the individual. Return to sport is typically a minimum of 9 months postoperatively, provided the functional goals are achieved. It is recommended that athletes participate in an injury prevention programme for as long as they continue to participate in sport. There are a number of prevention programmes available, but they should incorporate plyometric, balance and strengthening exercises and be performed for at least 10 minutes before every sport session.

Anterolateral reconstruction

The anterolateral structures of the knee are a subject of much debate. It is recognised that intra-articular ACL reconstruction may be inadequate to control the rotary instability seen during the pivot shift manoeuvre in all cases, and additional anterolateral extra-articular stabilisation may address this. It is hoped that addition of anterolateral extra-articular stabilisation may also reduce ACL graft rupture. Historically, however, such procedures were thought to be associated with over-constraint, stiffness and lateral osteoarthritis. These problems may have been due to excessive tensioning, postoperative cast immobilisation and co-existing chondral or meniscal injuries and seem not to be relevant to modern techniques. Nonetheless, anterolateral procedures are not currently recommended routinely. Indeed, the indications are yet to be fully defined but may include conditions associated with high graft failure or residual rotational instability rates:

- Participation in pivoting/contact sports
- High-grade pivot shift
- Hyperlaxity
- Revision ACL reconstruction
- Young patients
- Medial meniscectomy
- Injury to anterolateral structures/Segond fracture

With the recent interest in the description of an anterolateral ligament as a discrete structure, anterolateral ligament reconstructions are now performed by some surgeons in an attempt to address these issues. The authors' preferred approach, however, is to perform a modified lateral extra-articular tenodesis, which has been shown to be biomechanically superior. This is achieved through a lateral incision by using a 1 cm wide central strip of iliotibial band, approximately 10 cm in length. It is detached proximally but left attached to Gerdy's tubercle distally. The proximal end is tunnelled deep to the LCL. It is secured to the lateral distal femur proximal and posterior to the lateral epicondyle with a ligament staple, with the knee held at 30° flexion and neutral rotation, and with light tension, approximately 20N. The remaining free proximal end is then folded back distally superficial to the LCL and sutured to itself. The defect in the iliotibial band is closed.

Recommended references

Burnham JM, Malempati CS, Carpiaux A et al. Anatomic femoral and tibial tunnel placement during anterior cruciate ligament reconstruction: Anteromedial portal all-inside and outside-in techniques. *Arthroscopy Techniques*. 2017;**6**:275–282.

Frank CB, Jackson DW. Current concepts review – The science of reconstruction of the anterior cruciate ligament. *J Bone Joint Surg Am*. 1997;**79**:1556–1576.

Lutz C. Role of anterolateral reconstruction in patients undergoing anterior cruciate ligament reconstruction. *Orthopaedics & Traumatology: Surgery & Research*. 2018;**104**:S47–S53.

Salmon LJ, Russell VJ, Refshauge K et al. Long-term outcome of endoscopic anterior cruciate ligament reconstruction with patellar tendon autograft. *Am J Sports Med*. 2006;**34**:721–732.

Williams A, Ball S, Stephen J et al. The scientific rationale for lateral tenodesis augmentation of intra-articular ACL reconstruction using a modified 'Lemaire' procedure. *Knee Surg Sports Traumatol Arthrosc*. 2017;**25**:1339–1344.

Williams RJ, Hyman J, Petrigliano F et al. Anterior cruciate ligament reconstruction with a four-strand hamstring tendon autograft. *J Bone Joint Surg Am*. 2004;**86**:225–232.

Woo SL, Kanamori A, Zeminski J et al. The effectiveness of reconstruction of the anterior cruciate ligament with hamstrings and patellar tendon: A cadaveric study comparing anterior tibial and rotational loads. *J Bone Joint Surg Am*. 2002;**84**:907–914.

Posterolateral corner reconstruction

Preoperative planning

Indications

Isolated posterolateral corner injuries are uncommon. Low-grade isolated injuries can often be managed non-operatively. However, high-grade isolated injuries, as well as the more commonly seen combined injuries with cruciate ruptures, and those failing conservative management, require surgical treatment. Primary repair may be possible if treated within the first 3 weeks following injury, but results are often improved if augmented with reconstruction.

> ### Consent and risks
>
> - Approximately 10% persistent varus instability
> - Common peroneal nerve: Approximately 25% overall, but usually a result of the injury rather than surgery

Operative planning

A number of construct and graft options are described. Consensus is lacking about the optimal technique. The fibular-based technique using a free semitendinosus autograft described later, a modification of that described by Larson, is one that is commonly used and appears to produce comparable outcomes to more complex constructs.

Careful clinical examination is essential, both to ensure that posterolateral corner injury is not missed and to identify other associated injuries. Graft availability may be influenced by the requirement to perform additional reconstructions, or those performed previously.

Anaesthesia and positioning

These are the same as for ACL reconstruction.

Surgical technique

Landmarks
- Lateral epicondyle
- Gerdy's tubercle
- Fibular head

Incision and approach
The semitendinosus tendon is harvested as described for ACL reconstruction, noting that contralateral harvest may be required in the case of combined injuries.

The procedure can be performed through two small incisions, over the fibular head and lateral epicondyle, but the full approach is described here. A lateral longitudinal incision is made from the lateral epicondyle proximally, to midway between Gerdy's tubercle and the fibular head distally. Dissection is continued down to the iliotibial band. Three windows are created to expose the deep structures: the common peroneal nerve is exposed and released posterior to the biceps femoris tendon and protected throughout the remainder of the procedure; the tip of the fibula is exposed between the biceps tendon and iliotibial band and the femoral attachments of the LCL and popliteus tendon are exposed through a split in the iliotibial band centred on the lateral epicondyle.

Procedure
The free semitendinosus tendon is whip-stitched at both ends with heavy suture as for ACL reconstruction. A graft of length at least 16–19 cm is required.

A guide wire is inserted from anterolateral to posteromedial through the widest part of the fibular head, approximately 1–1.5 cm below the tip, and over-drilled to a diameter of 4–5 mm to accommodate the single hamstring tendon. The tendon is passed through the fibular tunnel so that the central portion is within the tunnel.

Two Beath pin guide wires are inserted into the lateral femoral condyle and directed anteromedially through the medial femur and skin of the medial thigh, one at the insertion of the LCL on the lateral epicondyle and the second at the insertion of the popliteus, which is found 18.5 mm anterior and distal to the former (**Figure 12.20**). It is important to direct the wires to avoid interference with the femoral tunnel of an associated ACL reconstruction. Inserting all femoral guide wires, to see their positions and avoid any clashes, before completing the reconstruction, may help with this. The femoral tunnels are then drilled to accommodate the free ends of the graft.

The end of the tendon exiting from the anterior end of the fibular tunnel will reconstruct the LCL while the posterior end will reconstruct the popliteus/popliteo-fibular ligament (**Figure 12.21**). The popliteo-fibular end of the reconstruction is secured first: it is passed deep to the iliotibial band and retrieved through the window at the femoral epicondyle, the whip-stitches are shuttled through the femoral tunnel at the popliteus insertion by pulling the Beath pin out through the medial thigh and the free end of the graft can then be pulled into the tunnel, aiming for at least 15 mm to be within the tunnel. It is secured with an interference screw in the femoral tunnel then tensioned to 10N by pulling on the remaining free end of the graft at 90° flexion and neutral rotation and secured with a screw from anterior

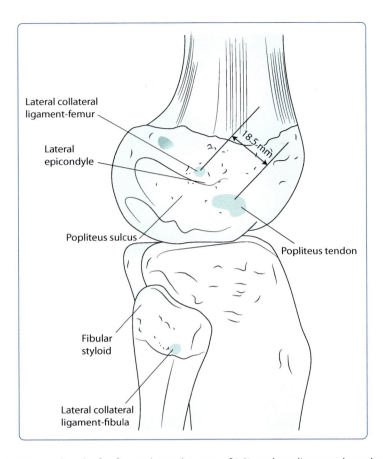

Figure 12.20 Landmarks for femoral attachments of LCL and popliteus on lateral condyle.

to posterior in the fibular tunnel. The remaining free end exiting the fibula anteriorly is then passed deep to the iliotibial band but superficial to the already secured popliteo-fibular part of the reconstruction and passed into the femoral tunnel at the LCL attachment in a similar fashion, thereby reconstructing the LCL. It is tensioned to 10N with the knee in extension and neutral rotation and secured in the femoral tunnel with an interference screw. The popliteo-fibular part of the graft should be tighter in flexion, while the LCL part tightens in extension.

Closure
The free whip-stitch ends are cut flush to the medial thigh skin and buried. The iliotibial band is closed with absorbable suture followed by the surgeon's chosen skin closure.

Postoperative care and instructions
Rehabilitation will often need to be tailored to the particular combination of injuries being addressed. In general, a period of protected weightbearing with the knee braced in extension for 6 weeks is employed. Passive range of motion from 0° to 90° can begin early, progressing to full flexion after 2–4 weeks. Quads exercises can start early, but hamstring activity should be avoided for the first 6 weeks. Progression to normal activity and sports will then follow a similar principle to ACL rehabilitation.

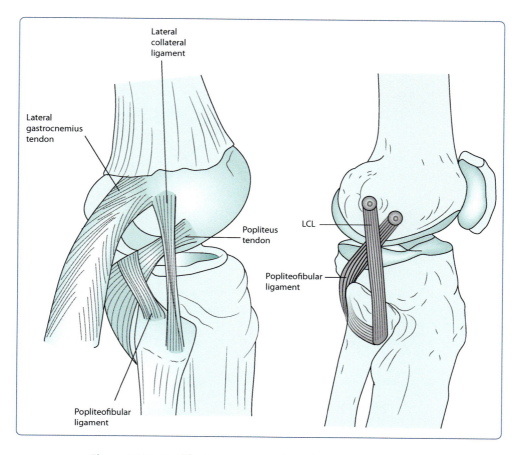

Figure 12.21 Modified Larson posterolateral corner reconstruction.

Recommended references

Crespo B, James EW, Metsavaht L et al. Injuries to posterolateral corner of the knee: A comprehensive review from anatomy to surgical treatment. *Rev Bras Ortop.* 2015;**50**:363–370.

Djian P. Posterolateral knee reconstruction. *Orthopaedics & Traumatology: Surgery & Research.* 2015;**101**:S159–S170.

Niki Y, Matsumoto H, Otani T et al. A modified Larson's method of posterolateral corner reconstruction of the knee reproducing the physiological tensioning pattern of the lateral collateral and popliteofibular ligaments. *Sports Medicine, Arthroscopy, Rehabilitation, Therapy & Technology.* 2012;**4**:21.

Posterior cruciate ligament reconstruction
Preoperative planning
Indications

Many isolated PCL ruptures will be successfully managed conservatively, particularly low-grade injuries; surgical reconstruction is indicated for persistent symptomatic instability (e.g. deceleration and slope/stair descent) despite conservative management and rehabilitation. Other surgical indications are combined injuries and refractory patellofemoral pain resulting from increased patellofemoral forces with posterior tibial translation.

Consent and risks

- Popliteal artery injury
- Posterior meniscal root injury – during placement of tibial tunnel
- Residual posterior laxity grade II or greater approximately 25%
- Osteoarthritis approximately 60% at 9 years

Operative planning

As with other ligament reconstructions around the knee, there are many options and controversies surrounding the optimal graft choice, construct and fixation. Both single- and double-bundle techniques can be used but the relative benefits of each continue to be debated. Single-bundle techniques typically aim to restore the larger anterolateral bundle. Graft choice may depend on previous surgery or combined injuries; autograft and allograft have both been used successfully. Later we describe the use of quadrupled hamstring graft, similar to that for ACL reconstruction, but consideration needs to be given to ensuring sufficient length of graft, which is longer than that for ACL reconstruction. Grafts with bone blocks may present challenges with graft passage because of the angle the graft needs to turn on exiting the tibial tunnel. For those reasons some surgeons will routinely use allograft as their primary graft choice.

Surgical technique

Incision

The procedure described next is performed arthroscopically. A posteromedial portal is placed to access the tibial attachment of the PCL. An accessory anterolateral portal may be used to position the femoral tunnel.

An incision over the medial proximal tibia is created as for hamstring harvest. If the hamstrings are being harvested this will be performed at the same time; if not then the anteromedial tibia is exposed to place the tunnel for PCL reconstruction.

Procedure

The free hamstring graft is harvested and prepared as for ACL reconstruction.

Following full diagnostic arthroscopy and treatment of any associated meniscal lesions, the femoral tunnel is created. The location of the femoral attachment on the medial wall of the notch is identified while visualising through the anterolateral portal. The larger anterolateral bundle is high on the medial wall and adjacent to the chondral surface of the medial femoral condyle. A point is marked at the intended guide wire insertion point so that when the tunnel is placed, matching the diameter of the graft, its edge will be adjacent to the chondral margin within the native femoral footprint (**Figure 12.22**). A Beath pin is inserted from the anterolateral portal and directed out through the anteromedial femur and thigh skin. The femoral tunnel is created in the same manner as described for hamstring ACL reconstruction: first drilled with a 4.5 mm drill to accommodate the suspensory button device, then over-drilled to match the graft diameter up to, but not through, the femoral cortex. A shuttle suture is pulled up through the tunnel and out the medial thigh using the Beath pin.

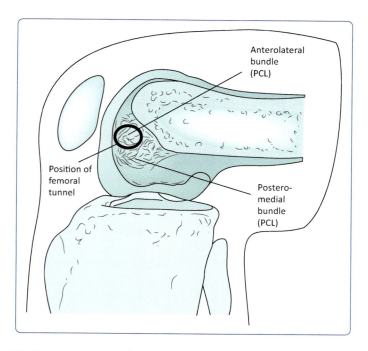

Figure 12.22 PCL footprint on medial wall of the notch, and position of femoral tunnel for single bundle reconstruction.

A posteromedial portal and arthroscopic cannula are placed. An arthroscopic shaver is used via the posteromedial portal, while visualising through the notch, to expose the tibial attachment of the PCL, taking care to face the shaver blade anteriorly to reduce risks to the popliteal neurovascular bundle. The tibial footprint is then visualised through the posteromedial portal while a guide wire is passed from the anteromedial tibia, approximately 6 cm below and at an angle of 50° to the tibial plateau, to exit at the planned tibial tunnel site. The tunnel is positioned at a ridge between the attachments of the anterolateral and posteromedial bundles, just proximal to the so-called 'champagne-glass drop-off' at the upper border of popliteus, and below the shiny white fibres at the posterior meniscal root attachment, which can be damaged if the tunnel is placed too high (**Figure 12.23**). Care must be taken to avoid posterior soft tissue penetration of the guide wire and risk to the popliteal neurovascular bundle; it must be directly visualised to penetrate the posterior cortex, and PCL-specific guides are available with protection devices to prevent over-penetration of the wire. The guide wire position can be confirmed with fluoroscopy. The tibial tunnel is drilled over the guide wire to match the diameter of the graft. Again, the tip of the guide wire must be visualised to prevent over-penetration with the drill; a curette placed in the posteromedial portal is used to cover the tip of the guide wire during drilling.

A rasp is used to smooth the proximal edge of the tibial tunnel aperture on the posterior cortex, to reduce graft abrasion at the tibial 'killer angle'. A second shuttle suture is passed into the knee through the tibial tunnel and retrieved through the anterolateral portal in order to pass the femoral shuttle suture back through the tibial tunnel. The suspensory button and attached graft are pulled up through the tibial and femoral tunnels. Passage of the graft around the

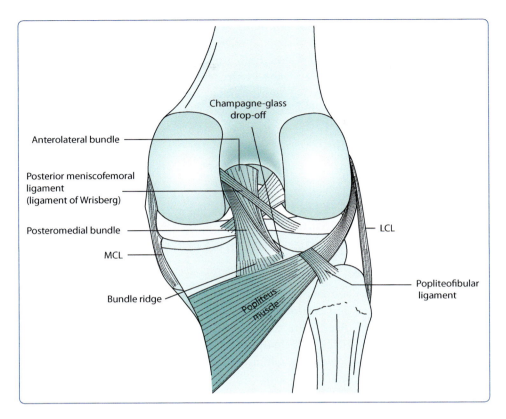

Figure 12.23 Tibial attachment of the PCL. The guide wire is positioned to exit at the bundle ridge.

angle of the tibial tunnel may be difficult; a trocar placed through the posteromedial portal can help to lever the graft out through the tunnel and work it around the angle toward the femoral tunnel. When passed out through the medial femoral cortex the suspensory button is flipped. The graft is tensioned at 90° flexion and with an anterior drawer applied to reduce the posterior tibial sag and secured in the tibial tunnel with an interference screw.

Postoperative care and instructions

PCL graft healing takes about double the length of time of ACL healing. Although individual surgeons may have their own preferred programmes and the precise rehabilitation may need to be tailored to associated injuries, the principles are for initial limited weightbearing, prevention of posterior tibial subluxation, focus on quadriceps strengthening and limitation of hamstring activity.

The patient remains non-weightbearing for the first 6 weeks, gradually increasing to full weightbearing thereafter. A static PCL brace (with a bolster behind the calf) in extension is used for the first 2 weeks before transitioning to a dynamic PCL brace to be worn at all times initially. Isometric quads activity is allowed immediately, and prone passive flexion is allowed once in the dynamic brace, limited to 90° for the first 6 weeks. From 6 to 12 weeks full passive range of motion is allowed, along with more intense quads strengthening, but weightbearing flexion remains restricted to 70°. After 12 weeks weightbearing flexion can increase and the brace can be weaned off, aiming for removal after about 4 months. Strengthening continues, allowing isolated hamstring activity at this time, followed by running and agility exercises after 5–6 months and a goal-directed sports-specific exercise programme with eventual return to sport after about 9 months.

Recommended references

Pache S, Aman ZS, Kennedy M et al. Posterior cruciate ligament: Current concepts review. *Arch Bone Jt Surg*. 2018;**6**:8–18.

Vaquero-Picado A, Rodríguez-Merchán EC. Isolated posterior cruciate ligament tears: An update of management. *EFORT Open Rev*. 2017;**2**:89–96.

Medial collateral ligament reconstruction

Preoperative planning

Indications

MCL injuries are common but will often be managed conservatively; a careful bracing regime may negate the need for reconstruction even after high-grade injuries. Reconstruction is indicated in multi-ligament or other combination injuries requiring surgical repair, in chronic instability which has failed conservative management and rarely following debridement of a Pellegrini-Stieda lesion. Occasionally, the ruptured end of the ligament may be incarcerated within the joint or displaced superficial to the pes (analogous to a Stener lesion) and will not be expected to heal without surgery. Primary repair is often possible if performed early but may need to be augmented depending on the quality of the repair and tissues.

Consent and risks

- Arthrofibrosis
- Saphenous nerve and its infrapatellar branch
- Recurrent instability/graft failure

Operative planning

Autograft, allograft and synthetics are all options for medial reconstruction. The main consideration when comparing different constructs is whether the posterior oblique ligament (POL) is also reconstructed. Careful examination for posteromedial corner injury, looking specifically for valgus laxity in full extension (also associated with cruciate injury) and increased external rotation due to excess anteromedial translation (in contrast to posterolateral injury where increased external rotation is due to posterolateral translation), may guide the need to include POL reconstruction, although whether this is included routinely remains a subject of discussion. The following description does include a limb to reconstruct the POL, although it is accepted that this may not necessarily be performed in all cases and there are other methods described to achieve this.

Surgical technique

Landmarks
- Medial epicondyle
- Medial proximal tibia
- Semimembranosus tendon

Incision and approach
The procedure can be performed through multiple smaller incisions but the full approach is described here. A curved medial longitudinal incision is made from the medial epicondyle to medial tibia about 6–7 cm below the joint line. Dissection is continued down to the sartorial fascia, which is incised in line with the skin incision, taking care not to damage the hamstring tendons. The semitendinosus tendon is harvested as per ACL reconstruction. The remaining native MCL is identified deep to the sartorial fascia and pes anserinus.

Procedure
The free semitendinosus tendon is whip-stitched at both ends with heavy suture as for ACL reconstruction. The tendon is looped over a suture or nylon tape and the diameter of the doubled graft measured. One limb of the graft will reconstruct the superficial MCL (sMCL) while the other will reconstruct the POL, in this case from a single femoral tunnel, although techniques with separate femoral tunnels are described.

The tibial attachments of the sMCL are identified (**Figure 12.24**). There are two sites of tibial attachment: the distal site is located approximately 6 cm below the joint line, deep to the pes anserinus, just anterior to the posterior tibial border; the proximal tibial attachment is located 12 mm below the joint line, in line with the semimembranosus attachment. A Beath pin is inserted at the distal site to exit the anterolateral tibia. It is positioned towards the posterior tibial border but so there is sufficient bone for a tunnel to be drilled without blowout of the posterior cortex.

The tibial attachment of the POL is identified 1–1.5 cm below the joint line at the posteromedial corner of the tibia (**Figure 12.24**), adjacent to the semimembranosus attachment. A second Beath pin is inserted aiming to exit the anterolateral tibia at Gerdy's tubercle.

The femoral tunnel site is identified next. The sMCL attachment is reported to be 3.2 mm proximal and 4.8 mm posterior to the medial epicondyle (**Figure 12.24**). A Beath pin is inserted at this point, directed anterolaterally to exit the femur and skin of the anterolateral thigh, being careful to avoid entering the intercondylar notch. Isometry is now checked by wrapping sutures around the Beath pins to connect the femoral and tibial guide pins in the proposed positions of the sMCL and POL reconstructions and putting the knee through a range of motion to assess the change in tension on the sutures. The sMCL should be isometric throughout, while the POL is lax in flexion but tightens in extension. The femoral pin position can be moved to improve isometry if necessary.

When the positions are confirmed, a tunnel to accommodate the looped end of the graft is drilled in the femur in the same way as for ACL reconstruction, for fixation with a cortical suspensory button device. A suspensory button with a loop length to place 2–2.5 cm of graft within the tunnel is selected. The graft is looped through the suspensory button device and

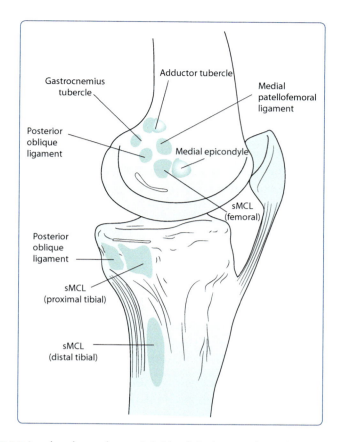

Figure 12.24 Landmarks on the medial side of the knee and attachment of the MCL.

pulled into the femoral tunnel via the Beath pin, and the button is flipped. After ensuring sufficient length on each end of the graft to perform the sMCL and POL reconstructions, with 2–2.5 cm of graft in each tunnel, the femoral end is secured with an interference screw.

The tibial tunnels are then drilled to an appropriate diameter and depth to accommodate the ends of the graft. One limb of the graft can then be pulled into the POL tunnel and the other into the sMCL tunnel via the whip-stitches and Beath pins. The POL reconstruction is tensioned at full extension and secured with an interference screw. The sMCL reconstruction is tensioned at 20° flexion with slight varus and secured at its distal attachment with an interference screw. The proximal tibial attachment site of the sMCL is finally secured with a ligament staple (**Figure 12.25**). Any lax and redundant posteromedial capsule can be tightened by suturing it to the POL reconstruction in full extension. The knee is put through a range of motion to determine a safe range for initial rehabilitation without placing undue tension on any repaired or reconstructed tissue.

Closure

The free whip-stitch ends are cut flush to the skin and buried. The cortical button's lead and flipping sutures are removed. The skin is closed in a standard fashion and a wool and crepe bandage applied.

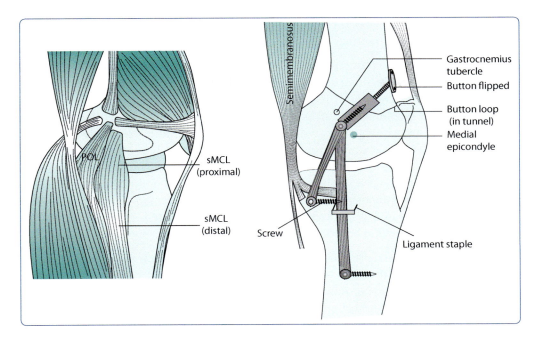

Figure 12.25 Completed MCL reconstruction.

Postoperative care and instructions

The patient mobilises non-weightbearing in a hinged brace for the first 6 weeks. Initial range of motion during the first 2 weeks is determined by the safe zone defined intraoperatively; this can be increased after 2 weeks. Simple quads exercises are started immediately. Weightbearing is gradually increased from 6 to 12 weeks. Further strengthening is allowed when gait has returned without significant limp, and eventual return to sport follows a goal-based regime.

Recommended references

Andrews K, Lu A, Mckean L et al. Review: Medial collateral ligament injuries. *J Orthop*. 2017;**14**:550–554.
DeLong JM, Waterman BR. Surgical techniques for the reconstruction of medial collateral ligament and posteromedial corner injuries of the knee: A systematic review. *Arthroscopy*. 2015;**31**:2258–2272.
Wijdicks CA, Griffith CJ, Johansen S et al. Injuries to the medial collateral ligament and associated medial structures of the knee. *J Bone Joint Surg Am*. 2010;**92**:1266–1280.

Multi-ligament injuries

The full details of multi-ligament knee injuries are beyond the scope of this book. As with all soft tissue knee surgery there are many controversies, but some reconstructive principles are worth noting here. These injuries are often high energy and associated with polytrauma; any life- or limb-threatening injuries must be identified and treated. If the knee is dislocated then it must be reduced urgently, and associated neurovascular injuries must also be identified and treated. A range-of-motion brace will usually be sufficient to maintain reduction. Care must be taken to identify the extent of the injury by thorough clinical examination, under anaesthesia if necessary, especially in cases where the knee has reduced spontaneously and plain radiographs may look normal. Definitive reconstructive procedures can then be planned.

The timing of definitive reconstruction remains a matter of debate. Some surgeons will routinely perform early reconstruction (within 3 weeks, second week is optimal) but indications for early reconstruction otherwise are irreducible dislocations, neurovascular injuries, posterolateral corner injury and associated fractures. Open surgery will be required in early cases because capsular injury will lead to arthroscopic fluid leak. Early repair of the medial and lateral/posterolateral structures is possible, especially avulsions, but improved outcomes are seen if augmented with reconstruction, particularly in mid-substance tears. The alternative approach is for delayed reconstruction (after 3 months) in the absence of indications for early reconstruction. A period of appropriate bracing can effectively downgrade the extent of the injury, allowing healing of the PCL and MCL in particular, and simplifying later reconstruction based on residual instability.

Whether the full reconstruction is performed in a single operation or a staged strategy is used largely depends on the experience of the surgeon and what the surgeon feels confident with, given the constraints of tourniquet time in these potentially long and demanding procedures. Either way, careful planning of the sequence in which the various steps of the reconstruction are performed is crucial, and the PCL, if being reconstructed, must be tensioned and secured before other reconstructions are completed in order to reduce the tibia under the femur (can be confirmed with fluoroscopy) and prevent fixed posterior translation that will occur if the ACL is tensioned without the restraint of a competent PCL.

Consideration will need to be given to the choice of grafts. Autograft, allograft and synthetics may all have their place, and harvest from the contralateral limb is common. It is widely accepted that synthetic grafts are a reasonable option for extra-articular reconstructions, and they may also be used for PCL reconstruction, although their use in ACL reconstruction is generally avoided for the reasons given earlier. Tunnels need to be positioned to avoid clashes. Placing the multiple required guide wires, which can then be checked with fluoroscopy prior to completing tunnel preparation, can be helpful in this regard.

Full range of motion must be confirmed at the end of the procedure. Rehabilitation depends on the specific injury pattern but a period of protected weightbearing and early passive restoration of motion in a hinged brace is preferable.

Recommended references

Buyukdogan K, Laidlaw MS, Miller MD. Surgical management of the multiple-ligament knee injury. *Arthrosc Tech*. 2018;**7**:e147–e164.

Lachman JR, Rehman S, Pipitone PS. Traumatic knee dislocations: Evaluation, management, and surgical treatment. *Orthop Clin North Am*. 2015;**46**:479–493.

Moatshe G, LaPrade RF, Engebretsen L. How to avoid tunnel convergence in a multiligament injured knee. *Ann Joint*. 2018;**3**:93.

Osteotomy and soft tissue surgery of the knee

Although the technical aspects of osteotomy about the knee are considered elsewhere, and the full details of this topic are beyond the scope of this book, it is worth noting the relevance of such techniques in the context of soft tissue reconstruction. Malalignment and abnormal tibial slope are known to be risk factors for failure of ligament reconstruction. Indeed, in chronic instability, particularly in the presence of degenerative changes, corrective osteotomy may be the operation of choice to address the instability with or without additional ligament reconstruction.

Similarly, both correct alignment and stability are required for optimal outcomes of both meniscal repair/allograft transplantation and chondral regenerative procedures. Furthermore, an intact and functional meniscus is required for successful chondral surgery. This has led to the concept of a reconstructive ladder of knee joint preservation surgery, requiring alignment, stability, meniscus and chondral surfaces all be addressed to optimise outcomes. An assessment of these is especially important in failed reconstructive surgery; an osteotomy may be required before embarking on any further soft tissue procedures to avoid repeat failures.

Recommended references

Cantin O, Magnussen RA, Corbi F et al. The role of high tibial osteotomy in the treatment of knee laxity: A comprehensive review. *Knee Surg Sports Traumatol Arthrosc.* 2015;**23**:3026–3037.

Harris JD, Cavo M, Brophy R et al. Biological knee reconstruction: A systematic review of combined meniscal allograft transplantation and cartilage repair or restoration. *Arthroscopy: The Journal of Arthroscopic and Related Surgery.* 2011;**27**:409–418.

Tischer T, Paul J, Pape D et al. The impact of osseous malalignment and realignment procedures in knee ligament surgery: A systematic review of the clinical evidence. *Orthop J Sports Med.* 2017;**5**:2325967117697287.

Viva questions

1. What equipment is required to perform a diagnostic arthroscopy?
2. Define the anatomy of the posterior knee arthroscopy portals.
3. Which structures are at risk in the posterior portals for knee arthroscopy?
4. What are the indications for meniscal repair?
5. Which techniques do you know for meniscal repair?
6. How are discoid lateral menisci classified?
7. What treatment do you use for a discoid lateral meniscus?
8. Which associated anatomical findings worsen a tight lateral retinaculum?
9. What are the advantages and disadvantages of arthroscopic over open lateral release?
10. What are the common indications for cartilage reconstruction surgery?
11. Describe the procedure of microplasty to the medial femoral condyle.
12. What are the advantages of autologous chondrocyte implantation over microplasty?
13. How are the cells provided for autologous chondrocyte implantation?
14. What risks do you describe to a patient consenting to ACL reconstruction?

15. Describe the anatomy of the pes anserinus.
16. How are the hamstrings harvested for an ACL graft?
17. What is the minimal acceptable graft thickness for ACL reconstruction?
18. Where are the isometric points for the origin of insertion of an ACL graft?
19. What position is the knee held in while an ACL graft is tensioned and fixed?
20. Describe your postoperative regimen after an ACL reconstruction.

13 Surgery of the Ankle

Matthew Welck, Laurence James and Dishan Singh

Ankle arthrodesis	367	Surgery for Achilles tendinopathy	377
Ankle arthroplasty	371	Surgery for peroneal tendinopathy	381
Ankle arthroscopy	374	Viva questions	383

Movement	Range of motion
Dorsiflexion	0°–20°
Plantarflexion	0°–45°

Position of arthrodesis
- Neutral flexion
- 0°–5° valgus
- 5°–10° external rotation

Ankle arthrodesis
Preoperative planning
Indications
- Arthropathy failing conservative management
- Failed arthroplasty
- Tumour reconstruction
- Sequelae of infection, particularly tuberculosis
- Avascular necrosis of talus
- Neuropathic joint
- Neurological conditions (resulting in instability)

Contraindications
- Infection
- Degeneration of subtalar and midfoot joints

> ### Consent and risks
>
> - Failure of fusion: Less than 2%
> - Malpositioning (poorly tolerated, particularly equinus, varus and internal rotation)
> - Metalwork prominence: May require further surgery
> - Nerve injury is rare
> - Progression of arthritis of surrounding joints
>
> The patient must understand that walking will not return to normal. There is a significant reduction in walking speed and increase in energy expenditure compared with normal.

Operative planning

Planning of the position of fusion is vital. The position is:

- 0° dorsiflexion
- 0°–5° valgus hindfoot (varus positioning restricts midtarsal mobility)
- 5°–10° external rotation (Note: Observe contralateral limb)

Posterior displacement of the talus allows for greater ease of 'rollover' at the end of the stance phase. Avoid residual anterior displacement.

Anaesthesia and positioning

These are performed as for ankle replacement.

Surgical technique

Arthrodesis can be performed arthroscopically (see 'Ankle arthroscopy' p. 374) or open. Arthroscopic ankle arthrodesis has been shown to have equivalent union rates with shorter hospital stay; however, it is more difficult to correct deformity. Open ankle arthrodesis is usually via an anterior approach (see 'Ankle arthroplasty' p. 371). The lateral transmalleolar approach may be used if soft tissues determine it, or if the subtalar joint is also to be arthrodesed (tibio-talo-calcaneal arthrodesis). Where possible the fibula is preserved for an isolated ankle arthrodesis to provide increased surface and vascularity for fusion and to enable potential conversion to arthroplasty in the future. Internal fixation is with crossed or parallel screws and/or plates for isolated ankle arthrodesis. Screws, plates or intramedullary nails are used for tibio-talo-calcaneal fusion. It is essential to obtain good hold and adequate compression (**Figure 13.1**). Thorough preparation of all joint surfaces is vital. This is achieved by removal of remaining articular cartilage and exposure of subchondral bleeding cancellous bone to aid biological union.

For surgical principles of joint surface preparation, see Chapter 14.

Ankle arthrodesis

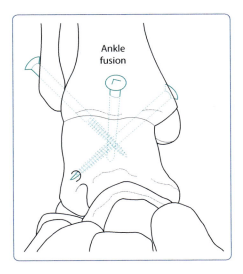

Figure 13.1 Arthrodesis with screw fixation.

Lateral transmalleolar approach

Landmarks
- Tip, anterior and posterior border of fibula
- Base of fourth metatarsal
- Anterior to sural nerve

Dissection
A longitudinal incision is made directly over the lateral aspect of the fibula, of sufficient length to avoid tension on the soft tissue flap. Distally the incision is angled toward the base of the fourth metatarsal to allow greater access to the ankle joint (and subtalar joint if required).

Procedure

> **Structures at risk**
> - Peroneal tendons
> - Sural nerve

Subperiosteal dissection of the fibula is carried out, protecting the peroneal tendons posteriorly and distally at all times. This also serves to protect the sural nerve. The joint line is identified, using an image intensifier, and is marked on the skin. The fibula is cut obliquely with a saw (superolateral to inferomedial ending at the level of the tibial plafond) and finished with an osteotome. The free distal end of the fibula is then reflected inferiorly and freed of soft tissues and ligamentous attachments, and it is excised. Care is taken not to divide the peroneal tendons at the tip of the distal fibula during excision. Capsulotomy then allows access to the tibiotalar surface. Continued dissection distally will expose the subtalar joint if required. The bone of the distal fibula can then be used to harvest cancellous bone graft and the surgeon's choice of fixation is performed. For an isolated ankle fusion, with good quality bone, cannulated screws can be used. For poorer quality bone, or if the subtalar joint is to be included, a retrograde tibio-talo-calcaneal nail is a better choice (**Figure 13.2**).

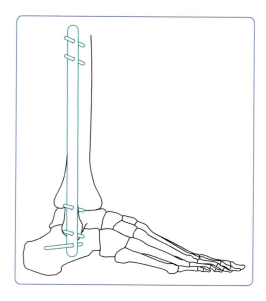

Figure 13.2 Arthrodesis with nail fixation.

Closure

A layered closure is followed by the surgeon's choice of skin closure for open techniques. Nylon to skin is used to close arthroscopic fusion portals.

Postoperative care and instructions

Thromboembolism should be prevented by early mobilisation and the addition of chemical or mechanical measures in patients at increased risk.

Early mobilisation is non-weightbearing, with the aid of crutches. Radiographic signs of union are sought before unprotected full weightbearing is allowed; this often takes around 3 months.

Recommended references

Buck P, Morrey BF, Chao EY. The optimum position of arthrodesis of the ankle. *J Bone Joint Surg Am.* 1987;**69**:1052–1062.
Hendrickx RP, Stufkens SA, de Bruijn EE, Sierevelt IN, van Dijk CN, Kerkhoffs GM. Medium- to long-term outcome of ankle arthrodesis. *Foot Ankle Int.* 2011;**32(10)**:940–947.
Kitaoka HB, Patzer GL, Felix NA. Arthrodesis for the treatment of arthrosis of the ankle and osteonecrosis of the talus. *J Bone Joint Surg Am.* 1998;**80**:370–379.
Mann RA. Arthrodesis of the foot and ankle. In RA Mann and MJ Coughlin, eds. *Surgery of the Foot and Ankle.* St. Louis, MO: Mosby Year Book, 1993.

Mann R, Rongstad AM. Arthrodesis of the ankle: A critical analysis. *Foot Ankle Int*. 1998;**19**:3–9.
Scranton PE. An overview of ankle arthrodesis. *Clin Orthop Relat Res*. 1991;**268**:268–296.
Townshend D, Di Silvestro M, Krause F et al. Arthroscopic versus open ankle arthrodesis: A multicenter comparative case series. *J Bone Joint Surg Am*. 2013;**95(2)**:98–102.

Ankle arthroplasty
Preoperative planning
Indications
Total ankle arthroplasty is indicated in painful conditions that have failed conservative management. The most frequent indications are:

- Osteoarthritis (often post-traumatic)
- Inflammatory arthritis and other arthropathies
- Average age 68 years, from latest National Joint Registry

Contraindications
- Ankle joint infection
- Avascular necrosis of a large part of the talar body
- Severe deformity that would not allow for good biomechanical function and cause early failure (traditionally felt to be greater than the 15° varus/valgus deformity, although experienced arthroplasty surgeons now sometimes exceeding this)
- Poor soft tissue envelope
- Heavy manual occupation
- Neurovascular compromise (e.g. Charcot neuroarthropathy)

Consent and risks
- Loosening: Failure rates variably reported usually between 1% and 2% per year.
- Malpositioning.
- Fracture: Most common is medial malleolus. Up to 10% though they fare well with appropriate identification and management.
- Wound problems.
- Pain and stiffness: 5%.
- Deep vein thrombosis (DVT)/pulmonary embolism/infection: 1%.

Operative planning
Assessment of the soft tissues, as well as vascular and neurological examination, are mandatory on the day of surgery. Recent weightbearing radiographs must be available. These may include long leg alignment films if there is any proximal deformity that needs to be taken into consideration.

Availability of the implants and operative sets must be checked by the surgeon. Prophylactic antibiotics are administered on induction (the antibiotic of choice depends on local policy).

Anaesthesia and positioning

Anaesthesia is usually general, regional or combined. A thigh tourniquet is used. The supine position is used with appropriate padding where necessary. Occasionally, a sandbag under the ipsilateral buttock allows for greater ease of surgery. The knee should always be exposed and prepared (with a germicidal solution) to allow for intraoperative orientation of the implant.

The ankle should be sufficiently mobile for appropriate movement intraoperatively. Some rest the calf on a support to facilitate this. Waterproof drapes are used with adhesive edges to provide a seal to the skin.

Surgical technique

Landmarks

These should be marked preoperatively:

- Tendons (tibialis anterior, extensor hallucis longus, extensor digitorum longus)
- Dorsalis pedis (Note: This is absent in 10% of the population.)
- Cutaneous branches of the superficial peroneal nerve (variable course)

Incision

The anterior approach to the ankle is used. The skin is incised in the midpoint between the medial and lateral malleoli – from 3 cm above, extending 5 cm below the palpable ankle joint and avoiding cutaneous nerves where encountered.

The superficial peroneal nerve is often encountered and should be freed and marked with a coloured loop. Care must be taken to avoid excess traction on this during the operation.

Dissection

> **Structures at risk**
>
> - Dorsalis pedis artery
> - Deep peroneal nerve

The extensor retinaculum is divided in the line of the incision. We tend to create medial and lateral flaps of the retinaculum as we are opening it, in order to facilitate closure and prevent bow stringing of the tibialis anterior tendon. Large skin flaps are avoided to reduce the risk of necrosis. The approach is then developed either between the extensor hallucis longs (EHL) and the extensor digitorum longus (EDL) or (more commonly) between the tibialis anterior and the EHL. The key is protecting the dorsalis pedis artery and deep peroneal nerve – identification (and protection) of these structures more proximally, before they cross at the ankle joint itself, may be required. A longitudinal capsulotomy is then performed.

Procedure

Several ankle prostheses are commercially available, and the individual operative technique should be referred to. Although the designs vary, the principles include minimal soft tissue handling and bone resection, correction of deformity at the ankle, press fit between bone and implant, ligament and tendon balancing and correction of any concomitant foot deformity. In general terms, an extramedullary guide is placed on the anterior surface of the tibia. Pins are used to fix the cutting guide to the tibia. The tibia is cut in the correct coronal, sagittal and rotational planes. The talar cut is then usually referenced from the tibial cut. This ensures parallel cuts in the distal tibia and talar dome, without altering the joint line height – approximately 2–3 mm is resected from each surface. Guides then size the tibial and talar components, and accurate anterior and posterior chamfer cuts are made to the talus. Trial components and a spacer (to assess stability and range of movement) are used prior to actual prosthesis placement.

Pitfalls to avoid include:

- Varus/valgus positioning of tibial and talar cutting guides, which can also lead to abnormal sagittal plane tilting – early loosening
- Anterior/posterior placement of talar or tibial components – early loosening
- Notching of medial and lateral malleoli during tibial cuts – fracture
- Failure to balance the foot underneath the ankle replacement (e.g. a rigid flat foot under an ankle replacement will cause early failure)

Newer-generation systems are uncemented with a predominance of fixed bearing implants. Commonly used prostheses include Infinity, Box, Zenith and STAR (Scandinavian Total Ankle Replacement).

Postoperative care and instructions

This usually includes non-weightbearing and immobilisation in a cast for 4–6 weeks. The patient is then transitioned into a removable boot and begins weightbearing and exercises. A return to work (and driving) would be expected after 3 months. Follow-up is recommended at 6 weeks, 6 months and 1 year after surgery. Continuation of follow-up is typically at 5 years, 10 years, 15 years and then at yearly intervals. The patient should be cautioned to return to the clinic if there is pain or functional deterioration.

Recommended references

Carachiolo B. Design features of current total ankle replacements: Implants and instruments. *J Am Acad Orthop Surg*. 2008;**19**:530–540.

Hopgood P, Kumar R, Wood PL. Arthrodesis for failed ankle replacement. *J Bone Joint Surg Br*. 2006;**88**:1032–1038.

Saltzman CL, Mann RA, Ahrens JE et al. Prospective controlled trial of STAR total ankle replacement versus ankle fusion: Initial results. *Foot Ankle Int*. 2009;**30(7)**:579–596.

Spirt AA, Assal M, Hansen ST Jr. Complications and failure after total ankle arthroplasty. *J Bone Joint Surg Am*. 2004;**86**:1172–1178.

Wood PL, Deakin S. Total ankle replacement: The results in 200 ankles. *J Bone Joint Surg Br*. 2003;**85**:334–341.

Zaidi R, Cro S, Gurusamy K et al. The outcome of total ankle replacement: A systematic review and meta-analysis. *Bone Joint J*. 2013;**95-B(11)**:1500–1507.

Ankle arthroscopy

Preoperative planning

Indications

- Osteochondral defect
- Undiagnosed ankle pain in the young
- Osteoarthritis
- Removal of loose bodies
- Synovectomy or synovial biopsy
- Impingement syndromes (bony and soft tissue, anterior and posterior)
- Arthrofibrosis (e.g. post-traumatic)
- Fracture
- Meniscoidal lesions
- Septic arthritis

Contraindications

- Infection of overlying skin
- Lack of proper instrumentation
- Gross osteoarthritis is a relative contraindication
- Severe oedema

Consent and risks

- Nerve injury: Less than 1%
- Vascular injury: Less than 1%
- Infection: Less than 1%; risk is very low, so prophylactic antibiotics are not recommended

Operative planning

It is vital that the patient is examined before transfer to theatre. This allows for identification and marking of structures vulnerable to damage during portal insertion intraoperatively. These include:

- Tibialis anterior and EHL tendons
- Dorsalis pedis artery and associated deep peroneal nerve
- Traction on second and fourth toes usually demonstrates medial and lateral branches of the superficial peroneal nerve
- Saphenous vein and nerve
- Medial and lateral malleoli

Recent radiographs and, where taken, magnetic resonance (MR) images should be available.

The equipment must be available; this should be checked by the surgeon. Usually, a 2.7 mm 30° arthroscope and 3.5 mm shavers are used; however, a 4 mm scope may be used in some circumstances (e.g. arthroscopic arthrodesis) to increase field of view. Water pressure is set at 50 mm Hg.

Anaesthesia and positioning

Anaesthesia is usually general with intraoperative local anaesthetic infiltration into the joint at the end of the procedure. A variety of techniques of patient positioning and joint distraction are available. For anterior arthroscopy, the authors' preferred technique involves the supine position, with the hip flexed and a well-padded support under the thigh. An ankle distractor is applied with the knee at 90° of flexion and the ankle in a neutral position. Adequate padding avoids damage to skin and neurological structures. Too much traction (>15 kg) and excessive time can lead to irreversible nerve damage.

The surgical field is prepared with a germicidal solution. Waterproof drapes are used with adhesive edges to provide a seal to the skin.

Surgical technique

The ankle joint is filled with 20 mL of saline to aid access and avoid chondral surface damage. Small longitudinal skin incisions are made, then blunt dissection (with a clip) is used to breech the ankle joint, thereby avoiding damage to the superficial nerves – unlike knee arthroscopy where a blade is passed directly into the joint.

Creation of portals

Structures at risk

- *Nerves*: Deep peroneal, superficial peroneal branches, sural, tibial
- *Arteries*: Dorsalis pedis, posterior tibial artery

A number of portal sites are described (**Figure 13.3**). The central anterior portal is best avoided because of a high risk of neurovascular damage.

- *Anteromedial portal*: This lies medial to tibialis anterior. The joint line is initially identified by palpation and then a white needle is inserted into the joint to confirm the level. It is helpful to mark out the tip of the medial and lateral malleoli in order to identify the ankle joint more proximal to these. The needle is directed slightly superiorly to pass over the talar dome. The arthroscope and introducing trochar should be able to be swept across the joint from medial to lateral.
- *Anterolateral portal*: This lies lateral to extensor peroneus tertius and the neurovascular bundle (dorsalis pedis and deep peroneal nerve), avoiding the superficial nerves marked out preoperatively. The light source within the joint can be used as a guide; this will also help to *identify the dorsal lateral branch of the superficial peroneal nerve which is at risk*. A white needle is inserted as outlined earlier. This helps ensure your instruments will come in from a suitable trajectory.

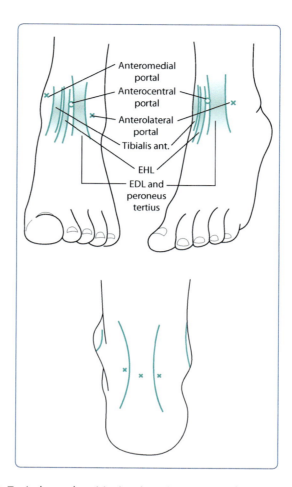

Figure 13.3 Typical portal positioning (anterior on top and posterior on bottom).

- *Posterolateral portal*: This is located lateral to the Achilles tendon 1 cm above the tip of fibula. The tip of the fibula is at the level of the subtalar joint. Insert prior to posteromedial portal – *risk of sural nerve damage*.
- *Posteromedial portal*: This is just medial to the Achilles tendon at the level of the posterolateral portal. Flexor hallucis longus is used to protect the *tibial nerve and posterior tibial artery – the main structures at risk*.

Posterior portals are not as frequently used (because of the increased risk of neurovascular damage) but are helpful in visualising the posterior ankle and subtalar joints.

Procedure

A systematic approach is essential if pathology is not to be missed. Initially the whole of the talar dome is inspected – ankle plantar flexion aids visualisation of the posterior dome. The talar neck is then examined. Pathology on the corresponding articulating surface of the tibia is also documented, as well as the anatomy of the anterior aspect of tibia. The medial and lateral gutters are then inspected. Key features to identify include:

- Medial malleolus
- Deltoid ligament
- Talar dome
- Tibial plafond
- Anterior inferior tibio-fibular ligament
- Posterior inferior tibio-fibular ligament
- Syndesmosis
- Lateral malleolus
- Anterior talofibular ligament

Closure

Non-absorbable suture is used to close the skin incisions.

Postoperative care and instructions

The patient is fully weightbearing – as tolerated – unless the patient has had a microfracture of an osteochondral defect, where range of movement is encouraged in a non-loading manner so as to protect the developing fibrocartilage plug.

Specific precautions are rarely required.

Recommended references

van Dijk CN, de Leeuw PA, Scholten PE. Hindfoot endoscopy for posterior ankle impingement. Surgical technique. *J Bone Joint Surg Am*. 2009;**91(Suppl 2)**:287–298.

Ferkel RD, Karzel RP, Del Pizzo W et al. Arthroscopic treatment of anterolateral impingement of the ankle. *Am J Sports Med*. 1991;**19**:440–446.

Ferkel RD, Zanotti RM, Komenda GA et al. Arthroscopic treatment of osteochondral lesions of the talus: Long-term results. *Am J Sports Med*. 2008;**36**:1750–1762.

Niek van Dijk C, van Bergen CJ. Advancements in ankle arthroscopy. *J Am Acad Orthop Surg*. 2008;**16**:635–646.

Tryfonidis M, Whitfield CG, Charalambous CP et al. Posterior ankle arthroscopy portal safety regarding proximity to the tibial and sural nerves. *Acta Orthop Belgica*. 2008;**74**:370–373.

Surgery for Achilles tendinopathy

Preoperative planning

There is an ever-increasing incidence of tendon problems, most commonly seen in recreational runners (racquet sports, track and field, volleyball and football) and competitive runners, who are 10 times more affected than age-matched controls.

Despite preventive measures, 7%–8% of top-level athletes experience the problem at some stage in their career.

Indications

There are three common patterns of Achilles tendon pathology:

- *Partial and complete ruptures*: There is a sudden onset of severe pain and marked disability. These ruptures are 10 times more common in males, with peak incidence in the 30s and 40s. Patients often describe hearing a 'pop' and feel an impact in the back of the leg or heel.

- *Non-insertional (mid-substance) tendinopathy*: This often has a gradual onset, classically with morning pain and stiffness that eases with activity and reoccurs at rest later. Associated with a sudden increase in activity, change of surface or change of footwear/poor footwear.
- *Insertional tendinopathy*: Degeneration and inflammation at the insertion of the Achilles tendon onto the calcaneus. This can be accompanied by a number of pathologies including retrocalcaneal bursitis, Haglund's disease (painful retrocalcaneal bursitis and a bony prominence), Achilles bursitis and enthesopathy.

Be aware of the systemic enthesopathies/rheumatoid arthritis and spondyloarthropathies.

This is an area where misdiagnosis is common and the differential diagnoses include:

- Posterior ankle impingement syndrome
- Accessory soleus
- Deep posterior compartment syndrome
- Sever's disease
- Stress fracture
- Inflammatory arthropathy
- Neurogenic referred pain

Contraindications

Active infection is a contraindication.

Consent and risks

- 12% complications (54% wound related)
- 88% return to function after a 6- to 12-month treatment programme

Operative planning

Non-operative management

Once the diagnosis has been made, consideration is given to whether operative treatment is the best option for the patient. These factors include:

- Age and activity level of patient.
- Ability to tolerate a rehabilitation regimen.
- *Gap size*: There have been reports of using the gap between tendon ends on dynamic ultrasound to help guide management. Some have used a gap of 5 or 10 mm in neutral or full equinus to drive surgical treatment, although there is no clear consensus on this.
- Traditionally the re-rupture rate was considerably greater with non-operative treatment; however, with the use of improved methods of non-operative treatment, the difference has narrowed.

Non-operative treatment of Achilles tendon rupture

Traditional techniques involved sequential non-weightbearing plasters, with lessening degrees of equinus. This had a high re-rupture rate. Recent studies support functional/

dynamic rehabilitation. This involves early weightbearing with a dynamic controlled range of motion.

Operative management

Anaesthesia and positioning
- General anaesthesia with local infiltration
- Thigh tourniquet
- Prone position with ankles resting on pillow

Surgical technique

There is much debate about open versus percutaneous repair. The open technique is described here, as an example. However, there is an increasing movement towards percutaneous repair techniques that reduce incidence of wound complications with little difference in strength of repair.

Landmarks
- Midpoint of the calcaneal tuberosity posteriorly where tendo-Achilles inserts
- Medial and lateral aspects of tendon traced proximally to bellies of gastrocnemius to identify aponeurosis

Incision

> **Structure at risk**
> - Sural nerve

A 5-10 cm incision is created (at the level of the defect) along the medial border of the Achilles tendon. This avoids the sural nerve and allows access to plantaris.

Dissection
- Directly deepen to paratenon
- Open paratenon and debride tendon
- Thick flaps are vital for healing

Procedure

It is necessary to address peritendinous adhesions and excise intratendinous lesions. A modified Kessler box suture is recommended. This consists of two standard Kessler sutures, at 90° to each other, ensuring the ends are tied inside not outside. It is best to use 1/0 PDS: this ensures good strength and slides easily. The repair is completed with a continuous epitendinous suture (3/0 Vicryl). A number of techniques are described where there is a large defect. This is usually for chronic ruptures with retraction. These include:

- *Turndown flaps*: This involves a centrally based fascial flap developed from the proximal segment and turned distally through 180° before suturing.

- *V-Y advancement*: A V-shaped incision is made in the aponeurosis. The limbs of the 'V' should be 1.5 cm longer than the gap to be filled. The intermediate segment is advanced distally, and the proximal segment is closed as a 'Y' in the lengthened position (**Figure 13.4**).

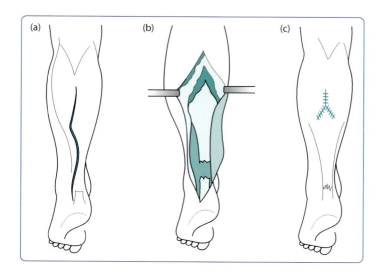

Figure 13.4 V-Y advancement for repairs with defect.

If the repair or augment is too compromised the flexor hallucis longus, the peroneus brevis or an allograft made of polyglycol or carbon fibre can be used.

Closure

Closure is performed in thick layers with a non-absorbable suture for the tendon repair. Absorbable suture is used for the paratenon and skin closure.

Postoperative care and instructions

Increasingly, functional regimens are also being used postoperatively. This involves early weightbearing and controlled range of motion.

Recommended references

Hufner TM, Brandes DB, Thermann H et al. Long-term results after functional nonoperative treatment of Achilles tendon rupture. *Foot Ankle Int*. 2006;**27**:167–171.

Kadakia AR, Dekker RG 2nd, Ho BS. Acute Achilles tendon ruptures: An update on treatment. *J Am Acad Orthop Surg*. 2017;**25(1)**:23–31.

Manoli A, Graham B. The subtle cavus foot. *Foot Ankle Int*. 2005;**26**:256–263.

Oyedele O, Maseko C, Mkasi N et al. High incidence of Os peroneum in cadavers. *Clin Anat*. 2005;**19**:605–610.

Soroceanu A, Sidhwa F, Aarabi S, Kaufman A, Glazebrook M. Surgical versus nonsurgical treatment of acute Achilles tendon rupture: A meta-analysis of randomized trials. *J Bone Joint Surg Am*. 2012;**94(23)**:2136–2143.

Surgery for peroneal tendinopathy

Preoperative planning

The peroneus longus originates from the lateral tibial condyle and head of fibula to insert on the first metatarsal base and medial cuneiform. The peroneus brevis originates from the middle one-third of the fibula and tibia to insert on the base of the fifth metatarsal. Remember, at the ankle the peroneus brevis is sandwiched between the bone and the peroneus longus – 'brevis to bone'.

Indications

A history of sprains is common. Other causes include trauma, inflammatory arthritides, fibula anatomy (shallow fibular groove, sharp lateral ridge), hypertrophied peroneal tubercle, lateral ankle instability and peroneus quartus (overcrowding). Developmental varus hindfoot alignment is associated with increased incidence of peroneal disorders:

- Tenosynovitis (a static mass on examination).
- Tendinosis (a mass moving with the tendon, through sheath).
- Tears (present with pain and weakness).
- Subluxation (palpation along the length of the tendons noting any deviation of their course).
- Os peroneum syndrome: Ossified in 20% population. Articulates with inferior margin of cuboid. May be degenerative/osteochondritis or fractured, leading to pain in the plantar/lateral aspect of the foot.
- Eventually pain-related functional weakness will lead to deformity.

Contraindications

Varus deformity related to underlying peroneal weakness rather than tendinopathy.

Consent and risks

- Sural nerve injury during dissection and skin closure
- Painful scar
- Late re-rupture/subluxation
- Fracture to tip of fibula/disruption of retinaculum
- Tendinous adhesions

Operative planning

Radiographs are helpful; however, magnetic resonance imaging and ultrasound show brevis flattening, thickening, nodules, tears, fluid in the peroneal sheath, dislocation and the retro-fibular groove anatomy in good detail (18% have a shallow or convex surface). The presence of fluid around a normal tendon on imaging indicates tenosynovitis.

Depending on the quality of proximal and distal tendon, orthoses (lateral posting) and physiotherapy are usually successful. Conservative management of peroneal subluxation has less than 50% success.

Anaesthesia and positioning

General anaesthesia with local infiltration, or spinal/epidural, can be used. The patient is positioned supine with a thigh tourniquet and a sandbag under the ipsilateral buttock or, more usually, the lateral position is used, with adequate supports and protection between leg pressure points.

Surgical technique

Landmarks

Landmarks are the tip of the fibula to the base of the fifth metatarsal.

Incision

A longitudinal incision is made parallel to the posterior border of the fibula. Distally, the incision is curved towards the base of the fifth metatarsal.

Dissection

Dissection is straight down, directly to the tendon sheath. Thick tissue flaps are reflected under minimal tension. The sheath is divided longitudinally and as posteriorly as possible, to aid repair and reduce scar tissue irritation when the tendons are mobilised under stress. Tendon hooks are used to isolate, deliver and clear individual tendons of adhesions.

Procedure

Surgical management for tendinopathy includes soft tissue procedures such as synovectomy, debridement or tubularization of tears. If greater than 50% of the tendon is intact, repair is advocated; if it is less than 50% tenodesis is recommended. Tendon transfer of flexor digitorum longus to peroneus brevis or an autograft using gracilis can maintain function.

Bony procedures include:

- *Deepening of the peroneal groove*: Using a 4.5 mm drill, a longitudinal hole is made in the posterior third of the tip of fibula, then the posterior cortex is 'stoved in' to deepen the peroneal groove. Some are now advocating this procedure to be done arthroscopically. The retinaculum is then repaired, and a calcaneal osteotomy can be performed if required. The tendons can also be rerouted behind the calcaneofibular ligament as an alternative to the deepening procedure.
- *Partial-thickness distal fibular osteotomy*: This is rotated posteriorly (Kelly procedure).
- *Distal fibular sliding graft* (Duvries modification): This can also be carried out (**Figure 13.5**).

Postoperative care and instructions

Tubularization of tears/bony procedures (4 weeks plaster of Paris, 4 weeks brace).

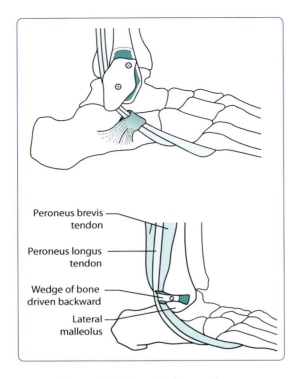

Figure 13.5 Bone block procedures.

Recommended references

Dombek MF, Catanzariti AR. Peroneal tendon tears: A retrospective review. *J Foot Ankle Surg.* 2003;**42**:250–258.

Manoli A, Graham B. The subtle cavus foot. *Foot Ankle Int.* 2005;**26**:256–263.

Oyedele O, Maseko C, Mkasi N et al. High incidence of Os peroneum in cadavers. *Clin Anat.* 2005;**19**:605–610.

Porter D, Torma J. Peroneal subluxation in athletes. *Foot Ankle Int.* 2005;**26**:436–441.

Viva questions

1. What are the indications for ankle arthrodesis?
2. What is the optimum position for ankle arthrodesis?
3. What are the treatment options for a 40-year-old man with symptomatic osteoarthritis of the ankle?
4. What are the pros and cons of ankle replacement versus ankle arthrodesis?
5. Describe the anatomy of the anterior approach to the ankle.
6. What complications do you warn the patient about prior to ankle replacement? What are their incidences?

7. What are the contraindications to ankle replacement?
8. Describe the portals used in anterior ankle arthroscopy.
9. How do you perform an ankle arthroscopy?
10. What are the complications of ankle arthroscopy, and how can they be minimised?
11. How would you fuse an ankle?
12. Describe the follow-up and complications you might expect following ankle arthrodesis.
13. What types of ankle arthroplasty are you aware of?
14. Describe the technique of ankle arthroplasty.
15. What are the two types of Achilles tendinopathy, and how do they differ?
16. What is meant by functional Achilles rehabilitation?
17. Describe the techniques for direct repair of the Achilles tendon.
18. How might you augment a tendo-Achilles repair, e.g. in a patient with tendon loss/shortening?
19. Describe an approach to the peroneal tendons.
20. How might you address peroneal tendon subluxation?

14 Surgery of the Foot

Yaser Ghani, Simon Clint and Nicholas Cullen

Principles of foot and ankle arthrodesis	385	Interdigital neuroma	408
		Lesser toe deformities	409
Hallux valgus correction	388	Lesser metatarsal (Weil's) osteotomy	414
First metatarsophalangeal joint cheilectomy	401	Fifth toe soft tissue correction (Butler's procedure)	416
First metatarsophalangeal joint arthrodesis	404	Hindfoot arthrodesis	417
		Calcaneal osteotomy	421
Ingrowing toenail surgery	406	Viva questions	424

Joint/Movement	Range of motion
Subtalar joint inversion	10°
Subtalar joint eversion	5°
Transverse tarsal joint adduction	20°
Transverse tarsal joint abduction	10°
Combined foot supination	30°
Combined foot pronation	15°
First metatarsophalangeal joint flexion	30°
First metatarsophalangeal joint extension	60°

Position of arthrodesis
- The positions of arthrodesis are covered in the relevant sections.

Principles of foot and ankle arthrodesis
Preoperative planning
Arthrodesis is a commonly used technique throughout the foot and ankle. Although the approach, position and fixation used are specific to each joint fused, the principles and techniques are common throughout the region and should be well understood. Individual arthrodeses will be dealt with in the relevant sections.

Indications

- *Painful arthropathy of a joint*: Given the large number of adjacent joints in the foot, it can be useful to localise the source of pain with a radiologically guided injection of the proposed joint preoperatively.
- *Deformity of a joint affecting the position of the remaining foot*: Often associated with congenital or acquired tendon or neuromuscular conditions.

Contraindications

- Active infection
- Critical ischaemia
- Multiple adjacent arthrodeses (relative contraindication)

Consent and risks

- *Prolonged postoperative treatment*: The joint must be immobilised until union and unprotected weightbearing avoided, which may take about 3 months in the hindfoot or ankle.
- *Infection and wound healing problems*: Dependent on surgical technique and soft tissue handling as well as patient factors.
- *Cutaneous nerve damage*: Given the subcutaneous and variable location of cutaneous nerves in the foot, inadvertent damage and subsequent painful neuroma formation can occur.
- *Non-union*: Absolute risk is dependent on technical and patient factors. Most patients have a 5%–10% risk of non-union and ongoing pain for most procedures. This is increased dramatically in smokers (up to sevenfold), those with poor perfusion, active infection or diabetes.
- *Malunion*: Technique dependent. Malunions may be symptomatic, requiring footwear adaptations or revision surgery, or may be asymptomatic and tolerated.
- *Development of arthropathy in neighbouring joints*: Common over time, but may represent the progression of unrecognised early joint disease.
- *Alteration of gait*: Dependent on number and location of arthrodeses.

Anaesthesia and positioning

General anaesthesia is usually required. A thigh tourniquet is required to allow exposure of the limb to above the knee. This allows accurate assessment of alignment. A supportive bolster under the calf is useful to allow free access to the foot.

Surgical principles

The principles for achieving successful arthrodesis are: (1) complete removal of cartilage and soft tissue that may prevent adequate fusion, (2) adequate compression across the fusion site, (3) optimal position of the joint and (4) adequate bone apposition until fusion is achieved. The general principles are to *mobilise the joint to allow correction of any deformity and complete access to the joint surfaces*. The surfaces are prepared, maintaining the joint shape and congruity while exposing bleeding cancellous bone. The joint is then held rigidly in the required position of arthrodesis.

Careful placement of incisions of adequate length is vital to prevent undue soft tissue damage and tension. Most joints are relatively superficial, so adequate soft tissue cover is vital.

The capsule and surrounding soft tissues need to be released to allow full access to the joint and to correct any deformity. Most deformities can be corrected with adequate mobilisation, but occasionally bone resection is required.

The joint surfaces need to be carefully prepared. First, any peripheral osteophytes should be removed to expose the true joint. Second, the cartilage and subchondral plate must be removed, maintaining the contour of the joint. This is best achieved with a variety of sharp chisels working in a methodical manner from superficial to deep. Power tools generate unwanted heat and should be avoided. As the joint is prepared, a laminar spreader is gradually advanced into the joint to open it up. Pituitary rongeurs and Kerrison laminectomy rongeurs are useful to access the deep recesses of the joint safely. Once all joint surfaces are removed, the surface area of bleeding bone should be increased by various methods. Using a chisel to cross-cut the surface and applying a slight twist on removal can produce bone 'petals' to good effect.

The joint should be positioned in the desired position and, if needed, provisionally held with a K-wire. A careful confirmation of the position with respect to the limb alignment and the rest of the foot must be undertaken to ensure a satisfactory outcome. It is unusual, unless bony destruction has occurred, to require a supplementary bone graft. If required, sufficient quantities can usually be harvested locally from the calcaneus, medial malleolus or proximal tibia without need to prepare the iliac crest.

Rigid fixation and compression of the joint must be achieved. This is usually done with some form of compression screw or screws. However, in certain situations other forms of fixation, such as staples, intramedullary devices or external fixations may be appropriate. Satisfactory compression can be tested by carefully inserting a fine chisel into the joint and twisting – there should be no give.

Careful, tension-free wound closure is critical. A soft tissue layer should be closed over the joint prior to skin closure. The joint is immobilised in a back slab to protect the fusion and soft tissues.

Postoperative care and instructions

The leg should be elevated until swelling has subsided. Mobilisation should avoid weightbearing on the joint. In the forefoot, a wedge-type shoe may be sufficient but may require a non-weightbearing cast. Unprotected weightbearing should be avoided until there is clinical and radiological evidence of union.

Recommended references

Glissan DJ. The indications for inducing fusion at the ankle by operation with description of two successful techniques. *Aust N Z J Surg.* 1949;**19**:64–71.

Hardy MA, Logan DB. Principles of arthrodesis and advances in fixation for the adult acquired flatfoot. *Clin Podiatr Med Surg.* 2007;**24**:789–813.

Hallux valgus correction

Preoperative planning

There are a multitude of procedures described for the correction of hallux valgus deformity, some considered historical and others in current use. In order to select the correct procedure for a specific patient, an understanding of the spectrum of hallux valgus deformities must exist.

> ### Indications and choice of procedure
> The presence of a bunion is not an indication for surgery.

The strongest indication for operative intervention in hallux valgus is pain. This pain is located over the bunion and usually only felt with shod feet. Pain present when barefoot or under the metatarsal head suggests another source of the pain should be sought. Footwear problems due to extreme deformities are a relative indication. Operating solely for cosmetic or fashion reasons is generally not recommended.

On examining the patient, the neurovascular status of the patient must be examined along with the overall hindfoot and foot alignment. Joint mobility is assessed: hypermobility of the first tarsometatarsal joint (TMTJ) is associated with an increased risk of postsurgical recurrence.

Contraindications

Patients with significant pre-existing degenerative change in the metatarsophalangeal joint (MTPJ) will usually not benefit from realignment surgery and should be offered arthrodesis (see 'First metatarsophalangeal joint arthrodesis', p. 404).

Patients with hypermobility or instability of the first TMTJ are likely to have a recurrence after a simple osteotomy. These deformities might be best treated with a first TMTJ arthrodesis combined with a lateral release (see 'Lapidus procedure', p. 399).

> ### Consent and risks
> There is considerable variation, depending on the specific procedure: details of operation-specific risks are detailed within the operative techniques discussed later. General complications are listed here:
>
> - *Foot shape*: Most procedures will result in a narrower forefoot with a straighter hallux. However, this may still preclude the wearing of many fashionable shoes.
> - *Stiffness*: Most procedures which violate the MTPJ are associated with varying degrees of postoperative stiffness. This can be particularly troublesome with the Scarf osteotomy due to the degree of soft tissue mobilisation.

- *Recurrence of deformity*: Usually associated with poor technique, attempting to push the indications of a procedure too far or not recognising complicating factors (laxity, increased distal metatarsal articular angle [DMAA], congruent joint, etc.).
- *Overcorrection and hallux varus*: Usually occur due to overenthusiastic soft tissue correction or excessive displacement of the capital fragment. Excessive medial eminence excision or the excision of the fibular sesamoid in a McBride release also predispose to hallux varus.
- *Nerve damage and neuroma formation*: Damage to the dorsomedial or plantar nerves is possible with most procedures and can cause painful neuroma formation.
- *Transfer metatarsalgia*: Anything that alters the relationship between the first and lesser metatarsals in the sagittal plane can lead to painful overloading of the lesser metatarsals, usually the second. This can occur in techniques that result in excessive shortening or elevation of the metatarsal head. It can also occur with defunctioning of the hallux, as occurs with a Keller procedure.

Operative planning

Radiology

All patients presenting with hallux valgus should have *weightbearing* anteroposterior (AP) and lateral radiographs of both feet obtained. Various radiographic angles and measurements are frequently used to define the anatomical location and magnitude of the hallux deformity which can aid surgical planning (**Figure 14.1a through d**). These include:

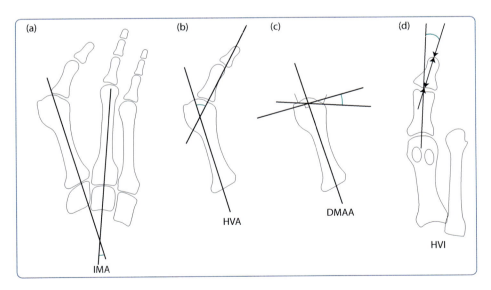

Figure 14.1 Radiographic assessment of hallux valgus. (a) Intermetatarsal angle (IMA). (b) Hallux valgus angle (HVA). (c) Distal metatarsal articular angle (DMAA). (d) Hallux valgus interphalangeus angle (HVI).

- *Hallux valgus angle (HVA)*: The angle between the anatomical axes of the first metatarsal and the proximal phalanx.

- *First-second intermetatarsal angle (IMA)*: The angle between the anatomical axes of the first and second metatarsals.
- *DMM*: The angle between a line drawn from the medial and lateral borders of the articular surface of the distal metatarsal and the anatomical axis of the metatarsal.
- *Interphalangeal angle*: The angle between the proximal and distal articular surfaces of the proximal phalanx of the hallux.
- *Hallux valgus interphalangeal angle (HVI)*: The angle formed between the long axis of the distal phalanx and the proximal phalanx and is usually less than 10°.
- *Joint congruity*: The medial and lateral borders of the joint surface of the metatarsal and phalanx are identified. The first MTPJ is said to be congruent if the lateral and medial borders of the two joint surfaces align. If they do not, the joint is incongruent (**Figure 14.2**).

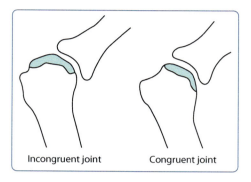

Figure 14.2 Assessment of first metatarsophalangeal joint congruity.

- *Presence of degenerative changes in the first MTPJ.*
- *Signs of first TMTJ instability*: These include opening up of the first TMTJ on the lateral view and widening of the gap between the first/second metatarsal bases.
- Congruent deformities require an osteotomy that incorporates rotation to correct the relationship of the articular surface to the axis of the metatarsal.
- Mild deformities can be corrected with a single metatarsal osteotomy (e.g. biplanar Chevron or modified Scarf – see later) with or without the addition of a phalangeal osteotomy (Akin osteotomy – see later).
- Severe deformities occasionally require a combined proximal and distal metatarsal osteotomy (see 'Proximal (basal) metatarsal osteotomy', p. 400).
- Most authors categorise incongruent hallux valgus based on broad categories of severity. Such categories are not absolute but act as general guidelines to help define the limits of certain procedures and to help in the selection of the correct treatment. *Table 14.1* shows typical figures.

Anaesthesia and positioning

All hallux valgus surgery can be performed under a regional (ankle) block or general anaesthesia. A bloodless field is provided by a thigh or ankle tourniquet. The patient is positioned supine and the whole foot and ankle prepared.

Table 14.1 Categorisation of hallux valgus severity

Angle measured	Normal	Mild	Moderate	Severe
HVA	<15°	15°–20°	20°–40°	>40°
IMMA	<9°	9°–11°	11°–16°	>16°
DMAA	<6°			

Source: After Coughlin MJ, Saltzamn CL, Anderson RB. *Mann's Surgery of the Foot and Ankle*. 9th ed. Philadelphia, PA: Mosby, 2007.

Surgical techniques

Given the huge range of surgical procedures described for hallux valgus, it is not within the scope of this book to describe them all. We shall therefore concentrate on those procedures commonly performed. Each procedure is described individually, but in practice, several techniques, such as the metatarsal osteotomy, Akin osteotomy and lateral soft tissue release, may be performed in combination.

First metatarsophalangeal joint soft tissue release

A soft tissue release attempts to balance out the soft tissues around the first MTPJ. With a valgus deformity, the medial tissues become attenuated and those on the lateral side contracted. The original McBride procedure was more extensive, including excision of the lateral sesamoid, and was associated with a high rate of hallux varus. The procedure has been altered so many times that the term 'modified McBride' is misleading and should be avoided.

A soft tissue release is rarely performed in isolation. However, it is part of many procedures so a detailed understanding is important.

Specific indications

- Incongruent, mild hallux valgus with normal, or near normal IMA
- In combination with another procedure (see later)

Consent and risks

- *Overcorrection and hallux varus*: Caused by excessive soft tissue release and excessive medial plication
- Excessive medial plication can also lead to joint stiffness
- *Nerve damage*: The common digital nerve is deep to the intermetatarsal ligament and can be damaged

Incision

Starting on the medial side, a medial longitudinal incision is made, centred over the metatarsal head and extending from the shaft of the proximal phalanx to the distal shaft of the metatarsal.

Dissection

> #### Structure at risk
> - Dorsomedial sensory nerve

Dissection is continued down to capsule and then a dorsal flap is carefully elevated to identify the dorsal nerve adherent to the capsule on the dorsomedial aspect. This is repeated on the plantar side, dissecting around the capsule to create a small pocket. A longitudinal capsulotomy is performed and any adhesions released.

Surgical technique

Unless a distal metatarsal osteotomy is also to be performed, the prominent medial eminence of the head can now be removed. This is done with a fine oscillating saw, aiming to cut in line with the medial shaft starting 2–3 mm from the medial sulcus (**Figure 14.3**).

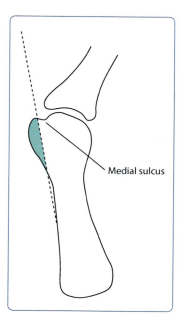

Figure 14.3 Excision of medial eminence of first metatarsophalangeal joint.

It is the authors' practice to use a separate incision for lateral release, however many surgeons use the same medial approach for the soft tissue release. Attention is now turned to the first web space. A 3 cm incision is centred between the metatarsal heads in the first web space then bluntly dissected down to the level of the heads. Inserting a laminar spreader or self-retainer between the heads allows identification of the lateral sesamoid and insertion of adductor hallucis into its lateral edge. Using a size 15 blade, the capsule is released from the dorsal aspect of the sesamoid then the blade is advanced to the insertion of adductor hallucis into the phalanx. The insertion of adductor hallucis is released from the phalanx then, working proximally, the remaining tendon is released from the sesamoid. Deep to this is the intermetatarsal ligament which runs from the second metatarsal to the lateral sesamoid, not the first metatarsal itself. This is carefully divided from the sesamoid, taking care to preserve the neurovascular bundle which lies directly underneath. The lateral capsule (metatarso-sesamoid ligament) is then incised longitudinally, after which the articular surface of the lateral sesamoid can be inspected and should be reducible underneath the metatarsal head. The retractor is removed and confirmation that the toe can be passively overcorrected is sought.

Returning to the medial side, the metatarsal head should be reducible onto the sesamoids. If too much resistance is encountered, a bony procedure is required to correct the deformity. Subsequent capsular plication is designed to take in excess capsule, not pull the sesamoid complex over.

Using an absorbable suture, the excess capsule is 'double-breasted' while holding the MTPJ flexed. This is done by passing a stitch through the dorsal capsule from outside in, medial to the extensor tendon and avoiding the identified nerve. The needle is then passed from outside the plantar capsule, just medial to the sesamoid then reversed to come from inside out. It is finished by exiting through the dorsal capsule, near the earlier entry point. As the suture is tightened, the dorsal capsule should double-breast over the plantar capsule. Plication is checked to ensure that it is not too tight by flexing and extending the joint.

Closure
The rest of the capsule is then closed with absorbable sutures prior to skin closure.

Scarf osteotomy
The Scarf osteotomy is a powerful and versatile osteotomy allowing correction of all of the axes of the hallux valgus deformity; *it is a technically challenging procedure* with a steep learning curve. It is named after a joiners' technique, used to connect two beams.

Specific indications
- Moderate or severe hallux valgus
- Hallux valgus with an increased DMAA
- Revision surgery

Specific contraindications
- Poor bone stock or osteoporosis increasing the risk of fracture

> ### Consent and risks
>
> - *Fracture*: Given the length of the osteotomy, fracture, either intraoperatively or postoperatively can occur (3%–5%).
> - *MTPJ stiffness*: Especially if the metatarsal is inadvertently lengthened.
> - *Malunion*: Care must be taken to ensure all cuts are in the correct direction in all three planes.
> - *Troughing*: This occurs when the shaft cortex of one fragment collapses into the cancellous bone of the other fragment (**Figure 14.4**). This results in elevation of the metatarsal head and rotation of the osteotomy. It is more common where there is poor bone stock. By ensuring the ends of the osteotomy are in dense metaphyseal bone, rather than the diaphysis, the risk can be reduced.

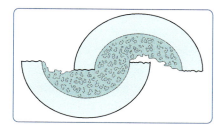

Figure 14.4 Troughing of Scarf osteotomy.

Incision

A medial approach, as described earlier, is performed. However, the incision continues proximally until approaching the TMTJ.

Dissection

> ### Structures at risk
>
> - Dorsomedial sensory nerve
> - Blood supply to first metatarsal head

Dorsally, the capsule and dorsal periosteum are released from the distal half of the bone, exposing the dorsal surface. Plantarwards, great care is taken to not damage the vascular leash entering the head on the plantar surface of the neck (**Figure 14.5**).

Surgical technique

The periosteum is only elevated from the proximal third, dissecting away from the neck. A minimal excision of the medial eminence is performed in line with the shaft, aiming to just expose cancellous bone. At this point it is advisable to draw out the planned osteotomy, on the medial aspect of the bone (see **Figure 14.5**). The longitudinal arm begins at a point

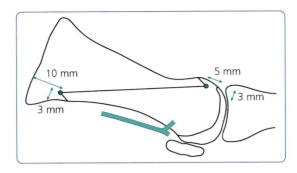

Figure 14.5 Scarf osteotomy and plantar vascular supply of the metatarsal head.

3 mm from the dorsal cortex, 5 mm proximal to the dorsal articular edge. This then extends proximally and plantarwards to a point 3 mm from the plantar surface and 10 mm from the TMTJ. Two horizontal 60° limbs are then added to the ends to exit the nearby cortices. The distal horizontal limb should be perpendicular to the second metatarsal shaft; we advise drawing a line connecting the medial point of origin of the distal first metatarsal cut running perpendicular to the second metatarsal shaft and on through the lateral rays. The metatarsal head that it passes through (usually the fourth) can be used as a reference for the cut. Palpating the fourth metatarsal head, another line is drawn on the dorsal surface, from the distal arm across the dorsal surface towards the fourth.

Once satisfied with the planned osteotomy, an oscillating saw is used to score the cortex for the longitudinal arm. After a starting point is made, the blade is angled plantarwards, in the plane of the shafts of the metatarsals. Maintaining this angle, the whole length of the longitudinal arm is cut, penetrating only the medial cortex; the lateral cortex is then softly cut in the same plane. Next, the distal arm is cut, maintaining the slight plantar angle and aiming for the fourth metatarsal head as planned. The proximal cut should now be cut parallel or slightly divergent to this – if the cuts converge, the osteotomy will not displace. The osteotomy should now be mobile. If not, all cuts are checked for completion and the two fragments gently freed with a MacDonald dissector, starting proximally.

The osteotomy is now displaced as required. This is facilitated by a 'push-pull' action, grasping the proximal fragment with a towel clip while pushing the distal fragment laterally. *The osteotomy should displace laterally and plantarwards.* The reduction is then held with a clamp. The reduction is checked by observing the position of the medial sesamoid: it should lie under the medial metatarsal head. Once the reduction is satisfactory, a K-wire is inserted along the lateral edge of the proximal fragment into the head and a stepped bone clamp will prevent displacement.

The osteotomy is secured with two screws – headless, variable pitch compression screws are ideal. The first screw should start from the dorsolateral aspect of the distal end of the proximal fragment and aim towards the medial sesamoid. *This must be intraosseous to avoid sesamoid damage.* A second screw can then be used in a dorsoplantar direction to secure the proximal extent of the osteotomy. The proximal screw should be bicortical.

After fixation, the prominent medial cortex of the proximal fragment can be bevelled flush with the shaft.

Closure

Closure of the capsule should be performed as described previously.

Akin osteotomy

Specific indications

- Hallux interphalangeus deformity, where the deformity occurs distal to the MTPJ
- In combination with a metatarsal osteotomy to correct residual phalangeal deformity

Specific contraindications

Akin osteotomy in isolation will not correct joint incongruity or an increased IMA so should not be used alone in these cases.

Incision

A medial longitudinal incision is performed, starting just proximal to the interphalangeal joint (IPJ) and extended past the medial eminence of the metatarsal. This can be incorporated into the incision for a metatarsal osteotomy if required.

Dissection

A longitudinal capsular incision is made and extended proximally to incise the periosteum of the phalanx. This is then carefully elevated, allowing the placement of retractors superiorly and inferiorly.

Surgical technique

> **Structure at risk**
>
> - Flexor hallucis longus tendon

If required, the medial eminence of the metatarsal can be excised, as earlier. The osteotomy is a closing wedge osteotomy, performed with an oscillating saw from the medial side; the lateral cortex is left intact. Particular care should be taken to avoid damage to the long flexor inferiorly. It is easy to overcorrect the deformity, so it is wise to underestimate the size of the wedge and check the result. The alignment of the osteotomy depends on the planned means of fixation (**Figure 14.6**).

If a staple is used, the first cut should be parallel to the proximal joint surface. The second cut is parallel to the base of the nail, aiming to converge before the lateral cortex, leaving it intact. The wedge is removed and the osteotomy closed. If there is resistance, the lateral cortex can be cautiously weakened with the saw, but should not be breached. Using the planned staple as a guide, entry holes are drilled using a fine K-wire and the staple inserted. After insertion the joint is inspected to ensure that it is not penetrated by the staple. Postoperative radiographs can be misleading in this regard because of the convex nature of the joint surface.

Hallux valgus correction

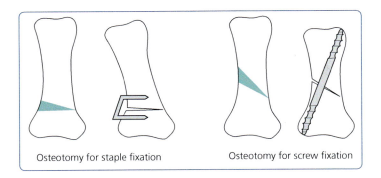

Figure 14.6 Akin osteotomy.

If a cannulated compression screw is to be used, the osteotomy will be angled to allow compression. A screw will be inserted over a guide wire passing from the medial edge of the proximal flair of the phalanx, exiting distally in the lateral cortex.

Closure
The capsule is closed with absorbable sutures prior to skin closure. A forefoot dressing is applied.

Chevron osteotomy
The chevron osteotomy is a relatively simple osteotomy for the correction of mild hallux valgus.

Specific indications
- Mild (and moderate – see later) hallux valgus deformity
- Congruent hallux valgus deformity as the osteotomy does not disturb the balance of the joint – using a biplanar chevron (see later)

Specific contraindications
Due to technical limits of the procedure, it should be reserved for deformities with an IMA less than 12°, HVA less than 30° and DMMA less than 15°. Attempting to push the indications further increases the risk of avascular necrosis of the capital fragment.

Consent and risks
- *Avascular necrosis of the capital fragment*: Up to 20% in some series. Probably technique dependent with increased avascular necrosis seen with extensive soft tissue stripping and release and with excessive displacements attempted.
- *Malunion*: If the osteotomy is angled too proximally, shortening of the first metatarsal will occur with translation. Similarly, if the osteotomy is angled dorsally the metatarsal head will be elevated. Both of these technical errors will alter the relationship of the first metatarsal head to that of the lesser metatarsals and may lead to transfer metatarsalgia.

Incision and dissection

A standard medial approach is made to the metatarsal head (see earlier).

Surgical technique

The medial eminence is resected in a plane parallel to the medial border of the foot, beginning at the sulcus. A lateral release is not routinely performed due to the increased risk of avascular necrosis. The chevron osteotomy is a V-shaped cut of *approximately 60° with the apex at the centre of the metatarsal head* (**Figure 14.7a**). Because the plane of the cuts is crucial, it can be useful to place a K-wire in this central point, running parallel to the sole of the foot and the distal articular surface of the metatarsal. This wire can then be used as a cutting guide to position the limbs of the chevron. The most crucial cut is the plantar limb, which must exit the plantar surface of the metatarsal in an extra-articular position to avoid damage to the sesamoid articulation. Several authors advocate a more horizontal plantar limb (see **Figure 14.7b**) to attempt to preserve the plantar blood supply (see 'Scarf osteotomy', p. 393). The dorsal limb is then cut at approximately 60° to the first cut. After completion of the cuts, the capital fragment can be translated laterally by up to 30% of its width to correct the hallux valgus.

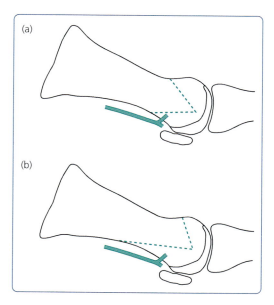

Figure 14.7 Chevron osteotomy. (a) Classic chevron osteotomy, risking damage to plantar blood supply to metatarsal head. (b) Modified chevron osteotomy to preserve plantar blood supply to metatarsal head.

If there is an increased DMMA, the joint can be reorientated by means of a biplanar chevron. By taking a small (1–2 mm) wedge from the superomedial and inferomedial aspect of the limbs, the fragment can be displaced laterally but rotated medially, correcting the DMMA as may be required in a congruent hallux valgus.

Although inherently a stable osteotomy, most surgeons hold the osteotomy with a K-wire or screw inserted from a dorso-proximal to plantar-distal direction. Care must be taken not to leave any fixation proud of the joint to avoid damage to the sesamoid articulation.

Closure

Capsular closure is as presented earlier.

Lapidus procedure

Specific indications

- Hallux valgus deformity in the presence of instability of the first TMTJ
- Moderate to severe incongruent hallux valgus deformity
- Salvage procedure for previous failed hallux valgus surgery
- Arthritis of the first TMTJ

Specific contraindications

Given the shortening of the first ray that occurs with Lapidus, the procedure should not be performed on patients with short first metatarsals.

Surgical technique

> ### Structure at risk
>
> - Tibialis anterior tendon

The Lapidus procedure involves first TMTJ arthrodesis; this should be performed with the previously described lateral soft tissue release, excision of the medial eminence and plication of the medial capsule. The medial incision for the MTPJ can be continued proximally to the TMTJ. Alternatively, a separate medial incision can be made centred over the joint. The joint is usually deep to a vein, crossing from dorsal to plantar, and some authors advocate preserving it to reduce postoperative swelling. The joint can be identified with the aid of a needle and opened to mobilise the joint. Care must be taken to avoid damage to the tendon of tibialis anterior, which lies on the inferomedial aspect of the joint. Using traction on the toe, the joint can be opened and preparation of the joint performed as detailed in 'Principles of foot and ankle arthrodesis' (p. 385). Once the preparation has begun, there is enough room to insert a laminar spreader.

Several authors describe a Lapidus procedure as a closing wedge arthrodesis. However, this is usually not required. By careful preservation of the joint shape, the base of the metatarsal can usually be displaced medially and slightly inferiorly with digital pressure, thereby reducing the IMA and overcoming the elevation of the metatarsal head caused by shortening of the joint. A good correction coincides with the appearance of a 'step' on the medial side. Once reduced, the joint is provisionally held with a K-wire before checking the position. If further correction is required, minimal resection of the inferolateral aspect of the metatarsal base is performed.

The arthrodesis can be secured by means of screws or a custom plate. To use screws, a 3.5 mm glide hole is drilled from the dorsum of the metatarsal, starting 15–20 mm from the joint and slightly laterally, aiming for the cuneiform. It is important to avoid aiming too plantarwards, which results in a poor hold on the cuneiform. The cuneiform is then drilled, using a 2.5 mm drill in standard AO fashion. Prior to inserting the screw, an oval groove in the transverse plane should be created (using a small burr or countersink) to accommodate the head of the screw and avoid breaking the dorsal cortical bridge. Once tightened, a second screw can be inserted from the cuneiform to the metatarsal, in a parallel sagittal plane to the first screw.

Closure
The soft tissues are closed over the fusion prior to skin closure.

Specific postoperative instructions
If satisfactory fixation is achieved and the patient is compliant, they may mobilise postoperatively in a forefoot-offloading wedge shoe for 12 weeks.

Otherwise a non-weightbearing cast can be used to protect the arthrodesis.

Proximal (basal) metatarsal osteotomy
The proximal metatarsal osteotomy is usually performed in combination with a lateral soft tissue release, excision of medial eminence and medial capsule closure, as described earlier.

Specific indications
Correction of moderate to severe hallux valgus is an indication, especially when associated with a large IMA. By making an osteotomy at the base of the metatarsal, larger corrections of IMA can be made than by operating more distally.

Specific contraindications
Congruent deformities (if used in isolation) – as the osteotomy does not alter the relationship between the anatomical axis of the metatarsal and the distal articular surface, it will not alter the DMMA. However, it may be of use when combined with a distal osteotomy to correct a congruent deformity with increased IMA (a double osteotomy).

Consent and risks
- *Malunion*: Any misorientation of the plane of the osteotomy can result in significant accidental misplacement of the metatarsal head.
- *Overcorrection*: Given the power of this osteotomy to realign the shaft, overcorrection and hallux varus can be troublesome, especially when combined with an aggressive lateral release.

Incision
A dorsal incision is made over the base of the metatarsal, avoiding any superficial cutaneous nerves.

Surgical technique

The osteotomy is ideally placed about 1 cm from the TMTJ in metaphyseal bone to provide a broad area for union. A dome osteotomy or closing or opening wedge osteotomies can be performed.

The lateral closing wedge will tend to shorten the metatarsal. There are various plates designed to fix the opening wedge osteotomies.

The coronal plane of the osteotomy is vital – It should be perpendicular to the plane of the metatarsal. If the blade is directed too medially, the head will be elevated; if directed too laterally, it will be depressed. In the sagittal plane, the blade should be positioned perpendicular to the sole then angled slightly proximally. Once cut, the osteotomy can provisionally be reduced and the position checked. If satisfactory the osteotomy is fixed with two screws or a screw and wire.

Keller procedure

This involves excision of the medial prominence of the metatarsal and the proximal third of the phalanx to relax the lateral structures and allow correction of the toe, which is then held with a temporary K-wire. Although once commonly performed, its generally unsatisfactory results have caused it to fall out of favour. The patient is left with a floppy great toe and, by defunctioning the hallux, is prone to overload their lesser rays with resultant pain. However, it can be considered in the older, minimally ambulatory patient who has footwear problems or in those patients whose soft tissues or general fitness precludes a more aggressive procedure.

General postoperative care and instructions

- The foot is dressed with a standard forefoot dressing, extending above the ankle.
- The foot is elevated for 72 hours to reduce swelling.
- The patient may mobilise, fully weightbearing, in a forefoot-offloading wedge shoe for 6 weeks.
- After skin wounds have healed, the patient is taught passive mobilisation of the MTPJ to reduce stiffness.

Recommended references

Barouk LS. Scarf osteotomy for hallux valgus correction. Local anatomy, surgical technique, and combination with other forefoot procedures. *Foot Ankle Clin.* 2000;**5**:525–558.

Barouk LS. *Forefoot Reconstruction*. Paris, France: Springer-Verlag, 2005.

Weil LS. Scarf osteotomy for correction of hallux valgus. Historical perspective, surgical technique, and results. *Foot Ankle Clin.* 2000;**5**:559–580.

First metatarsophalangeal joint cheilectomy

Preoperative planning

Hallux rigidus, or degenerative arthritis of the first MTPJ, is a common condition. Although in its early stages it can be managed with conservative measures, such as footwear and activity modifications, patients often require operative intervention. Cheilectomy, from the Greek for lip, *cheilos*, addresses both the pain and stiffness found in this condition.

Indications
- Mild to moderate degenerative changes in the first MTPJ with pain and stiffness, failing to respond to conservative management
- More advanced degenerative changes in a patient unwilling to lose joint movement (patient must be counselled that there may be improvement in movement but only limited improvement in pain)
- Prominent dorsal osteophytes causing footwear problems

Contraindications
Contraindications include advanced degenerative changes with loss of joint space.

Consent and risks
- *Failure or recurrence of symptoms*: Especially if the degenerative changes are more extensive than appreciated preoperatively or if insufficient resection is performed
- *Instability of first MTPJ*: Especially if resection exceeds 35% of joint surface
- Damage to dorsal cutaneous nerve and neuroma formation

Anaesthesia and positioning
- Regional or general anaesthesia
- Ankle or thigh tourniquet
- Supine on operating table

Surgical technique
Landmarks
- The MTPJ of the great toe is easily palpable
- Extensor hallucis longus (EHL) tendon

Incision
A 5 cm dorsal incision is made along the medial border of EHL centred over the first MTPJ.

Dissection
The underlying extensor hood is incised in line with the incision but leaving a cuff of tissue on the medial side of the tendon to avoid violating the tendon sheath and reducing the risk of adhesions.

The joint capsule is incised and the joint exposed by dissection medially and laterally. Alternatively, a medial approach, as described in first MTPJ arthrodesis, may be used.

Procedure

A full synovectomy is performed and any loose bodies removed. Flexing the joint fully allows inspection of the joint surface. In mild and moderate disease, the damage is usually limited to the dorsal aspect. Ideally, the resection should extend from just dorsal of the edge of the viable cartilage to just proximal of the dorsal prominence of the head. However, care should be taken to ensure that this resects 20%–30% of the joint (**Figure 14.8**).

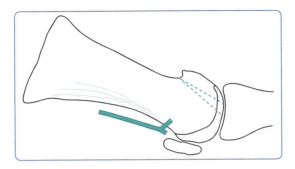

Figure 14.8 First metatarsophalangeal joint cheilectomy – minimum and maximum resection levels.

Note on resection level (**Figure 14.8**): A common cause for failure of cheilectomy is insufficient resection. *A minimum of 20% of the articular surface* must be removed, even if this includes normal joint surface, to ensure adequate movement. Exceeding 35% is likely to destabilise the joint.

The dorsal prominence is resected with a saw or osteotome and satisfactory dorsiflexion (ideally 60°) is confirmed. Any prominent osteophytes are removed from the dorsal phalanx and the medial and lateral aspect of the head, and the joint is irrigated to thoroughly wash out. Bone wax can be used sparingly to reduce bleeding and adhesions. Moberg osteotomy – proximal phalanx osteotomy. Once cheilectomy is carried out, the range of movement should then be assessed. If the cheilectomy fails to achieve between 30° and 40° of motion, then one can consider a proximal phalanx osteotomy. This is a dorsal closing wedge osteotomy popularized by Moberg in the adult population.

Closure

Careful closure of the capsule with interrupted Vicryl precedes skin closure. A forefoot dressing is applied to above the ankle.

Postoperative instructions

The foot is elevated for 48 hours. The patient fully weightbears on a postoperative shoe and aggressive active and passive mobilisation begins once skin healing has occurred.

Recommended reference

Coughlin MJ, Shurnas PS. Hallux rigidus. Grading and long-term results of operative treatment. *J Bone Joint Surg Am.* 2003;**85**:2072–2088.

First metatarsophalangeal joint arthrodesis

Preoperative planning

Once a patient has developed severe hallux rigidus, a cheilectomy is unlikely to address the problem. Although various arthroplasties are available, most either have limited long-term results or are associated with high failure rates. Arthrodesis of the joint provides a reliable solution to the pain of advanced arthritis of the joint.

Indications
- Painful arthropathy of first MTPJ not responding to conservative treatment and not suitable for less invasive treatment (e.g. cheilectomy)
- Severe first MTPJ deformity in the presence of degenerative changes
- Salvage of failed first ray surgery

Absolute contraindications
- Active infection
- Limb ischaemia or poor perfusion

Relative contraindication
This includes previous IPJ arthrodesis or pre-existing IPJ degenerative changes.

Consent and risks

(See also 'Principles of foot and ankle arthrodesis', p. 385.)

- *Malunion*: Excessive extension can cause defunctioning of hallux and transfer metatarsalgia. Excessive flexion can cause increased wear and pain in the IPJ. Excessive valgus can cause pressure on the second toe.
- Damage to dorsal cutaneous nerve and neuroma formation.
- *Unable to wear high heels after surgery*: This must be stressed to women considering operation.
- Minimum of 6 weeks protected weightbearing.

Anaesthesia and positioning
- Regional or general anaesthesia
- Ankle or thigh tourniquet
- Supine on operating table

Surgical technique

Landmarks
The MTPJ of the great toe is easily palpable.

Incision
A straight medial midline incision is made, centred over the MTPJ.

Dissection

This is continued straight down to the joint capsule, without developing flaps. The capsule is incised in line with the skin incision and freed dorsally over the metatarsal head and sufficiently around the phalangeal base to allow its surface to be delivered. Alternatively, the approach described for cheilectomy may be used.

Procedure

The surfaces are prepared in a manner outlined in 'Principles of foot and ankle arthrodesis' (p. 385). Given the joint's small size, it is not possible, or really necessary, to use a laminar spreader. Furthermore, the concave surface of the phalanx makes the use of chisels difficult; a curette or bone nibbler may be more useful. Various dome-shaped reamers may also be used, but care should be taken to avoid removal of excessive bone, which will lead to shortening.

Note about sagittal position of arthrodesis (**Figure 14.9**): several textbooks state a fixed value for the position of first MTPJ arthrodesis, e.g. 25°–30° extension. This can be confusing as it may be unclear if this refers to the angle relating to the floor or the metatarsal shaft. Furthermore, the angle to the metatarsal depends on the pitch of the metatarsal, i.e. whether the foot is planus or cavus. It is therefore preferred to arthrodese the joint in a relative position to a simulated floor. Using a flat surface to push up against the sole of the foot, assess the position of the pulp of the hallux with regard to the surface. If a finger can be pushed under the pulp, the toe is too extended. If there is no space for any flexion of the

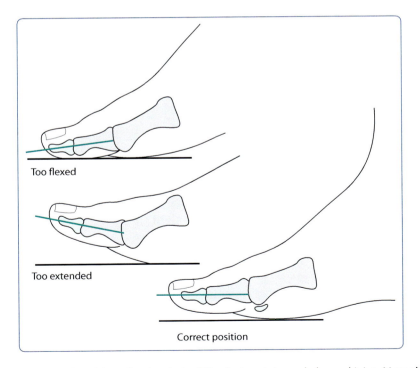

Figure 14.9 Coronal position of arthrodesis of the first metatarsophalangeal joint. Note that the phalanges are parallel to floor, allowing clearance of toe pulp.

IPJ, the position is too flexed. An ideal position allows a small amount of movement with downward pressure on the distal phalanx.

The joint is positioned as required and provisionally held with a K-wire. The sagittal position of the toe is then assessed with regard to a flat surface as outlined earlier. The coronal position should be of sufficient valgus to avoid the medial border of the toe rubbing upon the toe box of a shoe but not so much that there is impingement of the hallux against the second toe; 10°–15° HVA is usually appropriate. There should be no rotational deformity.

In primary surgery with good bone stock, the arthrodesis can be secured in various ways. A single-axial compression screw combined with a dorsal neutralising or compression plate or crossed screw techniques are commonly used. Our preferred method is the crossed screw technique using two crossed screws. The first is inserted with a lag technique to compress the joint; the second provides a de-rotational function. Alternatively, a custom-made plate may be used.

Closure
- Careful closure of the capsule with interrupted Vicryl precedes skin closure.
- A forefoot dressing is applied to above the ankle.

Postoperative instructions
The foot is elevated for 72 hours. A reliable patient can mobilise in a wedge shoe to offload the forefoot until evidence of clinical and radiological union. If there is concern about the compliance of the patient, a cast may be used.

Recommended references
Coughlin MJ, Saltzamn CL, Anderson RB. *Mann's Surgery of the Foot and Ankle*. 9th ed. Philadelphia, PA: Mosby, 2007.

Coughlin MJ, Shurnas PS. Hallux rigidus. *J Bone Joint Surg Am.* 2004;**86(Suppl 1)**:119–130.

Ingrowing toenail surgery
Preoperative planning
A multitude of operations exist to deal with ingrowing toenails, or onychocryptosis. Chemical ablation with phenol of either part or all of the nail matrix is associated with lower recurrence rates than surgical ablation in most series.

Indications
Indications include painful onychocryptosis or recurrent infections.

Contraindications
- Severe digital vascular compromise is an absolute contraindication.
- Active infection is a relative contraindication.

Recurrence may be better treated with total matrix ablation.

Ingrowing toenail surgery

> ## Consent and risks
>
> - *Recurrence*: Less than 5%
> - *Infection*: Superficial infection commonly dependent on postoperative care
> - *Phenol burns*: Rare

Anaesthesia and positioning

Toenail surgery can be effectively performed under digital block with or without additional sedation. A bloodless field is established with the use of a digital tourniquet secured with an artery forceps.

Surgical technique

The affected nail border is elevated from the nail bed and surrounding skin by blunt dissection with forceps. The nail border is then cut using a blade or scissors underneath the ungual fold (**Figure 14.10**). Grasping the fragment with an artery forceps and using a rotating movement, the nail border is carefully avulsed in its entirety, complete with the widened germinal base. The nail groove is then carefully curetted.

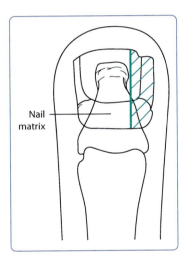

Figure 14.10 Partial matrix ablation – line of excision for nail border.

All blood is carefully cleared from the field and all exposed skin protected with petroleum jelly. A cotton bud is soaked in phenol and inserted along the exposed nail bed, under the ungual fold, and left for 60 seconds. This process is repeated once more then the whole area irrigated with copious amounts of saline. The tourniquet is released and a toe dressing applied.

Postoperative care and instructions

The foot is elevated for 48 hours then the dressings are reduced. The wound is then washed in tepid boiled salted water twice a day using a baby toothbrush, sweeping in a proximal to distal direction. When showering the patient is instructed to aim the spray directly over the wound.

Recommended references

Herold N, Houshian S, Riegels-Nielsen P. A prospective comparison of wedge matrix resection with nail matrix phenolization for the treatment of ingrown toenail. *J Foot Ankle Surg.* 2001;**40**:390–395.

Park DH, Singh D. The management of ingrowing toenails. *BMJ.* 2012;**344**:e2089.

Interdigital neuroma

Preoperative planning

Indications

Proven, symptomatic interdigital (Morton's) neuroma in the third (80%–90%) or second (10%–20%) web space failing to respond to conservative treatment.

Contraindications (relative)

- Vague symptoms or unusual location
- Other causes of metatarsalgia
- Lack of response to accurate injection of lesion

Consent and risks

- *Failure or recurrence*: Up to 20%, dependent on technique and diagnosis and closely related to short incision surgery
- *Scar pain* (especially with plantar incision)
- *Interdigital numbness*: Common but rarely troublesome
- *Vascular damage and digital ischaemia*: Risk if multiple web space explorations are undertaken

Anaesthesia and positioning

May be performed under general or regional anaesthesia. The patient is positioned supine with an ankle or thigh tourniquet to provide a bloodless field.

Surgical technique

Landmarks

The dorsal aspect of the affected web space is the landmark.

Incision

A longitudinal incision is placed over the dorsum of the foot, starting in the web space and extending 3–4 cm proximally. (An insufficient incision is commonly found in recurrent cases and is to be avoided.)

Dissection

> **Structure at risk**
> - Dorsal digital nerves

Taking care to avoid the dorsal digital nerves, dissection is carried down to the metatarsal heads and a laminar spreader is used between the metatarsal heads to place the transverse metatarsal ligament under tension. A Macdonald dissector is placed under the ligament which is then divided under direct vision. The laminar spreader is then advanced into the wound to open up the intermetatarsal space.

Procedure

> **Structure at risk**
> - Common digital artery

Plantar pressure will usually deliver the neuroma into the wound. Sometimes it will be obscured by a bursa which requires excision. Taking care to protect the common digital artery, the neuroma is retracted proximally and the two true digital nerves are divided. The nerve is then traced as proximally as possible and then divided under traction such that the cut end is proximal to the weightbearing area of the foot. The specimen should be sent for histology for confirmation of the diagnosis.

Closure

After release of the tourniquet, haemostasis is obtained. Skin is closed in a single layer and a forefoot bandage is applied.

Postoperative care and instructions

The patient should elevate the foot for 48 hours. They may mobilise, weightbearing as tolerated, in a postoperative flat shoe.

Recommended reference

Mann RA, Reynolds JD. Interdigital neuroma: A critical clinical analysis. *Foot Ankle*. 1983;**3**:238–243.

Lesser toe deformities

Preoperative planning

The decision-making process for correction of lesser toe deformities must take into account the type of deformity and whether it is fixed or flexible. A detailed examination of the deformity must be made in the awake patient prior to surgery. The position of the toe in the standing and lying position must be noted and any deformity assessed for a fixed component. Any subluxation or dislocation of the MTPJ must be identified. There is some confusion in the literature regarding toe deformity nomenclature. For the purposes of this book we have used the following terms:

- *Mallet toe*: A flexion deformity of the distal IPJ (DIPJ), often resulting in a callosity on the tip of the toe.
- *Hammer toe*: A flexion deformity of the proximal IPJ (PIPJ), often associated with hyperextension of the DIPJ and an accommodative hyperextension of the MTPJ.
- *Claw toe*: A term usually reserved for multiple toes and often associated with an underlying neurological condition. The primary deformity is one of hyperextension of the MTPJ with secondary flexion of the PIPJ.

Indications

- Painful lesser toe deformity not responding to conservative treatment
- Severe lesser toe deformity causing footwear problems and not responding to footwear modification

Contraindications

- Vascular insufficiency
- Local infection
- Undiagnosed underlying neurological condition (relative)

Consent and risks

- *Infection*: Less than 1%
- *Neurovascular damage*: Less than 1%.
- Vascular insufficiency of the digit following correction of a severe or long-standing deformity: may require further shortening or accepting a slightly flexed position
- Recurrence of deformity
- Swelling
- *Non-union of arthrodesis*: 20%–50% of PIPJ arthrodeses in some series formed a fibrous union, but this does not correlate with postoperative dissatisfaction
- *Malunion of arthrodesis*: Hyperextension of the joint or varus/valgus deformity often poorly tolerated
- Loss of movement or function of the toe, depending on procedure performed

Anaesthesia and positioning

Anaesthesia can be regional or general. If surgery is limited to the interphalangeal joints, a digital block can be used. A supine position is used, with the foot at the end of the table.

Surgical techniques

Percutaneous flexor digitorum longus tenotomy

Indication
Flexible mallet deformity.

Incision
Holding the toe to put the flexor tendon under tension, a size 15 blade (or tenotomy blade if available) is used to make a 2–3 mm incision over the DIPJ flexor crease.

Procedure

> **Structure at risk**
> - Neurovascular bundles

With the blade facing away from the neurovascular bundle, the tightened tendon is palpated with the blade and divided. The toe is then released to check the degree of correction.

Closure
Formal closure of the wound is not required.

Distal interphalangeal joint arthrodesis

Indication
A fixed mallet deformity is an indication.

Incision
An elliptical incision is made over the DIPJ and carried down to bone, excising the extensor tendon. Care is taken to avoid damage to the nail matrix distally.

Procedure

> **Structure at risk**
> - Neurovascular bundles

Facing the blade away from the neurovascular bundles, the collateral ligaments are divided, allowing deliverance of the condyles of the middle phalanx into the wound. Using a bone cutter, the condyles are excised at the metaphyseal flair. The articular surface of the distal phalanx is then decorticated. Under direct vision, the flexor digitorum longus tendon in the base of the wound is divided and the degree of correction is assessed. A double-ended K-wire is advanced in an antegrade direction through the distal phalanx, aiming to come out just below the nail bed. The joint is then reduced and the wire advanced into the middle phalanx to secure the joint.

Closure
The wound is best closed with non-absorbable mattress sutures to secure the skin and extensor tendon *en masse*.

Flexor tendon transfer (Girdlestone procedure)
The principle of this procedure is to recreate the action of the intrinsic muscles in flexing the MTPJ and extending the IPJs.

Indications
- Flexible hammer deformity
- Flexible claw toe deformity

Incision
A 5 mm transverse incision is made over the proximal flexor crease.

Procedure

Structure at risk
- Neurovascular bundles

Following blunt dissection down to the flexor sheath, the sheath is incised in a longitudinal manner. Of the three tendons seen, the flexor digitorum longus (FDL) is the central one. A percutaneous FDL tenotomy is performed at the level of the DIPJ (see earlier), and the FDL is delivered out of the proximal wound. The tendon is split into two halves along its length. On the dorsum of the toe, a longitudinal incision is made over the proximal phalanx. A small artery forceps is used to bluntly dissect down one side of the phalanx, remaining close to the extensor expansion, and exiting the toe through the plantar wound. The forceps are used to grasp one-half of the divided FDL tendon and deliver it to the dorsum, repeating the manoeuvre on the other side. Holding the MTPJ in about 20° flexion, both ends of the tendon are sutured to the extensor tendon, using an absorbable suture. The toe is released to ensure that the correction is being held. If there is judged to be some residual tightness in the MTPJ, a dorsal release may be performed (see later). A K-wire may be used to protect the repair.

Closure
Skin wounds are closed with appropriate sutures, usually non-absorbable suture material.

Proximal interphalangeal joint arthrodesis
Indication
Fixed hammer deformity or claw toe deformity is an indication.

Incision
An elliptical or a longitudinal incision is made over the PIPJ and carried down to bone excising the extensor tendon.

Procedure

Structure at risk
- Neurovascular bundles

Facing the blade away from the neurovascular bundles, the collateral ligaments are divided, allowing deliverance of the condyles of the proximal phalanx into the wound. Using a bone cutter, the condyles are excised at the metaphyseal flair. Sufficient bone must be removed to allow the toe to be straightened without undue tension on the tissues, especially the neurovascular bundles. The plantar plate is released from the middle phalanx allowing its base to be delivered. The articular surface is then decorticated using a nibbler. A double-ended K-wire is advanced in an antegrade direction through the middle and distal phalanges, aiming to come out just below the nail bed. The joint is then reduced and the wire advanced into the proximal phalanx to secure the joint.

Closure

The wound is closed with non-absorbable mattress sutures to secure skin and extensor tendon *en masse*. If the MTPJ remains extended, a dorsal release (see later) should be included to avoid a 'cock-up' deformity.

Metatarsophalangeal joint release

Indication

Hyperextension of the MTPJ with or without subluxation is an indication.

Incision

Structures at risk
- Dorsal veins
- Dorsal sensory nerve branches

A 3 cm incision is made in line with the metatarsal, centred over the MTPJ. If two adjacent joints are being addressed, the incision should be made in the web space. An attempt should be made to protect the dorsal veins and sensory nerves.

Procedure

Release of the joint should occur in a stepwise manner and stop when satisfactory release is achieved. The extensor digitorum longus (EDL) and extensor digitorum brevis (EDB) to the toe (EDL lies medial to EDB) are identified and their tightness assessed. If tight, the EDB may be divided but the EDL should be Z-lengthened. A dorsal capsulotomy is performed then, with the blade facing away from the neurovascular bundles, progressive capsular and collateral releases are performed both medially and laterally. In long-standing deformities, adhesions may exist between the plantar capsule and the metatarsal head which should be released. Once satisfactory release is achieved, the EDL should be repaired with absorbable suture and the wound closed. If, despite maximal release of the MTPJ, the joint cannot be reduced, *a metatarsal osteotomy should be considered*. (See 'Lesser metatarsal [Weil's] osteotomy', p. 414.)

Postoperative care and instructions

After all lesser toe surgery, the tourniquet should be released prior to waking the patient and the toe observed. If reperfusion is slow, releasing excessively tight dressings and hanging the foot over the side of the table usually allows the toe to reperfuse. If the toe remains white and a K-wire has been inserted, gently bending the arthrodesed joint will relieve excess tension on the blood vessels.

All patients can fully weightbear on a flat postoperative shoe. K-wires, if used, should be removed at 4–6 weeks.

Recommended reference

Coughlin MJ. Lesser-toe abnormalities. *J Bone Joint Surg Am*. 2002;**84**:1446–1469.

Lesser metatarsal (Weil's) osteotomy

Preoperative planning

Historically, the Helal osteotomy was a popular treatment for lesser metatarsal overload and subluxed lesser MTPJs. This has largely been replaced by the Weil osteotomy, as popularised by Barouk.

Indications

- Overload of a metatarsal head secondary to a relatively long metatarsal
- Reduction of a chronically subluxed or dislocated MTPJ

Contraindications

- Gross deformity of the joint
- Vascular insufficiency or infection

Consent and risks

- *Ongoing forefoot pain*: Often related to the use of an excessively long screw
- *MTPJ stiffness*: Some degree is very common
- *'Floating toe'*: Stiff hyperextension of the MTPJ preventing the toe from touching the floor
- *Infection*: Less than 1%
- *Avascular necrosis and non-union*: Rare
- *Neurovascular damage*: Rare

Anaesthesia and positioning
See 'Lesser toe deformities' (p. 409).

Surgical technique
Incision
A 4 cm incision is made over the metatarsal, or in the interspace if two adjacent osteotomies are to be performed.

Dissection

> **Structure at risk**
> - Neurovascular bundles

The extensor tendons are retracted out of the way and the dorsal capsule of the MTPJ released. Protecting the neurovascular bundles, the collaterals are released to allow the proximal phalanx to be displaced plantarwards.

Procedure
A Macdonald dissector or custom-made head elevator is inserted under the metatarsal head. Using a fine saw blade, an osteotomy is made, starting 2 mm below the dorsal surface of the head and continuing proximally, parallel to the sole of the foot (**Figure 14.11**). Using a fine osteotome or McDonald, the head fragment is freed up to allow it to retract proximally the desired amount. The fragment can then be fixed with a small screw, the length of which usually decreases from 14 mm in the second metatarsal to 11 mm in the fifth. The excess dorsal bone overhanging the head can then be trimmed to ensure that the proximal phalanx can freely dorsiflex.

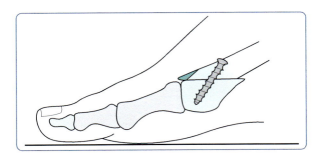

Figure 14.11 Orientation of Weil osteotomy of the lesser metatarsal and screw placement.

Postoperative care and instructions
The patient is asked to mobilise in a heel weightbearing shoe. Once wounds have healed, passive and active range-of-motion exercises can begin and the toe can be strapped down to prevent hyperextension.

Recommended references

Barouk LS. *Forefoot Reconstruction*. Berlin, Germany: Springer-Verlag, 2005.
Helal B. Metatarsal osteotomy for metatarsalgia. *J Bone Joint Surg Br*. 1975;**57**:187–192.
Trnka HJ, Mühlbauer M, Zettl R et al. Comparison of the results of the Weil and Helal osteotomies for the treatment of metatarsalgia secondary to dislocation of the lesser metatarsophalangeal joints. *Foot Ankle Int*. 1999;**20**:72–79.

Fifth toe soft tissue correction (Butler's procedure)

Preoperative planning

Indications

- Moderate or severe over-riding fifth toe with pain and callosity or footwear problems
- Failure of footwear adaptations and other conservative measures

Contraindications

Digital ischaemia or poor perfusion is a contraindication.

Consent and risks

- *Neurovascular damage and risk of toe ischaemia*: Reduced by careful dissection and avoidance of traction or manipulation of the toe
- *Recurrence of deformity*: Rare

Anaesthesia and positioning

Regional or general anaesthesia is required as digital anaesthesia is insufficient. The patient is positioned supine with an ankle or thigh tourniquet to ensure a bloodless field.

Surgical technique

Incision and dissection

Structure at risk

- Neurovascular bundles of the fifth toe

A double-racquet incision is drawn to ensure correct placement. The dorsal limb of the incision should follow the line of tension along the extensor tendon. The plantar limb should be longer and heading laterally (**Figure 14.12**). The skin is incised with care and the *neurovascular bundles identified and protected*.

Procedure

The tight extensor tendons are divided and then the joint capsule exposed. The tight dorsal capsule and usually the collateral ligaments require release. Sometimes the plantar capsule is adherent and needs to be dissected off. The toe should now assume the required position.

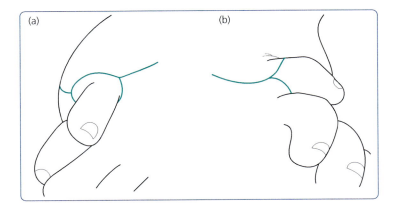

Figure 14.12 Butler procedure – position of skin incision. (a) Dorsal and (b) plantar views.

Closure

The skin is closed without tension. The dorsal incision assumes a V to Y position and the plantar incision a Y to V position. The tourniquet must be released to ensure adequate perfusion of the toe prior to the end of anaesthesia. No taping or splintage is required.

Postoperative care and instructions

The patient can mobilise fully weightbearing on a postoperative shoe.

Recommended reference

Cockin J. Butler's operation for an over-riding fifth toe. *J Bone Joint Surg Br.* 1968;**50**:78–81.

Hindfoot arthrodesis

Preoperative planning

The three joints of the hindfoot, the subtalar (ST), calcaneocuboid (CC) and talonavicular (TN) joints, can be arthrodesed individually or in combination, depending upon the indication. However, as all three joints work in unison, fusion of one will affect the others. As the normal hindfoot swings into varus during gait, Chopart's joints (TN and CC) are locked in position to provide a firm platform. Therefore, a subtalar fusion must avoid varus to leave Chopart's joints relatively mobile and avoid fixed supination of the foot. Similarly, fusion of the TN joint in isolation fixes the CC joint and greatly reduces the movement of the ST joint. Therefore, in arthrodesing one or more of these joints, attention to the position of all three must be taken.

The ultimate aim of any hindfoot fusion is to provide a pain-free, stable hindfoot and a foot that can be placed flat on the floor for weightbearing.

Indications

(See also 'Principles of foot and ankle arthrodesis', p. 385.)

- Painful arthropathy of one or more hindfoot joints secondary to degenerative, inflammatory or traumatic causes not responding to conservative management. In such cases, isolated fusion of the affected joint can be considered.

- Fixed deformity of the hindfoot not amenable to soft tissue correction and/or osteotomy. Historically, this was primarily for paralytic conditions, especially poliomyelitis. Hindfoot fusions are now more commonly performed for tibialis posterior dysfunction, rheumatoid arthritis and congenital neuromuscular disorders. In such cases, a double fusion of the TN and CC joints, or a triple fusion of all three joints is indicated.
- Gross instability of the hindfoot with bony destruction, as seen in rheumatoid arthritis or Charcot's joints in people with diabetes.

Contraindications

- Active infection or ischaemia of the limb is an absolute contraindication.
- A more proximal uncorrected deformity is a relative contraindication. It is difficult to judge hindfoot alignment if there is a more proximal deformity. Furthermore, if a proximal deformity is subsequently corrected, the hindfoot alignment may be rendered incorrect. It is therefore prudent to address proximal deformities first.
- Ipsilateral ankle fusion is a relative contraindication – the patient must be counselled that a combined ankle and hindfoot fusion will result in a loss of normal gait and possibly the need for footwear adaptations to walk.

Consent and risks

(See also 'Principles of foot and ankle arthrodesis', p. 385.)

- *Non-union*: The TN joint is especially prone to non-union. This is likely to be due to its curved surface and extensively cortical composition making adequate visualisation and preparation technically difficult. Obtaining adequate rigid fixation can also be difficult compared with the ST joint.
- *Malunion*: Due to incorrect positioning or fixation failure. A malunion preventing the patient from placing the foot flat on the floor, often with overload of the lateral border, is very poorly tolerated by the patient and often requires revision.

Anaesthesia and positioning

(See also 'Principles of foot and ankle arthrodesis', p. 385.)

For isolated subtalar fusion, a lateral decubitus position, with the operative side up, allows excellent access and visualisation. For TN or double/triple arthrodeses, a supine position is optimal. The use of a bolster under the calf allows free access around the foot.

Surgical technique
Landmarks

- *Utility lateral approach*: Tip of fibula and base of fourth metatarsal
- *Anterior approach*: EHL and tibialis anterior tendons
- *Anteromedial approach*: Tibialis anterior and posterior tendons

Incision

> **Structures at risk**
>
> - Sural nerve (utility lateral approach)
> - Superficial peroneal nerve (utility lateral approach)
> - Saphenous nerve and vein (anteromedial approach)

The incision(s) used will depend upon the joints to be addressed. For isolated TN arthrodesis, an anterior approach allows excellent visualisation. For isolated ST and/or CC joint fusion, a utility lateral approach is used. For a triple fusion, the utility lateral in combination with an anteromedial approach to the TN joint allows wide skin bridges (**Figure 14.13a and b**).

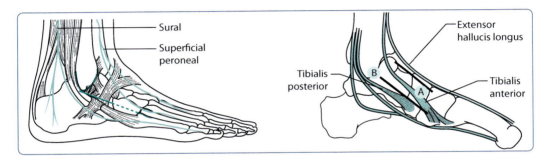

Figure 14.13 (a) Approaches for hindfoot arthrodesis – utility lateral approach. (b) Approaches for hindfoot arthrodesis – anterior (A) and anteromedial (B) approach to talonavicular joint.

The utility lateral approach allows excellent visualisation of the ST and CC joints. It is preferable to the traditional Ollier incision as there is less risk to the branches of the superficial peroneal nerve. A straight incision is made from the tip of the fibula towards the base of the fourth metatarsal. This should lie between the sural and peroneal nerves but care must be taken, especially distally. The incision can be stopped at the CC joint if access to only the subtalar joint is required.

The anterior approach is an extension of the approach used to access the ankle. A straight incision between the tendons of extensor hallucis longus and tibialis anterior is made over the TN joint and the extensor retinaculum carefully incised. This gives excellent access to the medial and lateral extents of the surprisingly broad TN joint.

Alternatively, if performing a triple fusion, an anteromedial incision between the tendons of tibialis anterior and posterior allows a wider skin bridge. Care must be taken of the saphenous vein and nerve, which lie in this plane. It is harder to access the far lateral extent of the TN joint through this incision, and access through the lateral incision may be required.

Dissection

The utility lateral incision is deepened to pass above the peroneal tendons to the subtalar joint. By releasing the insertion of extensor digitorum brevis and elevating this with a distally based flap, the sinus tarsi and CC joint can be visualised. In triple arthrodeses, after preparation of the CC and ST joints, the lateral aspect of the TN joint can be accessed from the lateral side.

Procedure

> **Structure at risk**
>
> - Tibial neurovascular bundle

Once exposed and mobilised, the selected joints should be meticulously prepared as detailed in 'Principles of foot and ankle arthrodesis' (p. 385). With regard to the TN joint, the full extent of the joint must be realised for successful fusion. It is easy not to prepare deep enough (one should see the spring ligament in the depth of the wound) or laterally enough. During subtalar preparation, the posterior facet is prepared first. When the tendon of FHL (identified by moving the toe) is visualised, preparation is deep enough. Great care should be taken, however, as deep to the FHL is the tibial neurovascular bundle. After preparation of the posterior facet, the medial facet can be prepared. Damage to the structures posterior to this, and the head of the talus superiorly, must be avoided. Once all of the required joints have been prepared, they need to be held in the required position of arthrodesis. For the ST joint, the optimum position is 5° of valgus. However, if there is rigidity of the midfoot from a long-standing deformity, 5° of valgus may not allow the foot to be placed flat on the floor. Therefore, the position of the weightbearing foot should be confirmed by using a flat surface prior to fixation of the ST joint. A varus position must be avoided.

The ideal position of arthrodesis of the TN joint is one of 'talar neutral' – that is, with the domed talar head central in the navicular. In this position, the long axis of the talus should pass through the long axis of the first metatarsal. Care must be taken not to extend or flex the TN joint, and the foot should be perpendicular to the tibia with the ankle in neutral. Again, the position of the foot flat on the floor must be checked and a suboptimal position may have to be accepted to achieve this. The CC joint position will be dictated by the other joints and therefore fixed last.

Various methods of ST joint fixation have been described. Our preferred method is to place a large-diameter (8 mm) cannulated compression screw from the posterolateral aspect of the calcaneum into the talus to cross the posterior facet at 90°. This avoids possible impingement problems from a screw inserted from the talar neck. The entry point is in a line down from the lateral margin of the Achilles tendon, just above the plantar skin of the heel. Too plantarwards or central an entry point may cause painful prominence of the screw head. Usually, a single screw is sufficient. The TN joint can be fixed using a retrograde screw from the medial edge of the navicular into the talar neck. Care must be taken to ensure a good bite is obtained medially without intruding upon the NC joint. Further fixation can be obtained with a screw from the anterior surface of the navicular. Screw fixation of the CC joint, antegrade from the anterior process of the calcaneum or retrograde from the cuboid, can sometimes be difficult, in which case compression staples or a low-profile plate can be used.

Closure

All wounds should be carefully closed, ensuring a good soft tissue layer is closed over the joints prior to skin closure. If an anterior approach has been used, the retinaculum must be carefully repaired. The leg is then placed in a back slab.

Postoperative care and instructions

(See also 'Principles of foot and ankle arthrodesis', p. 385.)

The patient is kept in a non-weightbearing cast for 6 weeks or until early radiological signs of union are seen. They can then begin to gradually increase their weightbearing. A cast should be retained for 3 months or until there is solid radiographical and clinical evidence of union.

Recommended reference

Davies MB, Rosenfeld PF, Stavrou P et al. A comprehensive review of subtalar arthrodesis. *Foot Ankle Int.* 2007;**28**:295–297.

Calcaneal osteotomy

Preoperative planning

Indications

A calcaneal osteotomy is rarely indicated in isolation. It is usually performed as part of a soft tissue correction of a hindfoot deformity to protect the reconstruction and reconstitute the mechanical axis of the hindfoot. Commonly used examples are a medial displacement osteotomy as part of a tibialis posterior reconstruction and a closing wedge or lateralising osteotomy as part of a pes cavus correction. Occasionally, an osteotomy may be used to correct a post-traumatic deformity of the calcaneum, but this is often done in combination with a subtalar arthrodesis as there is usually associated joint disruption.

Contraindications

- Active infection or critical ischaemia of the limb is an absolute contraindication.
- A more proximal uncorrected deformity is a relative contraindication. It is difficult to judge hindfoot alignment if there is a more proximal deformity. Furthermore, if a proximal deformity is subsequently corrected, the hindfoot alignment may become incorrect. It is therefore advisable to address proximal deformities first.

Consent and risks

- *Neurovascular damage*: The sural nerve is in the zone of the incision and must be avoided. On the medial extent of any osteotomy, the neurovascular bundle is close by and can be injured with aggressive use of power tools.
- *Malunion*: Usually due to technical errors in judging the degree of correction but also due to hardware failure.

- *Non-union*: Rare due to large surface area of cancellous bone.
- *Recurrence of deformity*: Especially if the deforming soft tissues are not correctly balanced or there is a progressive neuromuscular condition.

Anaesthesia and positioning

- General or spinal anaesthesia with a thigh tourniquet allowing exposure to above the knee to judge alignment satisfactorily.
- Most soft tissue procedures require access to both the medial and lateral sides of the hindfoot. Therefore, position the patient supine, with a removable sandbag under the ipsilateral buttock.

Surgical technique

The calcaneal osteotomy is usually performed first as part of any soft tissue correction of the hindfoot to avoid accidental damage to the correction.

Landmarks

- Anterior border of tendo-Achilles
- Junction of dorsal and plantar skin of heel

Incision

Structure at risk

- Sural nerve

Some authors advocate an oblique lateral incision over the line of the proposed osteotomy. Unfortunately, this coincides with the course of the sural nerve and puts it at risk. We therefore advise an extensile lateral incision, commonly used for calcaneal fixation, as the sural nerve is protected in the elevated flap. This also allows better visualisation of the calcaneum. The inferior limb of the incision runs along the junction of the plantar and dorsal skin. The superior limb extends superiorly in line with the anterior border of the tendo-Achilles (**Figure 14.14**).

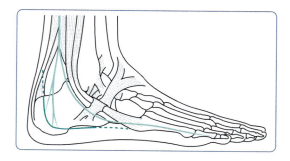

Figure 14.14 Extensile lateral approach to os calcis.

The extent of the exposure required is less than for calcaneal fixation, but the insertion of tendo-Achilles superiorly and plantar fascia inferiorly should be visualised.

Dissection

The incision is carried straight down to bone and the flap elevated in the subperiosteal layer with minimal trauma to the soft tissues.

Procedure

> **Structures at risk**
>
> - Tendo-Achilles
> - Plantar fascia

For both medial and lateral displacement and lateral closing wedge osteotomies, the angle of the osteotomy is the same, at about 45° to the plantar surface of the foot (**Figure 14.15**). It runs anterior to the insertion of tendo-Achilles to superior to the insertion of the plantar fascia. Trethowan bone levers are placed to protect these two structures and guide the osteotomy line. Using an oscillating saw, the lateral wall is cut and the saw advanced until it reaches the medial wall.

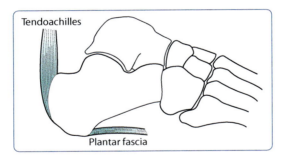

Figure 14.15 Alignment of calcaneal osteotomy.

The medial wall is cautiously weakened by bouncing the saw off the wall and the osteotomy completed using a broad osteotome *with care to avoid any pressure on the medial soft tissues*. Once completed, the osteotome is carefully twisted to mobilise the fragment and a dissector used to free the medial periosteum. The tuberosity fragment can then be displaced, either medially or laterally; this is performed with the ankle in a plantarflexed position. Displacement will depend upon the degree of correction required, 1 cm is usually sufficient. The position can usually be provisionally 'locked' by holding the foot in a plantigrade position. Once the surgeon is confident with the correction, a guide wire from a cannulated screw system can be inserted, under fluoroscopic guidance, from the lateral aspect of the tuberosity into the anterior fragment. Care must be taken to ensure that the wire enters the anterior calcaneum and does not penetrate medially. Once satisfied with the position, a single cannulated screw is sufficient to hold the osteotomy. Alternatively, a stepped plate may be used.

A lateral closing wedge can be added to the lateral displacement osteotomy, if required, to allow increased correction; the thickness of the wedge will depend upon the correction desired. Using minimal force, an attempt is made to close the wedge prior to fixation.

Closure

Closure of the flap must be meticulous and without tension. Deep Vicryl sutures and interrupted nylon sutures are satisfactory. The leg should be immobilised once the soft tissue component is completed.

Postoperative care and instructions

The leg should be elevated for 72 hours until swelling has subsided. The leg is then placed in a non-weightbearing cast for a duration usually dictated by the soft tissue correction. The osteotomy usually heals within about 6 weeks.

Recommended references

Dwyer FC. Osteotomy of the calcaneum for pes cavus. *J Bone Joint Surg Br.* 1959;**41**:80–86.
Evans D. Calcaneo-valgus deformity. *J Bone Joint Surg Br.* 1975;**57**:270–278.
Trnka HJ, Easley ME, Myerson MS. The role of calcaneal osteotomies for correction of adult flatfoot. *Clin Orthop Relat Res.* 1999;**365**:50–64.

Viva questions

1. Describe how you can maximise the union rate for a midfoot arthrodesis.
2. In the context of hallux valgus deformity, what is congruency, and how does it affect your decision-making process?
3. What radiographs do you use to assess hallux valgus deformity, what angles do you measure and how does this influence your choice of operation?
4. What surgical approach do you use for a first metatarsal osteotomy, and what are the important structures at risk?
5. Describe the blood supply to the first metatarsal head. How can your choice of hallux valgus procedure affect the blood supply?
6. What structures do you need to identify in performing a lateral release in a hallux valgus deformity?
7. In a Scarf osteotomy, what is 'troughing', and how does the design of your osteotomy influence occurrence?
8. Why is a Keller's procedure generally poorly tolerated by patients, and when would you consider performing one?
9. What are the key differences between a Weil's and a Helal's osteotomy of the lesser metatarsals?
10. What is the difference between a claw toe, mallet toe and a hammer toe?

11. Describe the mechanics of a Girdlestone tendon transfer for the lesser toes and when you would perform this.
12. How do you assess the severity of hallux rigidus, and how does this influence your treatment options?
13. What is the optimum position of arthrodesis of the first metatarsophalangeal joint (MTPJ), and how would you assess this intraoperatively?
14. Describe the anatomy of a toenail. How does this knowledge help in the treatment of ingrowing nails?
15. What is a Morton's neuroma, and where is it most commonly found?
16. How does movement of the subtalar joint in gait affect movement of the Chopart joints (talonavicular and calcaneocuboid)?
17. Describe your understanding of the concept of 'talar neutral', and why is this useful in assessing foot position?
18. What surgical approach do you use to reach the subtalar joint, what are the landmarks and what structures are at risk?
19. What structures are at risk during a calcaneal osteotomy?
20. When would you consider performing a lateralising calcaneal osteotomy?

15 Limb Reconstruction

Robert Jennings and Peter Calder

Principles of limb reconstruction	427	Principles of deformity correction	436
Surgical techniques	428	Innovation in limb lengthening and reconstruction	438
Femoral lengthening	433		
Tibial lengthening	434	Viva questions	441

Principles of limb reconstruction

When subjected to slow, steady traction, under the appropriate conditions, living tissue becomes metabolically activated and is able to regenerate. This 'tension-stress' effect was described by Professor Gavril Abramovich Ilizarov from Kurgan in western Siberia, who pioneered the field of limb reconstruction from the early 1950s and developed the highly successful techniques that are still in use today.

Callus, formed at a corticotomy site, can be distracted at speeds of up to 1 mm per day and, reliably, form new bone in the process of 'distraction osteogenesis'. Once the goal length is achieved, a period of consolidation is required before fixator removal. This takes approximately 30–40 days per centimetre of lengthening to prevent bowing or fracture. Anecdotally, the maximum, safe distraction possible per procedure is 20% of the original length of the bone being lengthened.

Distraction osteogenesis requires

- Stability
- Maintenance of blood supply
- A latency period (5–7 days)
- Appropriate rate of distraction (0.75–1 mm per day)
- Appropriate rhythm (frequency) of distraction (0.25 mm, 6–8 hourly)

Biomechanics

- Monolateral rail
  - Cantilever loading
  - Concentrated high stress on near cortex
- Circular frame
  - Beam loading
  - More even distribution of stress across cortices

Use of all-wire fixation across a diaphysis is less attractive, due to risks to soft tissues. Hence, hybrid fixation with half-pins and wires is preferred.

Methods to improve stability
- Wire
  - Increase diameter (1.8 mm for adult, 1.5 mm for child)
  - Increase tension (130 Nm for adult, 110 Nm for child)
  - Increase crossing angles (**Figure 15.1**)
  - Opposing 'olive' wires
  - Increase number of wires
- Half-pin
  - Increase diameter
  - Hydroxyapatite coating
  - Increase crossing angles (multiplanar)
  - Decrease distance of external construct to bone
  - Near and far positions (**Figure 15.2**)
  - Increase number
- Ring
  - Decrease diameter (Note: Allow at least 2 cm clearance for swelling)
  - Fix bone in middle (compromise with eccentrically positioned tibia)
  - Near and far positions
  - Increase number (including 'dummy' rings)
- Attachments
  - Use 'slotted' bolts – high surface area of contact with wire
  - Build ring to wire, if necessary – decrease bend on wire

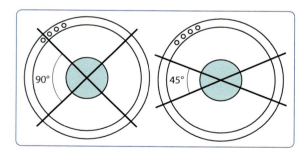

Figure 15.1 'Crossing angles': stability (a) greater than (b).

Surgical techniques
Preoperative planning
Indications
- Tibial/femoral lengthening
- Long bone deformity correction

Surgical techniques

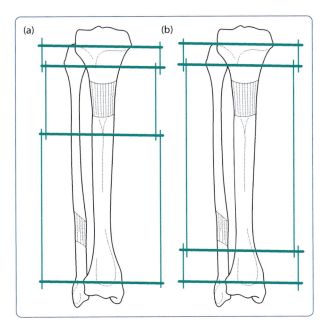

Figure 15.2 'Near and far' fixation: Stability (a) greater than (b).

Contraindications
- Non-compliant patient
- Adjacent joint instability
- Skin infection
- Significant soft tissue contractures
- Poor vascularity
- Pregnancy
- Smoker – relative

Consent and risks
- Duration of treatment must be emphasised (c. 40 days/cm)
- Pain: Post-surgical, chronic dull ache during distraction is common
- Pin site problems: Inflammation, soft tissue infection, osteomyelitis
- Joint stiffness or subluxation
- Soft tissue contractures
- Vascular injury
- Neurological injury: Perioperative; postoperative stretching
- Premature/delayed/non-union
- Hardware failure
- Late bowing
- Fracture
- Deep vein thrombosis/pulmonary embolism

Operative planning

Recent radiographs must be available. These should include full leg length views, in the anteroposterior plane, of both lower limbs with the patellae facing forwards and appropriate lateral views. The mechanical and anatomical axes need to be assessed on both legs. If both legs are 'abnormal', standard angles are used for calculations.

Leg length discrepancy

Assessment is made from history, examination and radiological findings. Care must be taken to differentiate true from apparent causes of leg length discrepancy.

Common causes of apparent leg length discrepancy

- Scoliosis
- Hip instability or dislocation
- Fixed hip adduction
- Fixed knee flexion
- Equinus deformity of the ankle

Angular deformity

Clinical and radiographical examination allows calculation of the centre of rotation of angulation (CORA; **Figure 15.3**). This is present at the intersection point of proximal and distal anatomical axes.

A decision is made as to whether the deformity requires surgical correction. This is based on the severity of deformity and the presence or absence of associated factors.

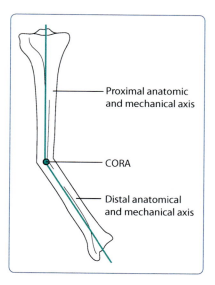

Figure 15.3 'CORA' (centre of rotation of angulation) – mechanical and anatomical axis.

Indications for surgical correction of angular deformity

- Mechanical axis deviation (MAD) (**Figure 15.4**)
- Rotational malalignment
- Translation
- Leg length discrepancy

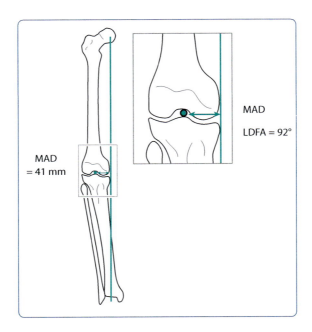

Figure 15.4 Mechanical axis deviation (MAD).

The next decision is the appropriate site for osteotomy. Osteotomy performed at the CORA will not result in translation (**Figure 15.5**); osteotomy away from the CORA will produce translation. Note: If the hinge is not on the bisector line (**Figure 15.6**) or the CORA is not on the anatomical axis, osteotomy at any level will result in translation.

Surgical technique

Wire insertion

- Aseptic 'no hands'/'Russian' technique
- Alcohol-soaked gauze used to coat and hold wire
- Low heat generation is ensured via short, intermittent bursts with the wire driver
- Wire tapped with mallet, when through contralateral skin

Half-pin insertion

- Stab skin incision
- Blunt dissection to bone

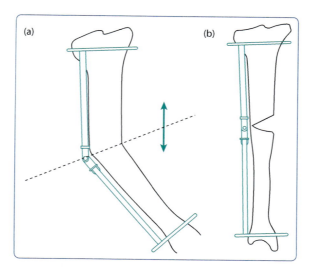

Figure 15.5 With the hinge placed along the 'bisector line of the CORA', there will be no translation.

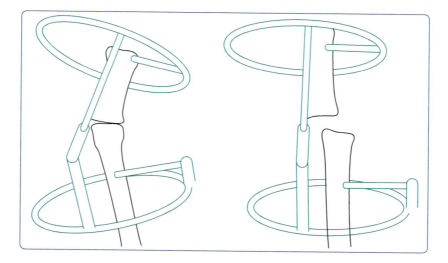

Figure 15.6 With the hinge placed off the 'bisector line of the CORA', translation will result.

- Soft tissue protecting drill guide
- Both cortices pre-drilled
- Low heat generation – intermittent drilling
- Saline to cool and wash out swarf (decreases infection risk)

Wire/half-pin placement
- 'Safe corridors' – avoid neurovascular structures
- Avoid crossing compartments, if possible
- Soft tissues on stretch, e.g. quadriceps in flexion, hamstrings in extension (helps postoperative mobility)

Corticotomy

- Low energy.
- Minimal incision, to admit osteotome.
- Periosteum incised and preserved, when possible.
- A row of holes are pre-drilled with a 4.8 mm drill, with saline used for cooling. This technique allows low heat generation, reducing corticotomy site bone necrosis.
- An osteotome is used to join holes, with a twist to break the posterior cortex.

Note: Latent period: 5–7 days; quarter turns: three to four times per day (0.75–1 mm/day).

Femoral lengthening

Preoperative planning

See 'Principles of limb reconstruction' (p. 427).

Surgical technique

Corticotomy

Landmarks

Junction of the proximal metaphysis and diaphysis – 1.5 cm distal to lesser trochanter.

Incision and dissection
- Image intensifier control
- Adequate longitudinal incision (to admit 8 mm osteotome)

Either

- *Anterior approach*: Between sartorius and tensor fascia lata (TFL), then through vastus intermedius and rectus femoris

Or

- *Lateral approach*: Through TFL and split vastus lateralis

Corticotomy technique as earlier.

Procedure

- Monolateral rail (**Figure 15.7**)
    - If no risk of joint subluxation
    - Three half-pins proximal and, at least, three distal to corticotomy
- Circular frame
    - If risk of joint subluxation
    - Span knee/pelvis
    - Arches/two-thirds rings to allow mobility
    - Same principles as earlier

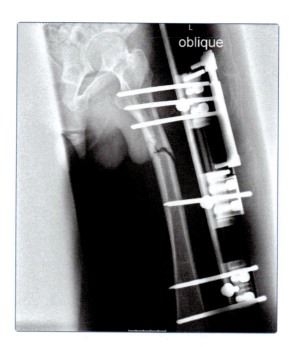

Figure 15.7 Radiograph of femoral limb reconstruction system (LRS) rail.

Tibial lengthening
Preoperative planning
See 'Principles of limb reconstruction' (p. 427) (**Figure 15.8**).

Surgical technique
Corticotomy
Landmarks
Junction of the proximal metaphysis and diaphysis, c.1.5 cm distal to tibial tuberosity.

Incision and dissection
- Image intensifier control
- Adequate longitudinal incision over anterior tibial crest (to admit 8 mm osteotome)
- Periosteum incised, then lifted off medially and laterally with blunt dissection
- Corticotomy technique as earlier

Procedure
- Two rings per bone segment (near and far)
- Two wires/half-pins per ring
- Four connecting, threaded rods between rings (**Figure 15.9**)
- Fibular osteotomy
  - Mid-diaphyseal avoids neurovascular structures
- Fix fibula (proximal and distal), to avoid joint subluxation

Tibial lengthening | 435

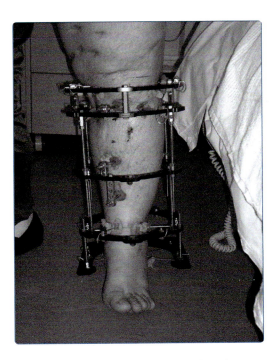

Figure 15.8 Tibial Ilizarov frame for lengthening.

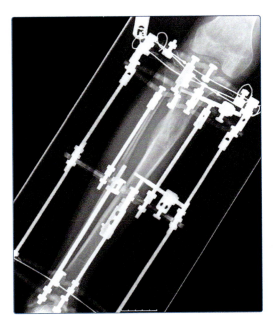

Figure 15.9 Radiograph of tibial Ilizarov frame for lengthening.

Principles of deformity correction
Preoperative planning
Operative planning

The initial decision is between acute and gradual correction of the deformity:

- Acute
  - Mild deformity
  - Opening or closing wedge
  - Plate and screws
  - Intramedullary (IM) nail
  - External fixation
- Gradual
  - More severe deformity
  - Less risk of neurological damage
  - Potential for revision of correction protocol
  - Distraction osteogenesis
  - Circular frame, e.g. Ilizarov or hexapod type (e.g. Taylor spatial frame [TSF])
  - Monolateral fixator: On convex side – distraction at osteotomy site (see **Figure 15.5**); on concave side – compression at osteotomy site therefore requires wedge excision

Surgical technique

Example: Simple, tibial diaphyseal deformity correction with a circular frame.

- Application of proximal and distal rings (see earlier; **Figure 15.10**)
- Osteotomy at CORA (see earlier)
- Ilizarov method
  - Inter-ring connections with hinges along bisector line of CORA (**Figure 15.11**)
- TSF method (**Figures 15.12** and **15.13**)
  - Inter-ring connections with six oblique, adjustable struts ('virtual hinge')

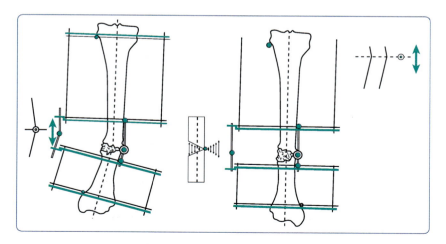

Figure 15.10 'Near and far' rings with osteotomy at centre of rotation of angulation (CORA), hinge along bisector line.

Principles of deformity correction | 437

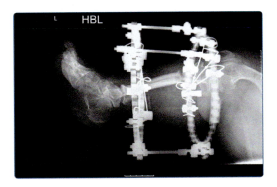

Figure 15.11 Radiograph of a simple Ilizarov frame construct used to correct deformity in a congenitally short tibia.

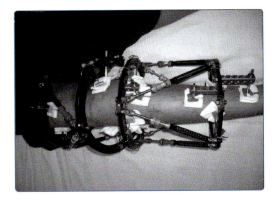

Figure 15.12 Tibial Taylor spatial frame.

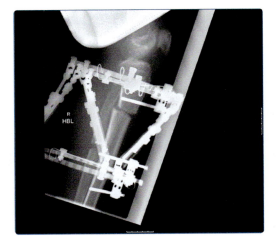

Figure 15.13 Radiograph of tibial Taylor spatial frame for deformity correction.

Online computer programme

- Requires: Postoperative radiograph measurements
  - Frame measurements (ring sizes/initial strut lengths)
- Delivers: Pre- and post-correction images
  - Corrective protocol

Postoperative care and instructions

- Latency period (5–7 days)
- Gradual correction period
- Consolidation period
- Removal of frame when clinically and radiologically appropriate

Innovation in limb lengthening and reconstruction

Complications associated with external fixation during limb reconstruction are common. These include pin-site infection, soft tissue tethering from the pins and wires resulting in pain, regenerate deformity from soft tissue forces or fracture following frame removal and patient intolerance of the frames during treatment.

Surgical techniques have changed in an attempt to minimise these complications. The use of intramedullary implants reduces fixator time and provides regenerate stability. Lengthening over a nail or lengthening followed by nailing still incorporates the use of an external fixator. The development of intramedullary lengthening nails eliminates the need for the external fixator. The initial designs utilised a ratchet mechanism that required rotation of the limb and bone segments to lengthen. A change in design was made where transcutaneous electrical energy drove a motor to improve control in lengthening. The latest and most popular implant is the Precice Intramedullary Lengthening Sysystem (NuVasive Inc., California). This is a magnet-operated telescopic internal lengthening device with an outer casing of titanium alloy (Ti-6Al-4V). A cylindrical rare earth magnet is connected to a gear box and screw shaft assembly within the nail. Two rotating rare earth magnets in an external remote controller (ERC)

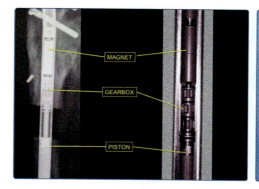
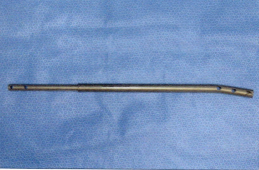

Figure 15.14 Precice lengthening nail.

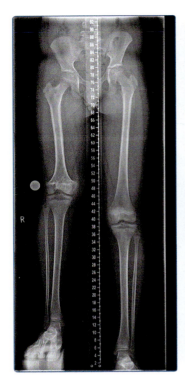 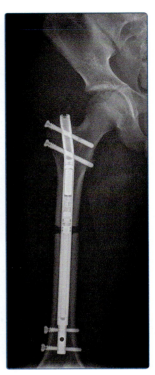

Figure 15.15 Growth arrest in a 12-year-old child.

are held over the magnet within the nail, resulting in rotation of the implant magnet which can either lengthen or shorten the nail with sub-millimeter accuracy. Early results are favourable confirming faster regenerate healing times, less complications, better cosmetic results and more favourable patient outcomes compared to lengthening using an external fixator (**Figures 15.14–15.17**).

Recommended references

De Bastiani G, Aldegheri R, Renzi-Brivio L et al. Limb lengthening by callus distraction (Callotasis). *J Pediatr Orthop*. 1987;**7**:129–134.

Cole JD, Justin D, Kasparis T et al. The intramedullary skeletal kinetic distractor (ISKD): First clinical results of a new intramedullary nail for lengthening of the femur and tibia. *Injury*. 2001;**32(Suppl 4)**: SD129–SD139.

Paley D, Herzenberg JE. *Principles of Deformity Correction*. Berlin, Germany: Springer, 2001.

Paley D, Herzenberg JE, Tetsworth K et al. Deformity planning for frontal and sagittal plane corrective osteotomies. *Orthop Clin North Am*. 1994;**25**:425–465.

Rozbruch SR, Ilizarov S. *Limb Lengthening and Reconstruction Surgery*. New York, NY: Informa, 2007.

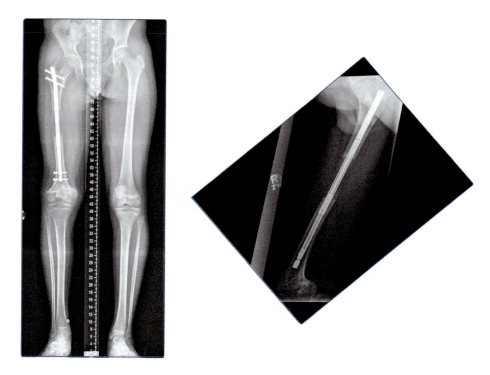

Figure 15.16 Completion of lengthening (8 cm).

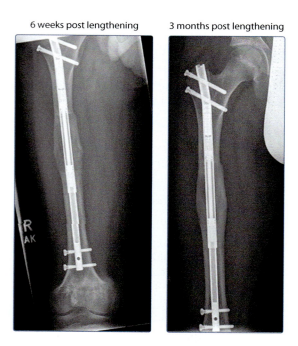

Figure 15.17 Consolidation (8 cm).

Viva questions

1. What are the causes of leg length discrepancy?
2. What problems are associated with leg length discrepancy?
3. How do you assess length discrepancy of the lower limbs?
4. What are the differences between true, apparent and functional leg length discrepancy?
5. What are the treatment options for leg length discrepancy in both adults and children?
6. What are the relative percentage contributions to normal growth of all of the lower limb physes?
7. How can you predict the magnitude of leg length discrepancy at skeletal maturity?
8. What are the problems associated with shoe raises?
9. What problems may occur as a consequence of acute shortening procedures?
10. Who was Professor Gavril Abramovich Ilizarov?
11. What problems may occur due to the leg lengthening procedure?
12. What are the prerequisite factors necessary for successful leg lengthening?
13. What are the reasons for leaving a 'latency period' prior to commencing distraction?
14. What are the advantages and disadvantages of lengthening intramedullary nails?
15. Give the causes of lower limb deformity.
16. How do you assess the degree of lower limb deformity?
17. Draw a 'Selenius graph'.
18. What options are available for correcting lower limb deformity in both adults and children?
19. What are the consequences of hinge misplacement when applying an Ilizarov frame for deformity correction?
20. What are the advantages of using a 'Taylor spatial frame' rather than an Ilizarov frame for deformity correction?

16 Paediatric Orthopaedic Surgery

Jonathan Wright, Russell Hawkins, Aresh Hashemi-Nejad and Peter Calder

Epiphysiodesis	443	Slipped upper femoral epiphysis: Osteotomy	462
Developmental dysplasia of the hip: Closed reduction	446	Tendo-Achilles lengthening	464
Developmental dysplasia of the hip: Open reduction	449	Congenital talipes equinovarus correction	469
Developmental dysplasia of the hip: Pelvic osteotomy	452	Surgical treatment of Perthes disease	473
		Principles of surgery in cerebral palsy	476
Developmental dysplasia of the hip: Proximal femoral osteotomy	456	Guided growth: Temporary hemiepiphysiodesis	479
Slipped upper femoral epiphysis: Pinning	459	Viva questions	481

Epiphysiodesis

Preoperative planning

Epiphysiodesis involves destruction of the physis to allow equalisation of leg length discrepancy (LLD) in children. As *most growth occurs around the knee*, the distal femoral and/or the proximal tibial and fibular physes are targeted depending on the predicted remaining growth.

Indications
- Predicted true LLD 2–5 cm at maturity
- May be used to treat LLD greater than 7 cm through lengthening of the short limb and epiphysiodesis of the long limb

Contraindications
- Apparent LLD
- LLD less than 1.5 cm
- Localised infection

- Tumour
- Closed physis

> **Consent and risks**
>
> - *Neurovascular injury*: Less than 1%
> - *Infection*: Less than 1%
> - *Fracture*: Less than 1%
> - *Angular deformity*: Less than 1%
> - *Residual LLD*: 80% patients within 1 cm

Operative planning

Various methods exist to determine the LLD at maturity and to guide the timing and type of epiphysiodesis (distal femoral and/or proximal tibial):

- *Green-Anderson growth remaining method*: Estimates growth potential in the distal femoral and proximal tibial physes at various skeletal ages separately for girls and boys.
- *Moseley straight-line graph*: A logarithmic representation of the Green-Anderson method.
- *Menelaus arithmetic method*: Assumes growth of 10 mm/year from distal femur and 6 mm/year from the proximal tibia and that girls reach maturity at 14 years and boys at 16 years.
- *Eastwood-Cole method*: A graphic representation of the arithmetic method but takes into account non-linear changes in LLD. Bone age is more reliable than chronological age in determining growth remaining and can be calculated using the Greulich and Pyle method. This involves comparison of a left hand and wrist radiograph with a known standard.

Anaesthesia and positioning

General anaesthesia is used, together with intravenous antibiotic prophylaxis. The patient is positioned supine with the knee slightly flexed over a small sandbag. A pneumatic thigh tourniquet is used. An image intensifier is required and a gonadal shield should be appropriately placed.

Surgical technique

Landmarks

The image intensifier is used to mark the orientation of the physis in the frontal plane and the midpoint of the physis in the lateral plane.

Approach

A 1–2 cm longitudinal incision is centred over the midpoint of physis medially and laterally. A larger incision is made laterally to identify and protect the common peroneal nerve if performing proximal fibular epiphysiodesis.

Dissection

Sharp dissection is continued down to bone.

Procedure

Physeal cartilage is removed using a 4.5 mm diameter drill under image guidance: A single entry point is made in the lateral cortex in line with the physis on the frontal view and at its midpoint on the lateral view. This minimises weakening of the cortex and the risk of subsequent fracture. The drill is advanced transversely along the line of the physis in the frontal view until the tip reaches its midpoint (**Figure 16.1**).

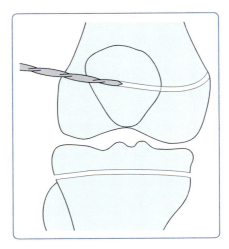

Figure 16.1 The trajectory of the drill should be checked periodically using the image intensifier to ensure obliteration of the physis.

Using the same entry point each time, the drill is tilted 30° first anteriorly then posteriorly and advanced to the halfway mark to remove a fan-shaped area of physeal cartilage (**Figure 16.2**). This technique is then repeated on the medial side. The swarf should be

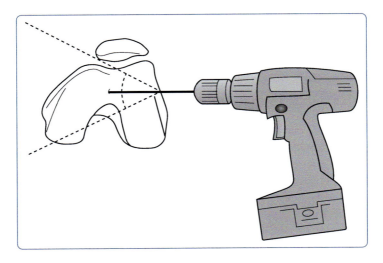

Figure 16.2 The drill is inserted in the mid-sagittal line of the femur then angled anteriorly and posteriorly by 30° using the same entry point.

inspected to ensure removal of physeal cartilage. Further curettage of the epiphyseal surface is performed to remove any remaining physeal cartilage.

Closure
A layered closure is used with absorbable subcuticular material to skin.

Postoperative instructions
- Mobilise full weightbearing with crutches for comfort for up to 2 weeks
- Radiographs at 3 months then periodically until maturity to assess physeal closure and leg lengths

Recommended references
Atar D, Lehman WB, Grant AD et al. Percutaneous epiphysiodesis. *J Bone Joint Surg Br.* 1991;**73**:173.
Eastwood DM, Cole WG. A graphic method for timing the correction of leg-length discrepancy. *J Bone Joint Surg Br.* 1995;**77**:743–747.
Menelaus MB. Correction of leg length discrepancy by epiphyseal arrest. *J Bone Joint Surg Br.* 1966;**48**:336–339.
Snyder M, Harcke HT, Bowen JR et al. Evaluation of physeal behaviour in response to epiphysiodesis with the use of serial magnetic resonance imaging. *J Bone Joint Surg Am.* 1994;**76**:224–229.

Developmental dysplasia of the hip: Closed reduction
Preoperative planning
Although often combined with an arthrogram and soft tissue releases, technically this remains a closed procedure as the capsule is not opened. Adductor and psoas releases are performed via an open medial approach, the technical details of which are provided in the section 'Developmental dysplasia of the hip: Open reduction' (p. 449).

The optimum timing of reduction is subject to debate: Waiting for the capital femoral epiphysis to appear reduces the risk of avascular necrosis although, conversely, early reduction suggests a better long-term outcome.

Indications
- 6- to 18-month-old child with developmental dysplasia of the hip (DDH)
- Failed treatment with Pavlik harness

Contraindications
This is contraindicated in a child less than 6 months or older than 18 months.

Consent and risks
- Application of spica plaster in the human position; subsequent care must be explained to parents
- *Avascular necrosis*: 5%–10%

- *Re-dislocation*: Less than 5%
- *Further surgery*: 20%
- *Neurovascular injury and infection*: Less than 1% (if arthrogram and soft tissue releases performed)
- *Risk of conversion to open reduction*: 10%–20%; greater risk for high-riding dislocation

Operative planning

Imaging studies are requested depending on the expected presence of the ossific nucleus:

- Dynamic ultrasound if less than 6 months of age to determine alpha and beta angles, reducibility and capsular laxity.
- Plain anteroposterior (AP) pelvis and frog lateral radiographs if older than 6 months. Note any delayed appearance of ossific nucleus, Shenton, Hilgenreiner and Perkins lines, acetabular index and Tonnis grade.

Anaesthesia and positioning

General anaesthesia is used. The patient is positioned supine at the end of a radiolucent table, to allow image intensifier access. The surgeon stands between flexed, abducted and externally rotated hips.

Surgical technique

Examination under anaesthesia (EUA) and arthrogram are first performed to assess reduction and the need for adductor longus, gracilis and psoas release.

Landmarks

The landmark is the adductor longus muscle – palpable in the child's groin (**Figure 16.3**).

Procedure

A 22G spinal needle is introduced beneath the palpable adductor longus tendon in the groin and advanced cranially towards the ipsilateral scapular until the tip is felt to traverse the hip capsule. The position is confirmed with image intensifier before instilling 0.5 mL of diluted contrast.

The hip is reduced with a combination of flexion, abduction and anterior displacement without excessive force. Soft tissue releases should be considered if this does not occur easily. If the head appears to stand out from the acetabulum on the arthrogram, this suggests a block to reduction such as an infolded labrum. A conversion to open reduction may therefore be required.

The stability is assessed within the safe zones of flexion and abduction. Typically, a stable position is 90° of flexion and 30°–50° of abduction. Extreme positions increase the risk of avascular necrosis and must be avoided.

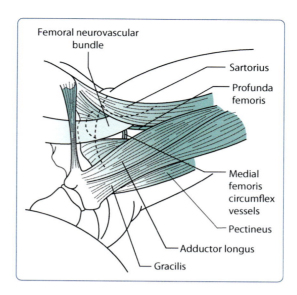

Figure 16.3 Adductor longus and its relationships.

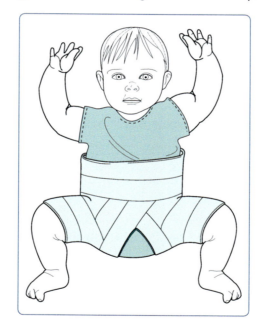

Figure 16.4 Child plastered in the 'human position'.

A well-padded spica plaster is carefully applied in the human position before final radiographic confirmation of reduction (**Figure 16.4**).

Postoperative instructions
- Plaster check prior to discharge
- Limited slice computed tomography (CT) at 2/52 to confirm maintenance of reduction

- Convert to abduction brace at 10/52
- Wean out of brace after further 6/52; depending on acetabular development, night-time bracing may continue for up to 1 year

Recommended references

Kalamchi A, MacEwen GD. Avascular necrosis following treatment of congenital dislocation of the hip. *J Bone Joint Surg Am.* 1980;**62**:87688.

Malvitz TA, Weinstein SL. Closed reduction for congenital dislocation of the hip. Functional and radiographic results after an average of thirty years. *J Bone Joint Surg Am.* 1994;**12**:177792.

Ramsey PL, Lasser S, MacEwen GD. Congenital dislocation of the hip: Use of the Pavlik harness in the child in the first six months of life. *J Bone Joint Surg Am.* 1978;**58**:1000–1004.

Severin E. Contribution to knowledge of congenital dislocation of the hip joint: Late results of closed reduction and arthrographic studies of recent cases. *Acta Chir Scand Suppl.* 1941;**63**:142.

Tennant SJ, Eastwood DM, Calder P, Hashemi-Nejad A, Catterall A. A protocol for the use of closed reduction in children with developmental dysplasia of the hip incorporating open psoas and adductor releases and a short-leg cast: Mid-term outcomes in 113 hips. *Bone Joint J.* 2016;**98–B(11)**:1548–1553.

Developmental dysplasia of the hip: Open reduction

Preoperative planning

Open reduction deals directly with soft tissue obstruction facilitating relocation of the hip without excessive force.

Indications

- Children 6–18 months with obstruction to closed reduction (psoas tendon, contracted capsule, ligamentum teres, transverse acetabular ligament and inverted limbus), an unstable safe zone, previous failed closed or open reduction
- Children presenting over 18 months

Contraindications

The procedure is contraindicated in children less than 6 months old.

Consent and risks

- Application of spica plaster; subsequent care must be explained to parents
- *Neurovascular injury*: Less than 1%
- *Infection*: Less than 1%
- *Avascular necrosis*: 5%
- *Re-dislocation*: 1%
- *Further surgery for dysplasia or LLD*: 10%–15%

Operative planning
Planning should include radiographs as per closed reduction.

Anaesthesia and positioning
General anaesthesia with intravenous antibiotics is used. The patient is positioned supine at the end of a radiolucent table. The surgeon stands between the patient's legs for a medial approach or on the operative side for an anterior approach. An image intensifier is required.

Surgical technique
A medial approach is used if the patient is less than 12 months old; an anterior approach, via a bikini incision, is preferred if the child is older.

Medial approach
Landmarks
The adductor longus tendon is a landmark – palpable in the groin, approximately 2 cm lateral to the labia/scrotum.

Incision
A 2.5 cm, vertical skin crease incision is centred on the palpable tendon of adductor longus.

Superficial dissection

> **Structures at risk**
> - Anterior and posterior divisions of obturator nerve

The fascia overlying the tendons of adductor longus and gracilis is opened along their length and fractional lengthening tenotomies are performed. Adductor magnus and brevis are exposed with blunt dissection. Branches of the obturator nerve are identified on the superficial surface of the adductor brevis and are protected.

Deep dissection

> **Structure at risk**
> - Medial circumflex femoral artery

The plane between the adductor magnus and brevis is dissected to access the lesser trochanter. A psoas tenotomy is performed under direct vision avoiding the medial femoral circumflex vessels which pass over the medial surface of the psoas tendon distally.

A medial arthrotomy is made above the vessels, and the acetabular attachment of the ligamentum teres is divided and used as a traction aid to relocate the femoral head. It is then sutured to the anterior inferior capsule.

Anterior approach

Landmarks
- Anterior superior iliac spine (ASIS)
- Pubic tubercle

Incision
The line of the inguinal ligament is marked between the ASIS and the pubic tubercle. A second line is then dropped vertically downwards from the ASIS. Next, a 5 cm bikini line incision is marked 2 cm inferior and parallel to the inguinal ligament, one-third of it medial and two-thirds lateral to the vertical line.

Superficial dissection

> **Structure at risk**
> - Lateral cutaneous nerve of the thigh

The interval between sartorius and tensor fascia lata is developed to reach the rectus femoris and gluteus medius.

Deep dissection
The interval between the rectus femoris and gluteus medius is dissected and the straight head of the rectus femoris is detached from the anterior capsule. It may then be retracted medially to allow psoas tenotomy and L-shaped anterior arthrotomy (see **Figure 16.5**).

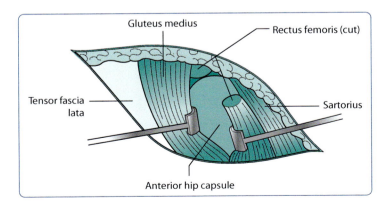

Figure 16.5 Anterior approach to the right hip.

Procedure

Obstructions to reduction are removed as necessary; pulvinar is extracted, the transverse ligament is released and the ligamentum teres excised if obstructive. Adductor releases are performed, via a separate groin incision, to facilitate reduction as required.

The redundant capsule is tightened with capsulorrhaphy following reduction. Using the image intensifier, the position of maximum stability is identified; the hip is placed in 30° of internal rotation, flexion and abduction and then each of these positions is removed in sequence to determine positioning in plaster and the need for future surgery.

Femoral osteotomy or an acetabular procedure may be undertaken concomitantly if severe dysplasia is present in an older child.

Closure

- Layered closure ensuring reconstruction of rectus femoris.
- Skin is closed with absorbable subcuticular material followed by a waterproof dressing.

A well-padded spica plaster is carefully applied in the stable safe zone of flexion and abduction before final radiographic confirmation of reduction. This should be in greater than 90° of flexion without forced flexion and abducted between 30° and 60°.

Postoperative instructions

- Plaster check prior to discharge
- Limited slice CT at 2 weeks to confirm maintenance of reduction
- Spica removal at 10 weeks and mobilisation allowed
- Follow-up at 3 months with radiographs

Recommended references

Ferguson AB Jr. Primary open reduction of congenital dislocation of the hip using a median adductor approach. *J Bone Joint Surg Am.* 1973;**55**:671–681.

Morcuende JA, Meyer MD, Dolan LA et al. Long term outcome after open reduction through an anteromedial approach for congenital dislocation of the hip. *J Bone Joint Surg Am.* 1997;**79**:810–817.

Wright J, Tudor F, Luff T, Hashemi-Nejad A. Surveillance after treatment of children with developmental dysplasia of the hip: Current UK practice and the proposed Stanmore protocol. *J Pediatr Orthop B.* 2013 Nov;**22(6)**:509–515.

Zadeh HG, Catterall A, Hashemi-Nejad A et al. Test of stability as an aid to decide the need for osteotomy in association with open reduction in developmental dysplasia of the hip. A long term review. *J Bone Joint Surg Br* 2000;**82**:17–27.

Developmental dysplasia of the hip: Pelvic osteotomy

Various techniques exist for pelvic osteotomy in DDH, and an account of them all is beyond the scope of this chapter. Therefore, only the Salter and Pemberton types are described further.

Salter osteotomy
Preoperative planning
Indications

- Acetabular dysplasia; acetabulum faces anterolaterally causing deficient anterior coverage in extension and deficient superior coverage in adduction

- Congruent hip
- 18 months to 6 years (as it requires flexibility of symphysis pubis)

Contraindications

- Bilateral DDH (uncovers contralateral hip)
- Congruent reduction not achievable on EUA arthrogram

Consent and risks

- *Overall risks*: Less than 5%
- *Neurovascular injury*: 1%
- Limited weightbearing/crutches
- *Infection*: Less than 1%
- *LLD*: Gains 1 cm with Salter osteotomy
- Triradiate cartilage growth arrest (Pemberton osteotomy)
- Failure of graft
- Hardware breakage
- Residual dysplasia (retroversion)
- *Secondary degeneration*: Lateralisation of joint increases joint reaction force (Salter)
- Further surgery (removal of hardware, salvage procedures)

Operative planning

Congruency confirmed with EUA arthrogram.

Anaesthesia and positioning

General anaesthesia is used, together with intravenous antibiotics. The patient is positioned supine with an ipsilateral sandbag in a position suitable for image intensifier access.

Surgical technique

Anterosuperior coverage is achieved at the expense of posterior coverage by flexing the acetabular fragment. Typically, the lateral centre edge angle will increase by 10°. It is performed via an anterior approach (see 'Developmental dysplasia of the hip: Open reduction', p. 449) extending the bikini incision proximally over the iliac crest to allow splitting of the iliac apophysis and subperiosteal exposure of the ilium to reach the sciatic notch.

Procedure

Structures at risk

- *Sciatic nerve*: Rang retractors are placed in the sciatic notch keeping them closely applied to bone to protect the nerve
- Devascularization/denervation of abductors

An osteotomy is performed between the sciatic notch and midway between the ASIS and anterior inferior iliac spine (AIIS) using a Gigli saw. This should appear to be parallel to the acetabular surface on AP images. Hinging on the symphysis pubis, the acetabulum is rotated anteriorly and laterally to gain coverage while avoiding retroversion.

A wedge of bone from the iliac wing is inserted perpendicular to the weightbearing axis. The 'winking sign' should be noted on an image intensifier (foreshortening of ipsilateral obturator foramen) and the position held with two threaded Schantz pins across the osteotomy. Image guidance is used to advance the pins proximodistally beginning just proximal to the ASIS and aiming for the triradiate cartilage (**Figures 16.6** and **16.7**).

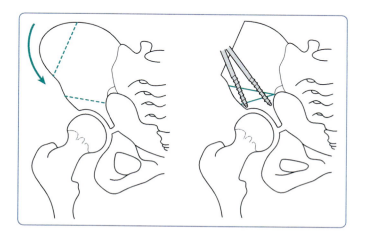

Figure 16.6 Salter osteotomy.

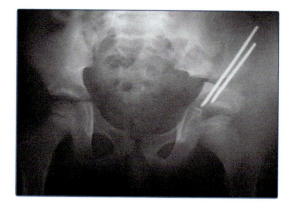

Figure 16.7 Radiograph showing left Salter osteotomy and 'winking sign'.

Closure

- Layered closure ensuring repair of the iliac apophysis
- Absorbable subcuticular material to skin

Postoperative instructions

Plaster spica for those under 6 years of age. Limited weightbearing with crutches for 6–8 weeks if over 6 years of age.

Pemberton osteotomy
Preoperative planning
Indications
- Double diameter dysplastic acetabulum
- Congruent hip
- Open triradiate cartilage
- Close to normal range of motion
- No degeneration
- Normal proximal femoral morphology
- Paralytic hip disorders/Ehlers-Danlos syndrome (posterior coverage is maintained, conferring stability)

Contraindications
- Poor range of motion (flexion, abduction and internal rotation will be further diminished)
- Closed triradiate cartilage
- Congruent reduction not achievable
- Centre of rotation of head and acetabulum coincide

For consent and risks/preoperative preparation/anaesthesia and positioning, see 'Salter osteotomy' (p. 452).

Surgical technique

The Pemberton osteotomy reduces the volume of a large-diameter acetabulum making the centre of rotation of both femoral head and socket coincident. The acetabulum is displaced forwards and laterally hinging on the triradiate cartilage (**Figure 16.8**). The autograft is stable and fixation is therefore not required. The approach and exposure are performed as per the Salter osteotomy.

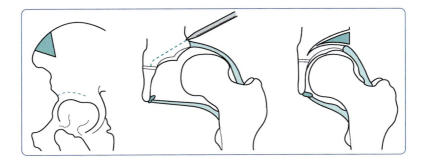

Figure 16.8 Pemberton osteotomy.

Procedure

The osteotomy is made 10–15 mm superior to the AIIS passing a curved osteotome posteriorly to reach the ilioischial and iliopubic limb of the triradiate cartilage (midway between sciatic notch and posterior acetabular rim). The acetabulum is hinged on the triradiate to improve coverage. Corticocancellous graft is harvested from the iliac wing and inserted into the osteotomy site. Posterior stability negates the need for internal fixation.

Closure

This is the same as per Salter osteotomy.

Postoperative instructions

Instructions are the same as per Salter osteotomy.

Recommended references

Colemann SS. The incomplete pericapsular (Pemberton) and innominate (Salter) osteotomies. *Clin Orthop.* 1974;**98**:116–123.

Pemberton PA. Pericapsular osteotomy of the ilium for treatment of congenital subluxation and dislocation of the hip. *J Bone Joint Surg Am.* 1965;**47**:65–86.

Salter RB. Innominate osteotomy in the treatment of congenital dislocation and subluxation of the hip. *J Bone Joint Surg Br.* 1961;**43**:518–539.

Thomas SR, Wedge JH, Salter RB. Outcome at forty five years after open reduction and innominate osteotomy for late presenting developmental dysplasia of the hip. *J Bone Joint Surg Am.* 2007;**89**:2341–2350.

Developmental dysplasia of the hip: Proximal femoral osteotomy

The varus derotation osteotomy (VDRO) is the most common type performed for DDH.

Preoperative planning

Indications

- Persistent dysplasia following DDH (coxa valga, anteversion)
- Congruent reduction in abduction and internal rotation
- Reasonable sphericity (lateral portion of head intact)

Contraindications

- Limited range of motion (abduction and internal rotation)
- Active infection
- Pelvic procedure more appropriate (centre-edge angle [CEA] <15°)
- Previous avascular necrosis is a relative contraindication with less predictable results
- Be aware that VDRO will compound an existing negative LLD

Consent and risks

- Plaster spica if under 6 years
- Limited weightbearing with crutches if over 6 years
- Bleeding
- Neurovascular damage: 1%
- *Infection*: Less than 1%
- *Delayed/non-union*: 1%–5% (greater risk with increasing age)
- *Failure of hardware*: Less than 1%
- Incomplete correction
- *LLD*: Inevitable with closing wedge varus osteotomy
- Joint degeneration
- Further surgery (removal of hardware, complex arthroplasty)

Operative planning

An EUA and arthrogram is performed to confirm adequate range of motion and concentric reduction; greater than 15° abduction is required for a varus femoral osteotomy. The type of fixation device and degree of fixed angle are decided (e.g. blade plate/Coventry pin and plate; 90° or 130° angle).

Anaesthesia and positioning

- General anaesthesia
- Supine with ipsilateral buttock sandbag
- Intravenous antibiotic prophylaxis
- Image intensifier

Surgical technique

A lateral approach to the subtrochanteric region of the proximal femur is used to avoid compromise to the vascular supply to the femoral head.

Landmarks

The predicted trajectory of the chosen device along the femoral neck is planned and marked using the image intensifier.

Incision

A 10 cm longitudinal wound is used, running along the lateral aspect of the proximal femur from the metaphyseal flare of the greater trochanter to the proximal femoral diaphysis.

Superficial dissection

The longitudinal incision is continued through superficial fat and the fascia lata, in line with the skin incision.

Deep dissection

> ### Structures at risk
>
> - Perforating branches of profunda femoris artery: These should be identified and cauterised where necessary.

The posterior insertion of vastus lateralis is detached from the posterior intermuscular septum and reflected anteriorly to expose the lateral surface of proximal femur. The periosteum is incised longitudinally and elevated at the site of the predicted osteotomy.

Procedure

Beginning from the lateral cortex just inferior to the flare of the greater trochanter, a guide wire is passed up the femoral neck, under image control, without breaching the physis. The trajectory should aim to restore a normal neck-shaft angle of 130°.

The wire is measured and over-drilled before insertion of the cannulated lag screw. Under image guidance, the proximal osteotomy is made perpendicular to the shaft in the subtrochanteric region using an oscillating saw.

The second osteotomy is made beginning at the same entry point on the lateral cortex with the saw tilted inferiorly creating a medially based wedge with a lateral apex. The medial cortex is then completed using an osteotome. A guide wire is inserted transversely into the anterolateral cortex distal to the future position of the plate.

The leg is adducted to close the varus osteotomy, and the guide wire is used as a joystick to externally rotate the distal shaft into a satisfactory position on fluoroscopy (**Figure 16.9**). Congruent alignment of the lateral cortices should be checked to ensure seating of the plate. The plate is applied over the lag screw, and the distal shaft is reduced onto the plate and held with a Hey-Groves clamp while maintaining correct orientation. Four bicortical screws are inserted to fix the plate before removal of the guide wire. The degree of correction and position of hardware are confirmed with imaging.

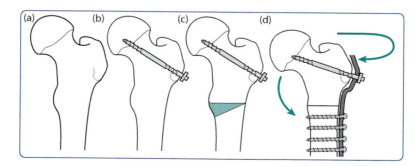

Figure 16.9 Stages in varus derotation osteotomy. (a) Valgus, anteverted proximal femur. (b) Screw placed under image guidance. (c) Medially based closing wedge osteotomy performed from lateral side. (d) Varus producing osteotomy closed and held with plate following derotation.

Closure
- Layered absorbable closure of vastus lateralis then fascia lata
- Subcuticular absorbable material to skin

Postoperative instructions
- Mobilise partial weightbearing
- Increase weightbearing status at 6–8 weeks after union confirmed clinically and radiographically

Recommended references
Blockey NJ. Derotation osteotomy in the management of congenital dislocation of the hip. *J Bone Joint Surg Br.* 1984;**66**:485–490.

Kasser JR, Bowen JR, MacEwen GD. Varus derotation osteotomy in the treatment of persistent dysplasia in congenital dysplasia of the hip. *J Bone Joint Surg Br.* 1985;**67**:195–202.

Williamson DM, Benson MKD. Late femoral osteotomy in congenital dislocation of the hip. *J Bone Joint Surg Br.* 1988;**70**:614–618.

Slipped upper femoral epiphysis: Pinning

Manoeuvres to reduce the epiphysis are associated with a high incidence of avascular necrosis (40%); pinning *in situ* therefore aims to prevent further displacement, promote physeal closure and minimise future secondary degeneration.

Slips are described as stable if weightbearing is possible or unstable if weightbearing is not possible even with crutches.

Preoperative planning

Indications
- Grades I–II slip (Southwick angle <60°)
- Bilateral pinning is performed if there is
  - Evidence of bilateral slip
  - Endocrinopathy
  - Younger end of age spectrum (10 years – girls, 12 years – boys)

Contraindications
- Advanced avascular necrosis
- Active infection

Consent and risks
- Limited weightbearing/crutches
- Avascular necrosis: 0%–5% but higher if unstable slip
- *Chondrolysis*: 10% (greater risk for African Caribbeans, females and poor technique)
- *Fracture*: Less than 1%
- *Infection*: Less than 1%

- Failure of hardware
- Further slip (associated with inadequate screw advancement)
- *LLD*: 1.5 cm difference on average
- Joint degeneration
- Further surgery (removal of hardware/osteotomy/arthrodesis/complex arthroplasty)

Operative planning

- An AP and Billings lateral of both hips – it is bilateral in 25% of cases (**Figures 16.10** and **16.11**)
- Endocrine workup if at younger end of age spectrum

Anaesthesia and positioning

- General anaesthesia is used.
- Patient is positioned supine on a radiolucent table; care is taken when transferring, preparing and draping the unstable hip to prevent further displacement.
- Intravenous antibiotic prophylaxis is given.
- Image intensifier.

Surgical technique

An aspiration of the hip is first performed under image guidance for pain relief and to decompress the retinacular vessels.

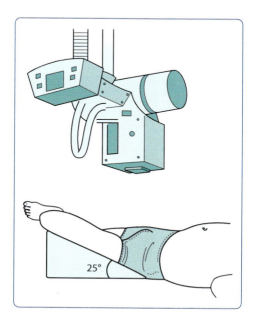

Figure 16.10 Patient positioning for Billings lateral radiograph. The hip is abducted, externally rotated and elevated 25° on a foam wedge.

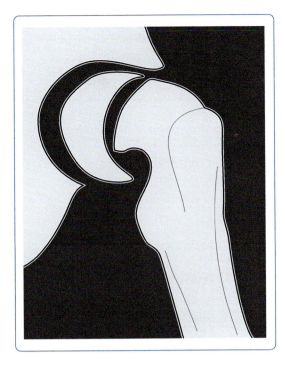

Figure 16.11 Billings lateral radiograph showing slip.

Landmarks
The image intensifier is used to delineate the joint and proximal femur.

Incision
As pinning is performed percutaneously, the planned trajectory of the screw is marked in two planes using the image intensifier bearing in mind the course of important neurovascular structures. The entry point of the screw should not be distal to the lesser trochanter as this creates stress risers and increases the incidence of fracture. Preoperative marking also limits the number of guide wire passes necessary to achieve a satisfactory screw position, further decreasing the chance of guide wire misplacement and minimising the risk of fracture. Because the epiphysis is relatively posterior and inferior to the neck, a more anterior entry point is required. Optimal screw position should avoid the posterior neck and posterior superior epiphysis to preserve the blood supply to the femoral head and minimise the risk of avascular necrosis.

Dissection
Tissues are dissected bluntly down to bone.

Procedure
A guide wire is passed under image intensifier control to avoid malposition and joint penetration. After measuring and over-drilling the wire, a partially threaded 6.5–7.5 mm

diameter cannulated screw is inserted. A reverse cutting thread is used for easier subsequent removal. Despite an increase in shear strength across the physis using multiple screws, the use of a single screw diminishes the risk of chondrolysis and avoids the disproportionate complication rate of multiple screws.

The passage of guide wire, drill and screw should be performed under image guidance to avoid joint penetration. The screw tip should reach the centre of the epiphysis, 5 mm from the articular surface with a minimum of three to four threads crossing the physis to provide adequate fixation. At completion, live screening of the hip is performed to ensure solid fixation of the epiphysis and confirm screw position.

Closure
Subcuticular absorbable material is used to close the stab incision.

Postoperative instructions
Range-of-motion exercises are begun on the first postoperative day. Mobilisation is then:

- Fully weightbearing with crutches for 2–3 weeks if slip is stable
- Partial weightbearing until healed if unstable

Assessment is carried out at 6–8 weeks for clinical and radiological evidence of union and to ensure that there has not been any further slip. Sporting activities are prohibited until physeal closure occurs. Following physeal closure, screw removal is recommended.

Recommended references
Givon U, Bowen JR. Chronic slipped femoral epiphysis: Treatment by pinning *in situ*. *J Pediatr Orthop B*. 1999;**8**:216–222.
Loder RT, Aronson DD, Dobbs MB et al. Slipped capital femoral epiphysis. *Instr Course Lect*. 2001;**50**:555–570.
Loder RT, Richards BS, Shapiro PS et al. Acute slipped capital femoral epiphysis. The importance of physeal stability. *J Bone Joint Surg Am*. 1993;**75**:1134–1140.
Phillips SA, Griffiths WEG, Clarke NMP. The timing and reduction of the acute unstable slipped upper femoral epiphysis. *J Bone Joint Surg Br*. 2001;**83**:1046–1049.

Slipped upper femoral epiphysis: Osteotomy
An open reduction with osteotomy serves to restore the head-neck angle with subsequent improvement in hip biomechanics. This aims to provide good future function, minimise or delay the onset of painful secondary degeneration, and normalise proximal femoral anatomy for future hip replacement. Osteotomy can be performed at various levels (intracapsular and extracapsular neck, intertrochanteric and subtrochanteric) with greater correction achievable at the site of deformity (more proximally). Although these proximal osteotomies have been associated with a greater risk of avascular necrosis, a Dunn or Fish cuneiform osteotomy performed with meticulous technique, as described later, can achieve excellent results.

Preoperative planning
Indications
- Slip greater than 60°
- Chronic/acute on chronic or unstable slip
- Open physis

Contraindications
Closed physis is a contraindication (Southwick intertrochanteric osteotomy may be more appropriate).

Consent and risks
- *Avascular necrosis*: 10%–48%
- *Chondrolysis*: 10%–12%
- *Infection*: Less than 1%
- Slip progression
- *LLD*: 1-2 cm shortening
- Further surgery (removal of hardware/complex arthroplasty)

Preoperative preparation
Preoperative AP and lateral radiographs are used to confirm the degree of slip and plan orientation of the osteotomy. Slings and springs are used preoperatively for 3 weeks if acute or acute on chronic.

Anaesthesia and positioning
- General anaesthesia
- Intravenous antibiotic prophylaxis
- Supine on radiolucent table
- Image intensifier

Surgical technique
Landmarks and approach
The osteotomy is performed via an anterior approach (see 'Developmental dysplasia of the hip: Open reduction', p. 449). Particular care must be taken not to disturb the posterior capsule or forcefully manipulate the slip to preserve vascularity to the femoral head.

Procedure
Following longitudinal capsulotomy, the epiphysis must be correctly identified as the anteriorly displaced neck may be mistaken for it. Two osteotomies are required:

- First, an osteotomy is performed perpendicular to the neck at the level of the physis taking more anteriorly to create a wedge. The aim is to leave a convex surface for later

reduction and shorten the neck by 3–4 mm. Over-shortening will lead to instability. Care must also be taken to avoid driving instruments into the posterior capsule, compromising the blood supply.
- Second, an osteotomy is made in the long axis of the neck to remove the bony beak on the side of the slip, again taking care not to breach the posterior capsule. Any remaining callus is carefully removed with a spoon from the posterior capsule.

Shortening the neck, removing the beak and elevating the posterior capsule allows tension-free reduction of the epiphysis. The epiphysis is reduced onto the neck by placing the leg in flexion, abduction and internal rotation. If insufficient bone has been removed, the epiphysis will not reduce easily, and posterior structures will be placed under tension increasing the risk of avascular necrosis. Shortening and wedging of the neck should cause the epiphysis to overlap the neck anteriorly giving a mushroom appearance. Restoration of the Shenton line and a valgus head-neck angle of 20° should be ensured using the image intensifier.

While an assistant maintains position, a lateral stab incision is made according to the predicted trajectory of cannulated screw followed by blunt dissection down to the lateral cortex of the proximal femur. A guide wire is then advanced across the osteotomy to hold the epiphysis. Images are checked in two planes to confirm a satisfactory position before definitive screw insertion. Similar to pinning *in situ*, the entry point should not be below the lesser trochanter, and screw tips should be 5 mm short of the articular surface.

Dynamic screening allows confirmation of both a solid fixation and satisfactory positioning of hardware.

Closure
- Layered closure including capsular repair with absorbable material
- Subcuticular absorbable material to skin

Postoperative instructions
- Bed rest with slings and springs for 5 days
- Mobilise 15 kg weightbearing 8 weeks; increase weightbearing status at 8 weeks, after confirming union clinically and radiographically

Recommended references
Dunn DM, Angel JC. Replacement of the femoral head by open operation in severe adolescent slipping of the upper femoral epiphysis. *J Bone Joint Surg Br.* 1978;**60**:394–403.
Fish JB. Cuneiform osteotomy of the femoral neck in the treatment of slipped capital femoral epiphysis. *J Bone Joint Surg Am.* 1984;**66**:1153–1168.
Loder RT. Unstable slipped capital femoral epiphysis. *J Pediatr Orthop.* 2001;**21**:694–699.
Vanhegan IS, Cashman JP, Buddhdev P, Hashemi-Nejad A. Outcomes following subcapital osteotomy for severe slipped upper femoral epiphysis. *Bone Joint J.* 2015;**97-B(12)**:1718–1725.

Tendo-Achilles lengthening
Preoperative planning
Various methods for tendo-Achilles lengthening (TAL) exist and may be used in conjunction with other procedures. Percutaneous methods such as the Hoke and DAMP (distal anterior, medial proximal; also called a White slide) technique and open methods such as the Baker

and Vulpius techniques are described (**Figures 16.12 through 16.14**). The choice depends on the cause, the individual patient and the surgeon's preference.

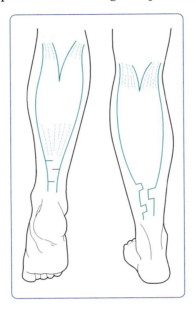

Figure 16.12 Hoke percutaneous tenotomy.

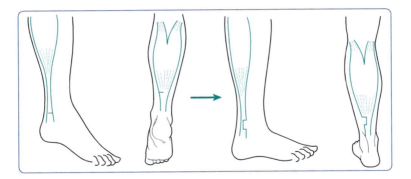

Figure 16.13 Distal anterior, medial proximal (DAMP) procedure.

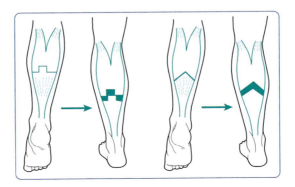

Figure 16.14 Two techniques of gastrocnemius recession: (a) Baker slide and (b) Vulpius technique.

Indications
- Fixed equinus deformity is defined as an inability to dorsiflex the ankle sufficiently to allow heel contact without compensation in the remainder of the limb or spine. Often, this correlates with dorsiflexion less than 5° and is seen in various conditions such as cerebral palsy, congenital talipes equinovarus (CTEV), congenital vertical talus, Charcot-Marie-Tooth (CMT), pes planus and intractable toe walkers.
- Failure of conservative treatment.
- To achieve stump coverage during Chopart's amputation for congenital malformation of the foot.

Contraindications
- Rigid bony deformity.
- Pseudoequinus: A false clinical appearance of equinus caused by plantarflexion of the mid- and forefoot (plantaris deformity).
- Medical co-morbidity is not a contraindication as percutaneous techniques can be performed under local anaesthesia.

Consent and risks
- The most predictable outcome following TAL is in patients with spastic hemiplegia. The least predictable scenario is seen with percutaneous procedures in patients with diplegia. The two most frequently encountered problems are over-lengthening and recurrence. The former tends to occur following percutaneous procedures on the conjoined tendon, whereas recurrence is associated with recession of the gastrocnemius or soleus aponeurosis.
- *Neurovascular damage*: The sural nerve in particular is at risk.
- *Percutaneous techniques*: 1%.
- *Open techniques*: 5%.
- Plaster immobilisation/limited mobility.
- Complete tendon rupture (percutaneous).
- Wound problems/infection (open): 1%.
- *Recurrence* (*Baker and Vulpius*): Less than 5%.
- *Over-lengthening leading to crouched gait*: More likely following percutaneous procedures and associated with uncontrolled lengthening in an older child.
- *Repeat lengthening*: More likely in a younger child and patients with hemiplegia.
- *Further surgery* (hamstring, psoas or selective gastrocnemius lengthening most often required in patients with diplegia).

Preoperative assessment
Silverskiold test under anaesthetic differentiates between pure gastrocnemius tightness (increased ankle dorsiflexion with knee flexion) and combined tightness of gastrocnemius and soleus (limited dorsiflexion in knee flexion and extension).

Anaesthesia and positioning
- General anaesthesia or local anaesthesia for percutaneous techniques
- Prone for open or supine for percutaneous techniques
- High pneumatic thigh tourniquet

Surgical technique
Percutaneous techniques
Both Hoke and DAMP procedures are used to treat combined gastrocnemius-soleus tightness. The advantages are improved healing and the option of local anaesthesia. However, these techniques are associated with an increased incidence of over-lengthening and inadvertent complete tenotomy.

Hoke technique

Structures at risk
- Tibial nerve – at risk proximally
- Sural nerve – laterally
- Flexor hallucis longus muscle – distally

Three points are marked on the tendo-Achilles at 1 cm, 3 cm and 6 cm from its calcaneal insertion. A number 15 blade scalpel is inserted longitudinally in the midline of the tendon at each marked level and then turned through 90° in the desired direction to perform the hemisection while the ankle is dorsiflexed to control the correction. The hemisections are performed on the medial half proximally and distally and the lateral half in the middle incision (see **Figure 16.12**).

DAMP technique
Two 1.5 cm skin incisions are made postero-medially, one 2 cm from the calcaneal insertion and another 5 cm proximal to it. The anterior two-thirds of the tendon is divided distally and the medial half to two-thirds proximally. (This is because of the 90° rotation of tendon fibres in the distal third of the leg.)

The tendon is divided progressively while tensioning the tendo-Achilles until it yields 5°–10° of dorsiflexion. The medial fibres slide over the lateral fibres, giving length in continuity with a thinned portion of tendon distally and a square cut proximally (see **Figure 16.13**).

Open techniques
These have the advantage of controlled lengthening but carry a greater risk of recurrence.

Incision

Structures at risk
- Sural nerve
- Short saphenous vein

A 7 cm longitudinal incision is made, 10 cm proximal to the calcaneal insertion positioned 1 cm medial to the midline to avoid the sural nerve.

Dissection

The sural nerve and short saphenous vein are retracted if encountered or may be avoided altogether by raising a full-thickness lateral flap. The paratenon is incised longitudinally in the midline to avoid the skin incision, and the medial and lateral edges of the gastrocnemius aponeurosis are exposed.

Baker slide procedure

Although considered a selective gastrocnemius lengthening, fibres of the soleus aponeurosis are also incised distally. However, this does not lead to over-lengthening as seen in procedures on the conjoined tendon owing to controlled lengthening and inherent stability.

The medial and lateral thirds of the aponeurosis are incised transversely 12 cm above the calcaneal insertion. A similar incision is then performed across the middle third at least 3 cm proximally to allow side-to-side contact after lengthening. A tongue and groove pattern is created by joining the proximal and distal cuts with two longitudinal incisions (see **Figure 16.14**). Dorsiflexion of the ankle allows slide-lengthening of the aponeurosis and reveals any remaining fibres that require incision.

The underlying muscle fibres of soleus are revealed as the aponeurosis is lengthened. Further lengthening should not be performed once 10° of dorsiflexion is achieved on the table, and 3/0 absorbable sutures are placed across the longitudinal portions of the aponeurosis.

Vulpius procedure

This is used to treat combined gastrocnemius-soleus tightness when plaster immobilisation is not desirable. Instead of a tongue and groove lengthening, an inverted 'V' incision is made in the aponeurosis of both the gastrocnemius and the soleus (see **Figure 16.14**).

Closure

- Tension-free layered closure with buried knots to avoid skin irritation
- Subcuticular absorbable material to skin

With the exception of the Vulpius technique, a below-knee plaster is applied in a plantigrade position. A dorsiflexed position must be avoided to prevent a calcaneus deformity.

Postoperative instructions

Mobilise weightbearing as tolerated in cast for 4 weeks if used. Convert to night-time splint at 4 weeks and continue for 6 months. Use guided physiotherapy to maintain position and prevent recurrence.

Recommended references

Baker LD. Surgical needs of the cerebral palsy patient. *J Bone Joint Surg Am.* 1956;**38**:313–323.

Borton DC, Walker K, Pirpiris M et al. Isolated calf lengthening in cerebral palsy. *J Bone Joint Surg Br.* 2001;**83**:364–370.

Graham HK, Fixsen JA. Lengthening of the calcaneal tendon in spastic hemiplegia by the white slide technique. *J Bone Joint Surg Br.* 1988;**70**:472–475.

Congenital talipes equinovarus correction

Ponseti technique

Preoperative planning

Indications

Flexible CTEV

Contraindications

- Rigid clubfoot
- Age over 7 years is a relative contraindication as results are notably worse

Consent and risks

- Neurovascular injury (any open procedure)
- Complete Achilles tenotomy
- Plaster impingement/skin ulceration
- Infection (open procedures)
- Stiffness
- Recurrent deformity: Long-term splintage required
- Deformity due to incorrect or incomplete correction, overcorrection or recurrence, e.g. cavus, rocker-bottom, longitudinal breach, flattening and lateral rotation of talus
- 1 cm limb shortening, 2 cm decreased calf girth and smaller shoe by one or half sizes are common sequelae

Do not expect a completely normal foot; although the Ponseti technique yields good clinical results, foot malformations still exist and can be seen radiographically.

Operative planning

The deformity can be graded using various methods. Dimeglio suggests a 20-point scoring system with four grades of severity which correlates with an increasing resistance to correction. The Pirani score helps to predict the need for Achilles tenotomy and is based upon the severity of deformity in the midfoot and hindfoot with a total maximum score of 6. Eighty-five per cent of patients with scores over 5 will require tenotomy.

Anaesthesia and positioning

No anaesthesia or sedation required unless the patient is extremely uncooperative. An assistant is essential.

Surgical technique

Casting is performed weekly, correcting all three components of the deformity in a predetermined sequence prior to additional operative procedures. At least three toe-to-groin casts are required over a period of 7–10 weeks depending on the severity of deformity.

Castings

- *Cavus*: Caused by a relative pronation of the forefoot due to a plantarflexed first ray. The first ray is elevated with pressure beneath the first metatarsal head to supinate the forefoot and align it with the varus hindfoot. Forced pronation of the foot is avoided as this will worsen the cavus.
- *Varus and adductus*: Correction of the abnormally internally rotated calcaneus is achieved by external rotation using the lateral talar head as the fulcrum. The cuboid and anterior calcaneus are displaced laterally by applying medial pressure to the navicular anterior to the ankle and pushing the posterior calcaneus medially by lateral pressure posterior to the ankle, ensuring the talar head does not externally rotate. In severe cases, the navicular may not fully reduce although abduction of the cuneiforms more distally will allow correction and the navicular-cuneiform joints will remodel. Once the calcaneocuboid alignment is restored with the anterior calcaneus lateralised, correction of varus can be achieved. The cast must be toe to groin with the knee in 90° of flexion to maintain abduction and external rotation. This will also treat any associated internal tibial torsion if present. Midfoot pronation must again be avoided to prevent cavus deformity and a midfoot breach.
- *Equinus*: With the hindfoot varus corrected, serial casts are applied in a progressively dorsiflexed position. This usually requires two to three casts to achieve 15° of dorsiflexion and 60° of external rotation. Dorsiflexion is achieved via pressure beneath the midfoot rather than the metatarsals to avoid rocker-bottom feet.

Additional procedures

Tendo-Achilles lengthening: If dorsiflexion of 15° is not achieved, then a percutaneous tenotomy under local anaesthesia is indicated. This is preferable to posterior ankle and subtalar capsulotomy as contraction of scar tissue in this region will lead to progressive loss of dorsiflexion.

Lateral transfer of the tibialis anterior tendon to the lateral cuneiform may be required for persistent supination.

Postoperative care and instructions

The final cast is left *in situ* for 3 weeks and then assessment made for residual equinus; 90% of patients will require Achilles tenotomy.

Denis Browne boots are worn full time for 2–3 months then at night only for 2–4 years or until age 7 years. These maintain 15° of dorsiflexion (to avoid equinus) and 60° external rotation (to prevent varus, adductus and in-toeing). High-top shoes are worn during the day to maintain position.

Periodic evaluation should be performed by an experienced clinician to assess the relationship between the hindfoot and forefoot, the attitude of the heel and range of ankle motion. Anteroposterior and lateral radiographs should also be obtained.

Extensive soft tissue release via the Cincinnati incision

Preoperative planning

Indications
- Failed Ponseti treatment: 50% may relapse at an average age of 2.5 years. Remanipulation and casting with or without Achilles tenotomy followed by splintage may be successful although extensive soft tissue releases are required in resistant cases.
- Rigid clubfoot.
- Walking on lateral border of foot/internally rotated gait.
- Posteriorly placed lateral malleolus (a reflection of uncorrected internal calcaneal rotation).
- Parallelism of talus and calcaneus on AP and lateral radiographs.

Contraindications
Contraindications include previous releases via alternative incisions.

Consent and risks
- Neurovascular damage (see later)
- Plaster immobilisation/impaired mobility/long-term splintage
- Residual deformity
- Recurrence and further surgery
- Wound irritation over the Achilles tendon, particularly rubbing on shoes
- Avascular necrosis of the talus
- Arthritis of the hindfoot and midfoot
- Ankle and subtalar stiffness

Preoperative assessment
- AP and lateral radiographs required for assessing the talocalcaneal angle
- Dimeglio and Pirani scores

Anaesthesia and positioning
General anaesthesia is used with addition of an intravenous prophylactic antibiotic. The patient is positioned prone with a high thigh tourniquet.

Surgical technique

Landmarks
The base of the first metatarsal, medial malleolus and lateral malleolus is palpable.

Incision (the Cincinnati incision)
An 8–9 cm extensile, transverse incision across the posterior ankle (at the level of the tibio-talar joint) is created. This begins at the base of the first metatarsal, curves below the medial malleolus, rises slightly to traverse the Achilles tendon and continues over the lateral malleolus to terminate distal and medial to the sinus tarsi.

Superficial dissection

Structures at risk
- Sural nerve laterally
- Superficial venous structures below the lateral malleolus

The proximal subcutaneous flap is raised off underlying tissues for around 3 cm to allow proximal visualisation.

Deep dissection

Structures at risk
- Posterior tibial nerve and vessels
- Deep tibiotalar portion of the deltoid ligament
- Medial and lateral plantar nerves

This begins laterally with incision of the calcaneofibular ligament and superior peroneal ligament to allow dissection of the peronei off the calcaneus without damaging them. The lateral talocalcaneal ligament and lateral capsule of subtalar joint are then released. The posterior tibial neurovascular bundle is retracted anteriorly to allow further release of the posterior ankle and subtalar capsule and the posterior talofibular ligament. Subsequent posterior retraction of the tibial neurovascular bundle allows division of the superficial tibiocalcaneal part of deltoid. The deep portion of the tibiotalar portion of the deltoid ligament is left intact to prevent excessive subtalar translation and flat foot deformity.

The tibialis posterior tendon sheath is opened along its length from above the medial malleolus to the navicular to allow Z-lengthening of the tendon at least 2.5 cm proximal to the medial malleolus. The nearby posterior tibial neurovascular bundle is protected to avoid its transection.

Dissection continues medially, into the arch of the foot, to release the lacinate ligament, the plantar aponeurosis and small plantar muscles, including abductor hallucis. Beneath the navicular, the master knot of Henry (intersection of the flexor hallucis longus [FHL] and flexor digitorum longus [FDL]) is taken down, taking care not to damage the medial and lateral plantar nerves on either side of it. The sheaths of the FDL and FHL are opened and tendon Z-lengthening performed to prevent flexion contracture of the toes when the ankle is dorsiflexed. This is done sufficiently proximally to allow the lengthened portions to be covered by tendon sheath. Conjoint lengthening is an alternative if the tendons are too small to perform Z-lengthening. This step may be unnecessary as toe contractures will often stretch out over time.

The talonavicular joint is freed to mobilise the navicular laterally and release all of its attachments; keeping hold of it via the distal end of tibialis posterior tendon will avoid handling the articular cartilage. The dorsal talonavicular ligament and the spring ligament can then be released. Release of the bifurcate ligament and the talocalcaneal interosseous ligament will allow external rotation of the anterior calcaneus.

Finally, the quadratus plantae is stripped off the calcaneus to release the long plantar ligament, the plantar calcaneocuboid ligament and inferior medial capsule of the calcaneocuboid joint without damaging the peroneus longus tendon. The extensive soft tissue releases should result in the plane of the foot being at 90° to the bimalleolar axis with the talus beneath the tibia and slight hindfoot valgus. If the mortise is not fully reduced, tibiofibular ligament release then tibiofibular syndesmosis release can be carried out if the talus is too wide anteriorly. Stabilisation with K-wires is the final stage, one passing along the medial column to hold the talonavicular joint and one across the lateral column to hold the calcaneocuboid joint.

Closure

Tendon sheaths over all over-lengthened tendons are closed. The medial and lateral extensions of the Cincinnati incision are closed, without tension, using absorbable sutures to the subcutaneous and subcuticular layers. The posterior, central portion of the wound is left open to heal by secondary intention. If blanching of wound edges following tourniquet release is noted, position in less dorsiflexion.

Apply plaster of Paris from the toes to the mid-thigh with a neutral or slightly plantarflexed foot and the knee flexed to 90°.

Postoperative care and instructions

The cast is changed at 10 days after surgery, to inspect the wound. It is removed, along with the K-wires, at 6 weeks. Denis Browne boots are prescribed for the next 12–18 months.

Physiotherapy (for mobility, to promote tarsal growth and preserve cartilage) is continued for at least 6 months.

Recommended references

Crawford AH, Marxen JL, Osterfield DL. The Cincinnati incision: A comprehensive approach for surgical procedures of the foot and ankle in childhood. *J Bone Joint Surg Am.* 1982;**84**:1355–1358.
Dimeglio A, Benshahel H, Souchet P et al. Classification of clubfoot. *J Pediatr Orthop B.* 1995;**4**:129–136.
McKay DW. New concept of and approach to clubfoot treatment: section II – Correction of the clubfoot. *J Pediatr Orthop.* 1983;**3**:10–21.
Pirani J, Outerbridge HK, Sawatzky B et al. A reliable method of clinically evaluating a virgin clubfoot. *21st World Congress of SICOT*, Sydney, Australia, 18–23 April 1999.
Ponseti I. *Congenital Clubfoot: Fundamentals of Treatment.* New York, NY: Oxford University Press, 1996.

Surgical treatment of Perthes disease

Perthes disease occurs as a result of a temporary cessation in the blood supply to the femoral head leading to avascular necrosis. It is commonly seen between the ages of 4 and 8 years although should be suspected from 2 to 12 years of age. Although more common in boys by a factor of four, it may be more severe in girls.

Presenting symptoms comprise hip or referred knee pain, stiffness, limping and a short leg. The disease progresses through the four phases of ischaemia (causing collapse and sclerosis), fragmentation, reossification and remodelling, which take place over a 4-year period.

However, development of the hip is frequently abnormal leading to incongruency, altered biomechanics and accelerated secondary degeneration. Prognosis is dependent on age and severity of disease at presentation, and treatment falls into the three broad categories of observation, containment and salvage, depending also on the phase of disease.

Preoperative planning

Indications

The type of treatment largely depends upon the capacity to remodel and therefore age. Below the age of 6 years, there is high potential for remodelling, and therapy therefore tends to be conservative. Above 8 years, further remodelling is limited and treatment is more aggressive in order to correct deformity and extend the longevity of the native hip.

Between the ages of 6 and 8 years, the indications for either a conservative approach or containment procedures depend upon bone age and remodelling potential, the presence of 'at-risk' signs for the viability of the femoral head and whether the hip is congruent or containable. The surgical options for containable hips are a varus osteotomy of the proximal femur and/or a Salter-type pelvic osteotomy.

Salvage procedures are indicated if hinge abduction occurs (**Figure 16.15**), where the overgrown and uncontained anterolateral portion of the femoral head abuts the lateral rim of the acetabulum. In this situation valgus extension osteotomy (VGEO) of the proximal femur is indicated, which will medialize the centre of rotation of the hip and make it congruent in the weightbearing position. The medial column must be of sufficient height after reossification and a better outcome is expected in younger patients where the

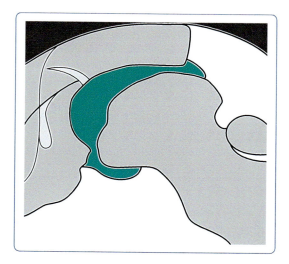

Figure 16.15 Hip arthrogram showing hinge abduction, where dye pools medially in abduction.

triradiate cartilage remains open. This will allow deformity correction, a better functional range of movement, improvement of leg length and abductor function.

Contraindications

Containment procedures are contraindicated if hips are not congruent or containable.

Consent and risks

The natural history of the disease must be explained to the child and parents. It should be emphasised that the aim is to improve symptoms and to achieve a spherical and contained femoral head to maximise and prolong native joint function. However, secondary degenerative changes may continue to occur at an unpredictable and accelerated rate ultimately leading to total joint arthroplasty or arthrodesis.

- An older presentation, particularly in girls, is associated with a worse outcome.
- Stiffness/contractures.
- Other risks pertain to the type of procedure being performed. See the relevant sections on DDH for the risks associated with pelvic and femoral osteotomies.

Operative planning

Various classification systems exist to guide treatment and predict the prognosis of Perthes disease.

Catterall grouped patients as I-IV, although large intra- and inter-observer error has been shown with this method. The Herring classification correlates with prognosis according to the degree of collapse of the lateral capital femoral epiphysis during the fragmentation phase using the AP radiograph of the pelvis.

The Stulberg classification (1-5) is made during the reossification phase and predicts the end result of Perthes disease dependent on the relative shapes of the femoral head and acetabulum. Increasing grade correlates with the likelihood of secondary osteoarthritis with Stulberg 5 hips likely to require total hip replacement before age 50 years.

Head at-risk signs include Gage's sign (a lytic 'rat bite' at the periphery of the physis), calcification lateral to the epiphysis, lateral subluxation of the femoral head and horizontal inclination of the physis.

Arthrography will determine the congruency of the hip in various positions and whether an appropriate range of movement is possible to perform the relevant femoral osteotomy (**Figure 16.15**). Significant abduction is required for a varus osteotomy and adduction for a valgus osteotomy.

Anaesthesia and positioning

- General anaesthesia
- Supine
- Intravenous prophylactic antibiotics

Surgical technique

- For varus osteotomy, the technique as described in the section 'Developmental dysplasia of the hip: Proximal femoral osteotomy' (p. 456) is used, employing the derotation component if required.
- For valgus osteotomy, a similar technique is used as for varus osteotomy, the difference being the orientation of the osteotomy to give a laterally based wedge to achieve the desired realignment.
- Pelvic osteotomy (see 'Salter osteotomy', p. 452).

Postoperative instructions

Instructions are as per the type of procedure performed. Regular periodic clinical and radiographic review is required to determine the presence of deterioration and the need for further surgery.

Recommended references

Bankes MJK, Catterall A, Hashemi-Nejad A. Valgus extension osteotomy for 'hinge abduction' in Perthes disease: Results at maturity and factors influencing the radiological outcome. *J Bone Joint Surg Br.* 2000;**82**:548–554.

Catterall A. The natural history of Perthes disease. *J Bone Joint Surg Br.* 1971;**53**:37–53.

Coates CJ, Paterson JMH, Catterall A et al. Femoral osteotomy in Perthes disease. Results at maturity. *J Bone Joint Surg Br.* 1990;**72**:581–585.

Herring JA, Kim HT, Browne R. Legg-Calvé-Perthes disease. Part I: Classification of radiographs with use of the modified lateral pillar and Stulberg classifications. *J Bone Joint Surg Am.* 2004;**86**:2103–2120.

Herring JA, Kim HT, Browne R. Legg-Calvé-Perthes disease. Part II: Prospective multicentre study of the effect of treatment on outcome. *J Bone Joint Surg Am.* 2004;**86**:2121–2134.

Principles of surgery in cerebral palsy

Preoperative planning

Cerebral palsy results from an insult to the immature brain and its effects are variable. It may be classified anatomically (hemiplegic, diplegic or total body involvement) or physiologically (spastic, athetoid, ataxic or mixed). The spastic form is most common; a combination of muscle weakness and spasticity leads to a progressive sequence of dynamic deformity, fixed contractures, bony deformity and joint subluxation or dislocation. Depending on the severity, intervention may be indicated at any point during this continuum to optimise energy consumption during gait, to perform activities of daily living, to facilitate standing or seated transfer and to maintain hygiene. Maximum function requires a straight spine over a level pelvis, congruent, mobile hips, mobile knees and plantigrade feet.

Cerebral palsy is typically treated in one of three phases:

- Dynamic contractures: Casting and/or botulinum toxin (BTX) injection
- Fixed contractures: Muscle balancing techniques such as releases, lengthening and transfers
- Bony deformity and joint incongruence: Osteotomies

Decisions around timing of surgery are difficult. Allowing maturation will improve certainty about the gait pattern and reduce the risk of recurrent deformity at the price of an increased chance of fixed deformities and multilevel operations being required. Surgery in the younger child may be less technically demanding but can lead to repeat surgery year on year. In addition, single-level operations may reveal further problems: a common example is a crouched gait occurring after Achilles tendon release due to unrecognised, concomitant tight hamstrings. Throughout all stages, physiotherapy helps to reduce fixed deformity and occupational therapy can adapt equipment to accommodate existing deformity.

Surgical techniques in muscle contractures

Botulinum toxin A injections

BTX A inhibits the release of acetylcholine from the nerve terminal at the neuromuscular junction, causing decreased muscle activity in a dose-dependent manner. It may be administered under local or general anaesthesia or sedation. It should be placed deep to the muscle fascia in a dose appropriate for the patient and the number of injection sites required. The injection volume must be sufficient to allow diffusion to endplate zones which may be scattered, particularly in the sartorius and gracilis.

Localise injection sites using palpation and anatomical knowledge; accuracy is improved with electrical stimulation or ultrasound guidance. Combine injection with casting, orthoses and guided physiotherapy to maximise the benefits.

Contraindications

- Myasthenia gravis
- Aminoglycoside antibiosis
- Non-depolarizing muscle relaxants
- Pseudobulbar palsy
- Gastro-oesophageal reflux or frequent chest infections

Consent and risks

- *Local*: Pain, temporary weakness in adjacent muscles
- *General*: Mild generalised weakness, urinary incontinence, constipation, dysphagia and aspiration pneumonia

Parents and patients should be warned of its temporary effect of 12–16 weeks and the risk of recurrence and further procedures.

Surgical technique

Muscle balancing techniques

Adductor psoas and gracilis release is commonly indicated for the classic flexion adduction contracture and scissoring gait seen in cerebral palsy. Muscle imbalance combined with infrequent weightbearing causes structural changes at the hip (increased anteversion, posterolateral acetabular dysplasia) leading to posterolateral migration, pelvic obliquity and scoliosis. This is more commonly seen in quadriplegic patients and releases are performed early (3–4 years) to prevent deterioration. Muscles should be released sequentially during the procedure and performed bilaterally to prevent a windswept deformity. Releases are also commonly combined with proximal varus femoral osteotomy at age 5 years.

Hamstrings may be released proximally or distally to improve flexion contracture at the knee. Equinus deformity at the ankle is very common and is treated with tendo-Achilles release (see section 'Tendo-Achilles Lengthening', p. 464 for details). Knee and ankle releases are performed in a walking child between 4 and 6 years old.

Another common problem is the thumb in hand deformity treated with adductor pollicis release and is performed in the older child. Tendon transfers such as tibialis anterior or tibialis posterior are often used in balancing the foot in combination with bony surgery.

Osteotomy and joint containment

Hip containment

Quadriplegic patients should be monitored regularly for hip subluxation and dislocation, which tends to occur between 18 months and 6 years. Hips at risk are those with limited abduction with uncovering of less than 50% on radiography. At-risk hips may be treated with adductor, psoas and hamstring release although a more aggressive approach may be considered. Subluxed hips (>50% uncovered) are treated with soft tissue releases and varus proximal femoral osteotomy.

Early dislocated hips may be treated with open reduction; however, this may not be possible and poor conformity between the head and acetabulum may lead to early failure. A varus derotational osteotomy with soft tissue releases and/or shortening may be more appropriate. This can be combined with pelvic osteotomy.

Late dislocations require either resurfacing or total joint arthroplasty; a large articulation is preferred to confer stability. Alternatively, a Girdlestone excision arthroplasty may be considered.

Triple arthrodesis of the ankle

Various foot and ankle deformities are seen in cerebral palsy such as planovalgus, equinovalgus, equinovarus and calcaneovalgus. Triple arthrodesis is indicated for symptomatic degeneration and uncontrolled deformity. Despite frequent complications such as residual deformity, pseudarthrosis, pain and progressive intertarsal and tarsometatarsal arthritis, the response to surgery is good.

Scoliosis surgery

Scoliosis is more common in quadriplegic and non-ambulatory diplegic patients. The risk of progression is related to age at presentation and hip problems. Curves are likely to reach 50° if present by age 5. Bracing is seldom preventive. Nutrition must be optimised preoperatively, and patients must be monitored closely postoperatively for respiratory complications.

Indications for surgery are curves greater than 40° or progression greater than 10° per annum. Ambulatory patients receive posterior fusion, whereas non-ambulatory patients require additional anterior fusion and pelvic fixation.

Recommended references

Gage JR. *The Treatment of Gait Problems in Cerebral Palsy.* Cambridge, United Kingdom: Cambridge University Press, 2004.

McCarthy JJ, D'andrea LP, Betz RR et al. Scoliosis in the child with cerebral palsy. *J Am Acad Orthop Surg.* 2006;**14**:367–375.

Owers KL, Pyman J, Gargan MF et al. Bilateral hip surgery in severe cerebral palsy. *J Bone Joint Surg Br.* 2001;**83**:1161–1167.

Ramachandran M, Eastwood DM. Botulinum toxin and its orthopaedic applications. *J Bone Joint Surg Br.* 2006;**88**:981–987.

Skoff H, Woodbury DF. Management of the upper extremity in cerebral palsy. *J Bone Joint Surg Am.* 1985;**67**:500–503.

Guided growth: Temporary hemiepiphysiodesis

Preoperative planning

Temporary hemiepiphysiodesis aims to produce a differential growth rate across a physis to allow correction of angular deformities. Several methods have been described to achieve this aim, including use of staples (Blount), percutaneous transphyseal screws (Metaizeau), or more recently the use of a two-hole tension band plate (e.g. 8-plate or Pediplate). This technique is most frequently used for coronal deformities about the knee, although use about other physes has been described.

Indications

Coronal plane deformity with an abnormal periarticular angle leading to abnormal/worsening mechanical axis alignment. Occasionally can be considered for correction of sagittal plane deformity (e.g. fixed knee flexion, as an alternative to capsular release).

Contraindications

- Active infection
- Untreated metabolic/nutritional cause for deformity 'sick physis'
- Insufficient remaining growth
- Non-compliance with follow-up
- Partial growth arrest

Consent and Risks

- Neurovascular injury
- Infection
- Fracture
- Physeal injury/growth arrest
- Over-/undercorrection
- Implant failure

Operative planning

Standardised long leg radiographs should be used for planning with leg lengths corrected using blocks and the patellae pointing forwards. Periarticular angles should be calculated to identify the location of the deformity. The tension band plate should be applied on the convexity of the deformity. Angular correction may be achieved at an average of 0.7° per month at the distal femoral physis and 0.5° per month at the proximal tibia.

Surgical technique

Anaesthesia and positioning

General anaesthesia is used with intravenous antibiotic prophylaxis. The patient is positioned supine on a radiolucent table with a thigh tourniquet. A sandbag or leg holder can be used to ensure the patella is pointing upwards.

Procedure

An image intensifier is used to position a 3 cm incision centred at the level of the physis in the coronal and sagittal planes. Sharp dissection is performed down to, but not through the periosteum. The guide wire is placed approximately 1 cm into the physis and the position checked on AP and lateral radiographs, ensuring that a true lateral view is obtained.

A suitably sized two-hole plate is passed down the guide wire and positioned, ensuring it is rotated to lie perpendicular to the physis on the lateral view. Two guide wires are placed through the centre of each hole to check the screw will not penetrate the physis or the joint. A cannulated drill is used to open the cortex and a screw is placed in each hole, either side of the physis. The guide wires are removed prior to final seating of the screws.

Closure

A layered closure is used, using absorbable subcuticular material to skin.

Postoperative instructions

- Full weightbearing is permitted immediately with crutches for comfort.
- Radiographs are performed at 3 months and then at regular intervals to monitor correction.
- Implant removal is required once correction has been achieved to prevent overcorrection.

Recommended references

Ballal MS, Bruce CE, Nayagam S. Correcting genu varum and genu valgum in children by guided growth: Temporary hemiepiphysiodesis using tension band plates. *J Bone Joint Surg Br.* 2010;**92(2)**:273–276.

Blount WP, Clarke GR. Control of bone growth by epiphyseal stapling: A preliminary report. *J Bone Joint Surg [Am]*. 1949;**31–A**:464–478.

Metaizeau JP, Wong-Chung J, Bertrand H, Pasquier P. Percutaneous epiphysiodesis using transphyseal screws (PETS). *J Pediatr Orthop.* 1998;**18(3)**:363–369.

Stevens PM. Guided growth for angular correction: A preliminary series using a tension band plate. *J Pediatr Orthop.* 2007;**27**:243–259.

Viva questions

1. What are the clinical signs of hip instability in the newborn?
2. What are Hilgenreiner and Perkins lines, and what is their relevance?
3. What are the relative advantages and disadvantages of the anterior and medial approaches to the paediatric hip in developmental dysplasia of the hip?
4. Describe the Smith-Petersen approach to the paediatric hip?
5. What are the indications for varus proximal femoral osteotomy in developmental dysplasia of the hip?
6. How does a varus proximal femoral osteotomy affect range of hip movement and leg lengths?
7. What structures are at risk during a Salter pelvic osteotomy?
8. What are the indications and contraindications of the Pemberton pelvic osteotomy?
9. What is the ideal screw position when pinning a slipped upper femoral epiphysis? What risks are associated with this procedure?
10. What are the indications for prophylactic pinning of the contralateral hip in slipped upper femoral epiphysis?
11. How does the blood supply to the femoral head change throughout childhood?
12. What are the treatment options for avascular necrosis following slipped upper femoral epiphysis?
13. What is your approach to the treatment of Perthes disease in a 7-year-old child?
14. What classification systems do you know for grading the severity and predicting the prognosis of Perthes disease?
15. What are the component deformities of club foot, and which structures are tight?
16. Which structures are at risk during extensive soft tissue release of congenital talipes equinovarus via the Cincinnati approach?
17. How would you distinguish between a tight tendo-Achilles complex and gastrocnemius tightness?
18. What methods can you describe to determine when epiphysiodesis should be performed?
19. How much growth per year can be expected from each of the four main physes in the lower extremity in adolescence?
20. What is your approach to the orthopaedic assessment and treatment of the child with cerebral palsy?

17 Amputations

Heledd Havard, William Aston and Rob Pollock

Above-knee amputation	483	Hindquarter amputation/hip disarticulation	493
Below-knee amputation	487	Viva questions	494
Lesser toe amputation	488		
Foot/ray amputations	490		

Following are ideal amputation stump lengths, including the shortest and longest to allow adequate prosthetic fitting and the increased energy expenditure by level.

Amputation	Ideal level – Shortest (S)/longest (L)	Increased energy expenditure
Transradial	Proximal 2/3 – distal 1/3 junction S – 3 cm distal to biceps insertion L – 5 cm above wrist joint	Not applicable
Transhumeral	Middle 1/3 of humerus S – 4 cm below axillary fold L – 10 cm above olecranon	Not applicable
Transfemoral	Middle 1/3 of femur S – 8 cm below pubic ramus L – 15 cm above medial joint line	Traumatic 68% Vascular 100%
Transtibial	8 cm for every 1 m of height S – 7.5 cm below medial joint line L – Allow adequate soft tissue coverage	Traumatic 25% Vascular 40% Bilateral amputations BKA + BKA 40% AKA + BKA 118% AKA + AKA >200%

Above-knee amputation

Preoperative planning

Indications

'Dead, dangerous or damn nuisance' (Apley). This essentially means that if a limb is not viable due to disease or trauma; a danger to the patient due to infection, crush injury or tumour; or nonfunctional as a result of a congenital abnormality or trauma and not amenable to other treatment modalities, then amputation should be considered.

Indications by percentage are:

- Peripheral vascular disease: 55%
- Diabetes: 25%

- Trauma: 10%
- Tumour: 5%
- Infection/congenital: 5%

Contraindications

Inability to gain consent in a well-orientated patient in time, place and person.

> ### Consent and risks
> - Neurological pain
> - Phantom limb sensation
> - Flap demarcation and necrosis necessitating stump revision or vac pump application
> - Dermatological problems related to the scar and the skin-prosthesis interface
> - Problems with prosthetic fitting related to the size/shape/length of the stump and the associated soft tissues
> - Joint contractures
> - Choke syndrome: Venous outflow obstruction in the distal part of the stump due to prosthetic constriction

Operative planning

Anteroposterior and lateral radiographs are used for templating to determine the necessary bone resection level, and clinical examination is vital to plan satisfactory soft tissue closure with skin that is sensate and that will heal normally. A priority is adequate blood supply to the soft tissues to enable this. Ideal and minimal resection levels should be taken into account (see p. 481). Flap lengths and their positioning may have to be altered to accommodate skin problems or tumour excision. By doing this it may be possible to prevent a more proximal amputation.

Anaesthesia and positioning

General anaesthesia is used, with the patient positioned supine. There is some evidence to suggest (and is the authors' preference) that epidural anaesthesia, local anaesthetic infiltration of the nerves prior to transection and good analgesia in the immediate postoperative period are effective in reducing the significant problem of postoperative neurological pain.

If a tourniquet can be used in the non-ischaemic limb then it should, but must be deflated prior to wound closure to ensure that adequate haemostasis has been achieved. A tourniquet should not be used in an ischaemic limb.

Surgical technique

Landmarks and incision

The bone transection point is marked as per planning/templating. Equal anterior and posterior flaps are marked on the thigh, with their apices at the midpoint medially and laterally, at the level of anticipated bony transection. The lengths of the flaps combined must be greater than the width of the limb.

An easy way to do this (**Figure 17.1**) is to pass a suture length around the limb at the level of transection. This length is then halved and placed around the anterior portion of the thigh at the transection level, then the medial and lateral apices of the flaps at the ends of the suture are marked. The suture is then halved in length again and measured distally from the transection point in the midline anteriorly and posteriorly to mark the maximal extent of the flaps. By marking a quadrant of a circle between each of these four points, two semicircular flaps of correct length are drawn onto the anterior and posterior aspects of the leg.

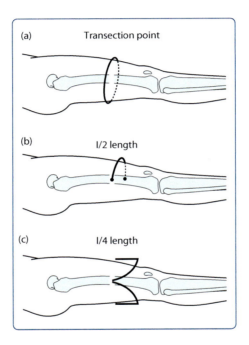

Figure 17.1 Amputation flap marking for equal anterior and posterior flaps. (a) Measurement of circumference of limb at bony transection point with a suture – length. (b) Marking medial and lateral apices. (c) Marking extent at flaps.

Superficial dissection

The incision follows the line as marked vertically down through the skin, subcutaneous fat and deep fascia to form the skin flaps. At all times careful soft tissue handling techniques should be used.

Deep dissection

The quadriceps muscle is divided, straight down to bone, in the line of the incision. The femoral canal is identified medial to the femur and the artery and vein ligated within it. These should be double tied proximally and if necessary a transfixion suture used. The periosteum is incised at the level of resection and the femur transected using a saw, ensuring protection of the soft tissues. A rasp is used to smooth the sharp edges of the cut bone and prevent high-pressure areas in the stump. The sciatic nerve is identified and transected, with a sharp blade under gentle traction, so that the end retracts proximally. Any cutaneous nerves encountered should also be transected in a similar fashion. The sciatic nerve has a significant artery running within it and therefore should be ligated, but this is not necessary for other nerves. The hamstring compartment is divided and the leg removed. The wound should be washed thoroughly and the tourniquet released to ensure adequate haemostasis.

Assessment of the flaps is carried out and any necessary trimming of muscle. In a non-ischaemic limb the quadriceps and the hamstrings can be sutured (myodesis) through drill holes, to the bone, under slight tension. The deep muscle fascia is sutured together over the end of the bone (**Figure 17.2**). A drain is inserted and the superficial fascial, fat and skin layers closed separately. The skin can be closed with absorbable or non-absorbable sutures as tissue healing should be normal.

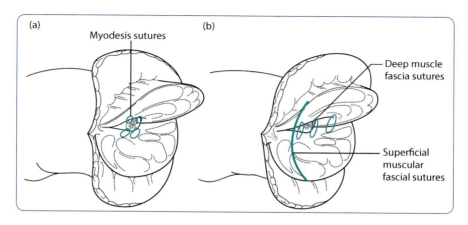

Figure 17.2 Femoral amputation stump – closure in layers: (a) myodesis sutures to bone and (b) muscle fascial layer closure.

In the ischaemic limb care should be taken to keep the skin and muscle flap as one myocutaneous flap and any tension on the tissues should be avoided, due to potential compromise of the vascular supply and therefore myodesis should not be used. Instead the muscle can simply be sutured to the periosteum (myoplasty) or the deep fascial layers of the muscle masses be sutured together over the end of the bone. Drain insertion and layered closure is as previously mentioned, except the skin should be closed under no tension and interrupted non-absorbable sutures used.

A suitable stump dressing should be securely applied, and this should remain in place for the first 5 days.

Technical aspects of procedure

In order to avoid large amounts of redundant soft tissue, the muscle flaps and skin flaps should be debrided as appropriate. However, a cylindrical, soft, well-padded soft tissue mass over the stump is desirable. In some cases, such as when atypical flaps are used, the stump may be left large on purpose to allow for possible skin demarcation and the potential for refashioning and closure. To avoid large dog-ears a stepwise approach to closing the flaps is advised, starting by opposing the middle of the flaps and subsequently halving the distance between sutures for each layer. Scars placed directly over bony prominences with little or no intervening soft tissue must be avoided as they will lead to scar adherence to the bone and skin breakdown.

Closure
Closure is as described earlier.

Postoperative care and instructions
- The drain is taken out when there is minimal drainage, typically 48–72 hours.
- Dressings to be changed, under aseptic precautions at 3–5 days, looking specifically for signs of infection or skin flap demarcation.
- Specialist physiotherapy referral for stump bandaging and rehabilitation should be made preoperatively and start as soon as the wound is satisfactory.
- Prosthetic referral can also be made preoperatively or postoperatively if appropriate.
- Definitive prosthetic fitting is often 4–6 months after surgery, when the stump has matured.
- A temporary prosthesis can be used within a week of surgery.

Below-knee amputation
Preoperative planning
Planning includes similar principles as for above-knee amputation with specific reference to the ideal stump lengths set out earlier (see p. 481).

Surgical technique
Landmarks and incision
In the non-ischaemic limb, equal flaps are marked out in a similar way to above-knee amputation; in the ischaemic limb a long posterior flap (**Figure 17.3**) is used as the posterior blood supply is significantly better.

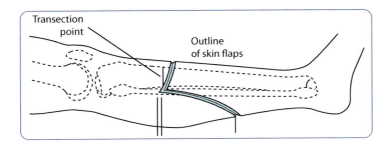

Figure 17.3 Tibial – long posterior flap.

Superficial dissection
This is the same as for above-knee amputation.

Deep dissection
Deep dissection is generally as for above-knee amputation. The anterior tibial artery and vein are encountered, with the deep peroneal nerve in the anterior compartment, the superficial peroneal nerve in the lateral compartment and the posterior tibial and peroneal artery and veins with the tibial nerve in the deep posterior compartment. Nerves and vessels should be ligated and/or transected as for above-knee amputation.

Technical aspects of procedure
The same rules regarding soft tissue reconstruction and closure apply in the ischaemic and non-ischaemic limb as for above-knee amputation.

The fibula should be transected obliquely approximately 2 cm proximal to the tibial transection and the ends smoothed.

Closure
Closure is as for above-knee amputation.

Postoperative instructions
These instructions are as for above-knee amputation.

Complications
Complications are as for above-knee amputation.

Lesser toe amputation
Preoperative planning
Similar principles as for above-knee amputation apply.

Surgical technique
Landmarks and incision
For an amputation at the base of the toe/proximal phalanx, a tennis racquet incision can be used (**Figure 17.4**). More distally the principle of a short dorsal and longer plantar flap is applied.

Dissection
Full-thickness myocutaneous flaps are created, down to periosteum. Division of the flexor and extensor tendons allows them to retract proximally. The neurovascular bundles are sought to allow transection of stretched digital nerves and tying off of the vessels. The bone

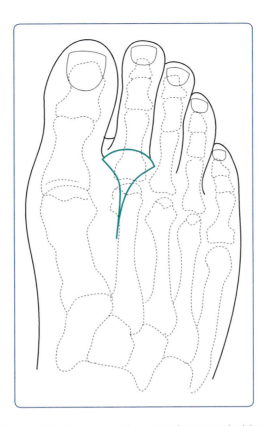

Figure 17.4 Toe amputation – tennis racquet incision.

is transected and smoothed off with a rasp. Care must be taken with closure of the muscle and fascia over the stump.

Technical aspects of procedure
When amputating the second toe it is best to try to leave as much of the proximal phalanx as possible to avoid drift of the hallux into valgus.

Hallux amputation
Amputation is as for lesser toe except a posteromedially based flap is used to swing into the defect.

Closure
Interrupted non-absorbable sutures are used.

Postoperative instructions
Dressings are changed, with aseptic precautions, at 3–5 days, looking specifically for signs of infection or skin flap demarcation.

Foot/ray amputations

Preoperative planning
Planning includes similar principles as for above-knee amputation.

Surgical technique: Dependent on type/level of amputation

Border ray amputation: First or fifth ray
Landmarks and incision
A tennis racquet incision is used, based on the metatarsal (**Figure 17.5**). With the proximal extent of the incision coming up to the level of the tarsometatarsal joint.

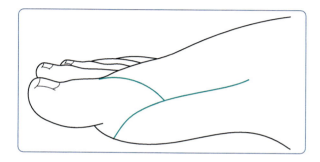

Figure 17.5 Tennis racquet incision for excision of first ray.

Dissection
Create one full-thickness flap, down to bone, to prevent devascularisation of the flap. Once the bone has been reached, subperiosteal dissection continues. The bone is transected, at the base of the appropriate metatarsal, sloping the cut to the shape of the foot and to minimise pressure on the skin. Tendons are cut under tension and allowed to retract, ligate arteries and transect nerves.

Technical aspects of procedure
Removal of the ray may be made easier if the metatarsophalangeal joint is disarticulated first and the metatarsal is removed separately. Note, during disarticulation of the first metatarsophalangeal joint, the penetrating branch of the dorsalis pedis should be preserved (approximately 1 cm distal to the joint).

Closure
A single layer of non-absorbable suture is used.

Central ray amputation
Landmarks and incision
Dorsal incision with tennis racquet is made around the toe.

Superficial dissection
Dissection is made from skin and fat to bone.

Deep dissection

Subperiosteal dissection is done. Transection of the base of the metatarsal leaving a remnant is technically easier than disarticulation at the cuneiform joints. Dissect out from proximal to distal removing the intrinsics either side.

Technical aspects of procedure

If two rays are to be removed then place the incision between the metatarsals. The second ray is relatively immobile and therefore if the third and fourth rays are to be removed then an osteotomy at the base of the fifth may be required to enable closure of the wound. Protected weightbearing for 4 weeks should be performed.

Closure

Closure is made with interrupted non-absorbable sutures.

Transmetatarsal (midtarsal) amputation

Landmarks and incision

A long plantar and shorter dorsal flap is used (**Figure 17.6**). The dorsal flap begins at the level of the intended transection and curves distally as comes medially. The plantar flap starts at the level of the metatarsal heads and curves to meet the dorsal incision medially and laterally.

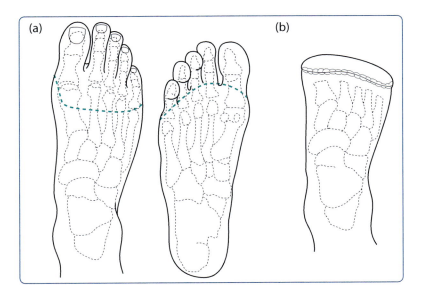

Figure 17.6 Transmetatarsal amputation: (a) Incision and (b) after closure.

Dissection

Skin and fat are incised in line with the skin. The metatarsophalangeal joints should be disarticulated and toes removed. The levels of transection of the metatarsals are marked and cut and edges smoothed. The tendons are stretched and cut so that they retract proximally. Similarly, the nerves are divided proximally, and the digital arteries ligated are then divided.

Technical aspects of procedure
Longer flaps are required medially, due to increased thickness of the foot.

Closure
Interrupted non-absorbable single-layer closure is all that is required.

Midfoot amputations

These amputations use the same principles as earlier. As opposed to a midtarsal amputation, these amputations do not leave any of the metatarsals behind. The Lisfranc amputation is at the level of the tarsometatarsal joints and the Chopart amputation at the level of the midtarsal joints. Lisfranc and Chopart amputations have a tendency to go into an equinovarus deformity with time.

Hindfoot amputation: Syme amputation

When considering performing a Symes amputation, a below-knee amputation must also be considered. A below-knee amputation gives a superior cosmetic result and enables better prosthetic fitting and subsequent function. However, what a Symes does provide is a short leg and a stump that can be used to mobilise short distances, such as going to the bathroom in the middle of the night, without having to hop or apply a prosthesis.

Landmarks and incision
A single posterior heel flap is used. The incision is from the tip of the lateral malleolus across the ankle joint to 2 cm below the medial malleolus. It continues vertically down around the heel, and back to the tip of the lateral malleolus (**Figure 17.7**).

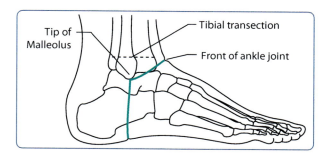

Figure 17.7 Syme amputation: Incision and tibial transection point.

Dissection
Skin and fat are incised in line with the skin. All structures are then transected down to bone. The talus is excised by placing the foot in equinus and sequentially dividing theanterior capsule, deltoid ligament and calcaneofibular ligament, taking care to preserve the posterior tibial artery. After division of the posterior capsule and the tendo-Achilles, the foot is removed by shelling out the calcaneus and preserving the posterior flap.

The distal tibia is transected 0.6 cm from the joint line, cut so that it will be parallel to the ground, and the edges rounded off (see **Figure 17.7**). The tendons are cut and allowed to retract proximally, as are the medial and lateral plantar nerves. The anterior tibial and posterior tibial arteries are ligated just proximal to the edges of the flap. The heal pad is brought forward, over the cut surface of the tibia, and sutured through drill holes on the anterior surface of the tibia.

Technical aspects of procedure
The skin flap should not be excessively trimmed as it may devascularize it. The dog-ears will resolve over time, with bandaging or further procedure.

Closure
A drain is inserted and the skin closed over it, using interrupted nylon sutures.

Postoperative care and instructions (for all foot/ray amputations)
- Partial or non-weightbearing is dependent on the procedure.
- Physiotherapy/prosthetic referral is recommended at an early stage.

Hindquarter amputation/hip disarticulation

When considering performing a hip disarticulation or hindquarter amputation, all patients should receive preoperative support including consultation with a psychologist, specialised amputee physiotherapist and prosthetist. The majority of patients will not progress to a prosthetic and the consequences of surgery will have a significant impact on their day-to-day living circumstances, with some unable to return to their home.

Indications
Indications include pelvic tumours including soft tissue lesions, primary bone tumours or large metastatic tumours that involve the neurovascular structures whereby limb salvage surgery is not feasible. The procedure can be curative or palliative but is highly morbid with high complication rates and generally poor functional outcome.

Contraindications
The inability to gain consent in a well-orientated patient in time, place and person is a contraindication.

Consent and risks
- Wound complications including flap demarcation/necrosis
- Neurological pain/neuroma formation
- Phantom limb sensation
- Need for VAC pump application with or without plastic surgery

Recommended references

Byrne RL, Nicholson ML, Woolford TJ et al. Factors influencing the healing of distal amputations performed for lower limb ischaemia. *Br J Surg.* 1992;**79**:73–75.

Falstie-Jensen N, Christensen KS, Brochner-Mortensen J. Long posterior flap versus equal sagittal flaps in below-knee amputation for ischaemia. *J Bone Joint Surg Br.* 1989;**71**:102–104.

Grimer RJ. Hindquarter amputation: Is it still needed and what are the outcomes? *Bone Joint J.* 2013;**95-B(1)**:127–131.

Hagberg E, Berlin OK, Renstrom P. Function after through-knee compared with below-knee and above-knee amputation. *Prosthet Orthot Int.* 1992;**16**:168–173.

Halbert J, Crotty M, Cameron ID. Evidence for the optimal management of acute and chronic phantom pain: A systematic review. *Clin J Pain.* 2002;**18**:84–92.

Harris RI. Syme's amputation: The technique essential to secure a satisfactory end-bearing stump. *Can J Surg.* 1964;**7**:53–63.

Hudson JR, Yu GV, Marzano R et al. Syme's amputation. Surgical technique, prosthetic considerations, and case reports. *J Am Podiatr Med Assoc.* 2002;**92**:232–246.

Malawer MM, Sugarbaker PH. *Musculoskeletal Cancer Surgery Treatment of Sarcomas and Allied Diseases.* London, United Kingdom: Kluwer Academic, 2001.

Pardasaney PK, Sullivan PE, Portney LG et al. Advantage of limb salvage over amputation for proximal extremity tumours. *Clin Orthop Relat Res.* 2006;**444**:201–208.

Viva questions

1. What are the indications for amputation?
2. What are the ideal amputation levels in long bones and why?
3. How does the surgical technique differ when performing an amputation on a limb with vascular disease?
4. How would you decide on the appropriate level for an amputation?
5. Describe above- or below-knee, or toe or foot/ray amputations.
6. How do you transect a nerve?
7. What are the complications associated with amputation? How can these complications be minimized?
8. What measures would you take to minimise postoperative pain?
9. How would you decide between a Syme and a below-knee amputation?

Index

AAOS, *see* American Academy of Orthopedic Surgeons
Abductor digiti minimi (ADM), 226
Abductor pollicis brevis (APB), 226
Abductor pollicis longus (APL), 161
Above-knee amputation, 483; *see also* Amputations; Below-knee amputation
  amputation flap marking, 485
  femoral amputation stump, 486
  postoperative care and instructions, 487
  preoperative planning, 483–484
  surgical technique, 484–487
Achilles tendinopathy, 377; *see also* Ankle surgery
  postoperative care, 380
  preoperative planning, 377–379
  surgical technique, 379–380
  V-Y advancement, 380
ACI, *see* Auto-logous chondrocyte implantation
ACJ, *see* Acromioclavicular joint
ACL, *see* Anterior cruciate ligament
Acromioclavicular joint (ACJ), 87, 99
Adhesive capsulitis, 97
ADM, *see* Abductor digiti minimi
AIIS, *see* Anterior inferior iliac spine
AIN, *see* Anterior interosseous nerve
Akin osteotomy, 396–397; *see also* Hallux valgus correction
AM, *see* Anteromedial

American Academy of Orthopedic Surgeons (AAOS), 258, 261
Amputations, 483; *see also* Above-knee amputation; Below-knee amputation
  foot, 490–493
  hip disarticulation, 493
  lesser toe, 488–489
  viva questions, 494
Anaesthesia in orthopaedic surgery, 1
  airway assessment, 2
  analgesia, 6–7
  analgesic ladder, 6
  cardiovascular assessment, 2–4
  enhanced recovery, 8
  fasting, 1–2
  intraoperative techniques, 5–6
  intravenous fluid therapy, 8
  local anaesthetic drug, 6
  myocardial infarction risk, 3
  oxygen therapy, 7–8
  postoperative care, 6–8
  preoperative assessment, 1–5
  respiratory assessment, 4–5
  viva questions, 9
Analgesic ladder, 6
Ankle arthrodesis, 367; *see also* Ankle surgery
  with nail fixation, 370
  postoperative care, 370
  preoperative planning, 367–368
  with screw fixation, 369
  surgical technique, 368–370
Ankle arthroplasty, 371; *see also* Ankle surgery
  postoperative care, 373
  preoperative planning, 371–372
  surgical technique, 372–373

Ankle arthroscopy, 374; *see also* Ankle surgery
  postoperative care, 377
  preoperative planning, 374–375
  surgical technique, 375–377
  typical portal positioning, 376
Ankle surgery, 367
  achilles tendinopathy, 377–380
  ankle arthrodesis, 367–370
  ankle arthroplasty, 371–373
  ankle arthroscopy, 374–377
  peroneal tendinopathy, 381–383
  viva questions, 383–384
Anterior cruciate ligament (ACL), 283, 330
Anterior cruciate ligament reconstruction, 342; *see also* Soft tissue surgery of knee
  anatomy of pes anserinus, 349
  anterolateral reconstruction, 352
  bone-patellar tendon–bone graft, 344–348
  graft harvest, 345
  hamstring graft, 348–351
  native femoral ACL footprint position, 346
  position of femoral tunnel placement, 346
  postoperative care, 351–352
  preoperative planning, 342–343
  site of tibial tunnel, 347
  surgical technique, 343–344
  suture loop retrieval, 347
Anterior inferior iliac spine (AIIS), 454
Anterior interosseous nerve (AIN), 228
Anterior superior iliac spine (ASIS), 451

Index

Anteromedial (AM), 345
Anteroposterior (AP), 2, 269, 389, 447
AP, *see* Anteroposterior
APB, *see* Abductor pollicis brevis
APL, *see* Abductor pollicis longus
Arthrodesis, 385; *see also* Foot surgery
  postoperative care, 387
  preoperative planning, 385–386
  surgical principles, 386–387
Arthrodesis in hand, 203; *see also* Hand surgery
  Chamay approach, 207
  distal interphalangeal joint fusion, 207
  incisions for access to dip joint, 206
  longitudinal split, 207
  operative planning, 204–205
  positions, 205
  postoperative care, 208
  preoperative planning, 203–204
  surgical technique, 205–208
Arthroplasty in hand, 209; *see also* Hand surgery
  postoperative care, 213
  preoperative planning, 209
  surgical technique, 210–212
  Swanson's implant, 210
Arthroscopic meniscal knee surgery, 328; *see also* Soft tissue surgery of knee
  acute meniscal tears, 328
  arthroscopic probe, 329
  bucket-handle tear surgery, 330
  discoid meniscus surgery, 331
  meniscal repair, 330–331
  postoperative care, 331
  preoperative planning, 328
  resection points, 330
  surgical technique, 328–331
  upbiter in posterior horn resection, 329
Arthroscopic procedures, 90; *see also* Shoulder surgery
  acromioclavicular joint excision, 92

arthroscopic soft tissue repair, 95–97
biceps tenotomy, 92–93
capsular release, 97
capsulolabral reconstruction, 96
rotator cuff repair, 93–95
side-to-side sutures, 95
subacromial decompression, 90–91
Arthroscopic subacromial decompressions (ASDs), 90
ASDs, *see* Arthroscopic subacromial decompressions
ASIS, *see* Anterior superior iliac spine
Auto-logous chondrocyte implantation (ACI), 340

Baker slide procedure, 465, 468; *see also* Tendo-Achilles lengthening
Below-knee amputation, 487; *see also* Above-knee amputation; Amputations
  complications, 488
  postoperative instructions, 488
  preoperative planning, 487
  surgical technique, 487–488
  tibial–long posterior flap, 487
Biopsy, 11; *see also* Tumours
  needle biopsy of bone, 11–14
  open biopsy of bone, 14–16
BMI, *see* Body mass index
Body mass index (BMI), 280
Bone cyst curettage, 17; *see also* Tumours
  postoperative instructions, 19
  preoperative planning, 17–18
  surgical technique, 18–19
Botulinum toxin (BTX), 476
  toxin A injections, 477
Bowers' procedure, 183; *see also* Wrist surgery
Brachial plexus surgery, 80; *see also* Peripheral nerve surgery

Fiolle Delmas approach, 82, 83
  infraclavicular approach, 82
  postoperative care, 83
  preganglionic, 81
  preoperative planning, 80–81
  supraclavicular approach, 81–82
BTX, *see* Botulinum toxin
Butler's procedure, *see* Fifth toe soft tissue correction

Calcaneal osteotomy, 421; *see also* Foot surgery
  alignment of, 423
  extensile lateral approach to os calcis, 422
  postoperative care, 424
  preoperative planning, 421–422
  surgical technique, 422–424
Carpal tunnel decompression, 63; *see also* Peripheral nerve surgery
  anaesthesia and positioning, 64
  consent and risks, 63
  contraindications, 63
  dissection, 66–67
  endoscopic decompression, 67
  extended incision for revision, 65
  extensile measures, 67
  incision, 64
  indications, 63
  operative planning, 64
  postoperative care, 68
  preoperative planning, 63
  release of flexor retinaculum, 66
  surgical technique, 64
  wrist and hand anatomy, 65
Carpometacarpal (CMC), 205
Carpometacarpal joint (CMCJ), 186
Cartilage reconstruction surgery, 339; *see also* Soft tissue surgery of knee
  femoral condylar defect repair, 341
  microfracture of medial femoral condyle, 341

postoperative care, 342
preoperative planning, 339–340
surgical technique, 340–342
CEA, see Centre-edge angle
Centre-edge angle (CEA), 456
Cerebral palsy surgery, 476; see also Paediatric orthopaedic surgery
  botulinum toxin A injections, 477
  muscle balancing techniques, 477–478
  osteotomy and joint containment, 478–479
  preoperative planning, 476–477
  surgical techniques, 477
Cerebrospinal fluid (CSF), 26
Cervical spine surgery, 25
  anterior approach to, 25–31
  deep dissection, 31, 34
  halo vest fixation, 36–41
  pin sites and baseplate positioning, 39
  posterior approach to, 31–35
  posterior approach to upper, 35–36
  safe zones for pin placement, 38
  superficial dissection, 30
  viva questions, 41
Chamay approach, 207
Charcot-Marie-Tooth (CMT), 466
Chevron osteotomy, 397–399; see also Hallux valgus correction
Choke syndrome, 484
Closed reduction, 446; see also Developmental dysplasia of the hip; Paediatric orthopaedic surgery
  adductor longus, 448
  child plastered in 'human position', 448
  postoperative instructions, 448–449
  preoperative planning, 446–447
  surgical technique, 447–448
CMC, see Carpometacarpal

CMCJ, see Carpometacarpal joint
CMT, see Charcot-Marie-Tooth
Common peroneal nerve (CPN), 280
Computed tomography (CT), 2, 35, 47, 269, 448
Congenital talipes equinovarus (CTEV), 466; see also Paediatric orthopaedic surgery
  correction, 469
  extensive soft tissue release, 471–473
  Ponseti technique, 469–471
CORA (centre of rotation of angulation), 430
CPN, see Common peroneal nerve
CR, see Cruciate retaining
Cruciate retaining (CR), 282
CSF, see Cerebrospinal fluid
CT, see Computed tomography
CTEV, see Congenital talipes equinovarus

DAA, see Direct anterior approach to the hip
DAMP, see Distal anterior, medial proximal
DDH, see Developmental dysplasia of the hip
Deep vein thrombosis (DVT), 280, 371
Deformity correction, 436; see also Limb reconstruction
  'near and far' rings, 436
  Ilizarov frame construct, 437
  postoperative care, 438
  preoperative planning, 436
  surgical technique, 436
  tibial Taylor spatial frame, 437
De Quervain's release, 162–165
Dermofasciectomy, 199–200; see also Dupuytren's surgery
Developmental dysplasia of the hip (DDH), 446; see also Paediatric orthopaedic surgery
  closed reduction, 446–449

  open reduction, 449–452
  pelvic osteotomy, 452–456
  proximal femoral osteotomy, 456–459
DEXA, see Dual-energy X-ray absorptiometry
Diagnostic shoulder arthroscopy, 85; see also Shoulder surgery
  anaesthesia and positioning, 86
  arthroscopic portals, 88
  closure and postoperative care, 90
  contraindications, 85
  operative planning, 86
  portals, 87
  positioning and traction, 87
  procedure, 88–90
DIP, see Distal interphalangeal
DIPJ, see Distal IPJ
Direct anterior approach to the hip (DAA), 241
Distal anterior, medial proximal (DAMP), 464
Distal femoral osteotomy, 309; see also Knee surgery
  lateral opening wedge, 311
  postoperative care, 313
  preoperative planning, 309–311
  surgical technique, 311–313
Distal interphalangeal (DIP), 197, 207
Distal IPJ (DIPJ), 410
Distal metatarsal articular angle (DMAA), 389
Distal radio ulnar joint (DRUJ), 161
Distal radio ulnar joint arthrodesis, 182; see also Wrist surgery
  postoperative care, 183
  surgical technique, 182–183
Distal ulna excision, 180; see also Wrist surgery
  approach to, 181
  Darrach's procedure, 182
  postoperative care, 182
  preoperative planning, 181
  procedures, 180
Distal ulna hemi-resection, 183; see also Wrist surgery

Distraction osteogenesis, 427
DMAA, *see* Distal metatarsal articular angle
DRUJ, *see* Distal radio ulnar joint
Dual-energy X-ray absorptiometry (DEXA), 262
Dupuytren's surgery, 193; *see also* Hand surgery
　dermofasciectomy, 199–200
　fasciectomy, 196
　fasciotomy, 193–194
　needle fasciotomy, 195
　postoperative care, 196, 199
　preoperative planning, 193
　Skoog's straight-line incision, 198
　surgical technique, 194–196, 197
　Z-plasty marked, 198
DVT, *see* Deep vein thrombosis
DXA, *see* Dual-energy X-ray absorptiometry

ECG, *see* Electrocardiogram
ECRB, *see* Extensor carpi radialis brevis
ECRL, *see* Extensor carpi radialis longus
ECU, *see* Extensor carpi ulnaris
EDB, *see* Extensor digitorum brevis
EDM, *see* Extensor digitorum minimi
Elbow, 117
Elbow arthroscopy, 154; *see also* Elbow surgery
　lateral portals for, 155
　medial portals for, 157
　postoperative care, 158
　preoperative planning, 154–155
　surgical technique, 155–158
Elbow surgery, 113
　aspiration/injection, 152–154
　elbow arthroscopy, 154–158
　landmarks for elbow aspiration, 153
　lateral collateral ligament reconstruction, 148–152
　open elbow arthrolysis, 137–142
　postoperative care and instructions, 154
　radial head replacement, 113–123
　tennis/golfer's elbow release, 142–148
　total elbow arthroplasty, 123–136
　viva question, 158
Electrocardiogram (ECG), 3, 44, 311
Enhanced recovery, 8
EPB, *see* Extensor pollicis brevis
Epiphysiodesis, 443; *see also* Paediatric orthopaedic surgery
　drill, 445
　postoperative instructions, 446
　preoperative planning, 443–444
　surgical technique, 444–446
EPL, *see* Extensor pollicis longus
ERC, *see* External remote controller
EUA, *see* Examination under anaesthesia
Examination under anaesthesia (EUA), 447
Excision hip arthroplasty (Girdlestone procedure), 267; *see also* Hip surgery
　postoperative care, 268
　preoperative planning, 267–268
　surgical technique, 268
Excision hip arthroplasty, 267
Extensor carpi radialis brevis (ECRB), 118, 161, 226
Extensor carpi radialis longus (ECRL), 116, 226
Extensor carpi ulnaris (ECU), 161
Extensor digitorum brevis (EDB), 413
Extensor digitorum communis (EDC), 118, 167, 143, 226
Extensor digitorum longus (EDL), 372, 413
Extensor digitorum minimi (EDM), 161, 227
Extensor hallucis longus (EHL), 372, 402
Extensor pollicis brevis (EPB), 162
Extensor pollicis longus (EPL), 161, 226
Extensor tendon repair, 213; *see also* Hand surgery
　anaesthesia and positioning, 216
　anatomy, 214
　consent and risks, 215
　contraindications, 215
　extensor tendon repair, 217, 218
　extensor tendon zones, 214
　indications and operative planning, 213–215
　postoperative care, 218–219
　pulvertaft weave, 218
　reinserting central slip, 216
　surgical technique, 216–218
External remote controller (ERC), 438

Fasciectomy, 196; *see also* Dupuytren's surgery
　postoperative care, 199
　Skoog's straight-line incision, 198
　surgical technique, 197
　Z-plasty marked out, 198
Fasciotomy, 193–194; *see also* Dupuytren's surgery
　needle, 195
　postoperative care, 196
　technique, 194–196
FCR, *see* Flexor carpi radialis
FCU, *see* Flexor carpi ulnaris
FDL, *see* Flexor digitorum longus
FDP, *see* Flexor digitorum profundus
FDS, *see* Flexor digitorum superficialis
Femoroacetabular impingement surgery, 268; *see also* Hip surgery
　postoperative care, 272
　preoperative planning, 268–270

Index

technique, 270–271
variants of, 269
FHL, see Flexor hallucis longus
Fifth toe soft tissue correction (Butler's procedure), 416; see also Foot surgery
  postoperative care, 417
  preoperative planning, 416
  surgical technique, 416–417
Fine needle aspiration (FNA), 12
Fiolle Delmas approach, 82, 83
First extensor compartment (De Quervain's) release, 162; see also Wrist surgery
  first dorsal compartment, 163–165
  preoperative planning, 162
  surgical technique, 164–165
First metatarsophalangeal joint arthrodesis, 404; see also Foot surgery
  coronal position of arthrodesis, 405
  postoperative instructions, 406
  preoperative planning, 404
  surgical technique, 404–406
First metatarsophalangeal joint cheilectomy, 401; see also Foot surgery
  minimum and maximum resection levels, 403
  postoperative instructions, 403
  preoperative planning, 401–402
  surgical technique, 402–403
Flexor carpi radialis (FCR), 163, 226
Flexor carpi ulnaris (FCU), 69, 128, 185, 226
Flexor digitorum longus (FDL), 412, 472
Flexor digitorum profundus (FDP), 204
Flexor digitorum superficialis (FDS), 71, 220
Flexor hallucis longus (FHL), 472
Flexor pollicis longus (FPL), 219
Flexor tendon repair, 223; see also Hand surgery
  bruner incisions to approach flexors, 222
  indications and operative planning, 219–221
  postoperative care and instructions, 224
  preoperative planning, 219
  surgical technique, 221–224
  zones of flexor tendon injury, 220
FNA, see Fine needle aspiration
Foot amputations, 490; see also Amputations
  postoperative care, 493
  preoperative planning, 490
  surgical technique, 490–493
  syme amputation, 492
  tennis racquet incision, 490
  transmetatarsal amputation, 491
Foot surgery, 385
  calcaneal osteotomy, 421
  fifth toe soft tissue correction, 416–417
  first metatarsophalangeal joint arthrodesis, 404–406
  first metatarsophalangeal joint cheilectomy, 401–404
  hallux valgus correction, 388–401
  hindfoot arthrodesis, 417–421
  ingrowing toenail surgery, 406–407
  interdigital neuroma, 408–409
  lesser metatarsal osteotomy, 414–415
  lesser toe deformities, 409–414
  principles of foot and ankle arthrodesis, 385–387
  viva questions, 424–425
FPL, see Flexor pollicis longus

Ganglion excision at wrist, 165; see also Wrist surgery
  ganglion of scapho-trapezial joint, 168
  preoperative planning, 166
  skin incision for, 167
  and stalk from scapholunate ligament, 168
  surgical technique, 166
Girdlestone procedure, 412; see also Excision hip arthroplasty

Hallux valgus correction, 388; see also Foot surgery
  akin osteotomy, 396–397
  assessment of first metatarsophalangeal joint congruity, 390
  categorisation of hallux valgus severity, 391
  chevron osteotomy, 397–399
  excision of medial eminence of first metatarsophalangeal joint, 392
  lapidus procedure, 399–400
  preoperative planning, 388–391
  proximal metatarsal osteotomy, 400–401
  radiographic assessment of hallux valgus, 389
  scarf osteotomy, 393–396
  surgical techniques, 391–393
  troughing of scarf osteotomy, 394
Hand surgery, 193
  arthrodesis in hand, 203–208
  arthroplasty in hand, 209–213
  Dupuytren's surgery, 193–200
  extensor tendon repair, 213–219
  flexor tendon repair preoperative planning, 219–224
  soft tissue reconstruction, 228–233
  synovial cyst treatment, 201–203
  tendon transfers, 224–228
  trigger finger surgery, 234–235
  trigger thumb surgery, 235
  viva questions, 237–238
Hindfoot arthrodesis, 417; see also Foot surgery
  approaches for, 419–421
  postoperative care, 421
  preoperative planning, 417–418
  surgical technique, 418

Index

Hip arthrodesis, 264; *see also* Hip surgery
  with cobra plate, 267
  postoperative care, 266–267
  preoperative planning, 264–265
  surgical technique, 265–266
Hip arthrography, 275; *see also* Hip surgery
  postoperative care, 276
  preoperative planning, 275
  surgical technique, 276
Hip arthroscopy, 272; *see also* Hip surgery
  arthroscopic debridement, 274
  entry to hip joint, 274
  postoperative care and instructions, 275
  preoperative planning, 272–273
  superolateral portals, 273
  surgical technique, 273–275
Hip resurfacing, 262; *see also* Hip surgery
  closure and postoperative care, 264
  extensive release of tip capsule, 263–264
  preoperative planning, 262
  surgical technique, 262
Hip surgery, 239
  excision hip arthroplasty, 267
  femoroacetabular impingement surgery, 268–272
  hip arthrodesis, 264–267
  hip arthrography, 275
  hip arthroscopy, 272–275
  hip resurfacing, 262–264
  primary total hip arthroplasty, 239
  revision total hip arthroplasty, 255–261
  viva questions, 277
Hoke percutaneous tenotomy, 465; *see also* Tendo-Achilles lengthening

ICU, *see* Intensive care unit
IM, *see* Intramedullary
Ingrowing toenail surgery, 406; *see also* Foot surgery
  partial matrix ablation, 407
  postoperative care, 407
  preoperative planning, 406–407
  surgical technique, 407
Intensive care unit (ICU), 44
Interdigital neuroma, 408; *see also* Foot surgery
  postoperative care, 409
  preoperative planning, 408
  surgical technique, 408–409
Interphalangeal joint (IPJ), 396
Intramedullary (IM), 436
Intravenous
  fluid therapy, 8
  opiates, 7
IPJ, *see* Interphalangeal joint

Jamshidi needle, 13

Knee arthrodesis, 317; *see also* Knee surgery
  postoperative care, 319
  preoperative planning, 317–318
  technique, 318–319
Knee arthroscopy, 321, 326–327; *see also* Soft tissue surgery of knee
  figure-four position, 328
  portals, 323
  postoperative care, 325
  preoperative planning, 321–322
  surgical technique, 322–325
Knee surgery, 279; *see also* Soft tissue surgery of knee
  distal femoral osteotomy, 309–313
  knee arthrodesis, 317–319
  patellofemoral replacement, 302–305
  postoperative care and instructions, 319
  primary total knee replacement, 279–293
  proximal tibial osteotomy, 313–317
  revision total knee replacement, 293–301
  unicompartmental knee replacement, 305–309
  viva questions, 320

Kocher approach, 117

Lapidus procedure, 399–400; *see also* Hallux valgus correction
Lateral collateral ligament (LCL), 149, 324
Lateral collateral ligament reconstruction, 148; *see also* Elbow surgery
  five millimetres of doubled tendon, 152
  humeral tunnels, 151
  operative planning, 149–150
  postoperative care, 152
  preoperative planning, 149
  surgical technique, 150–152
  ulnar tunnels, 151
Lateral patellar retinaculum release, 332; *see also* Soft tissue surgery of knee
  postoperative care, 334
  preoperative planning, 332
  surgical technique, 332–333
Lateral ulnar collateral ligament (LUCL), 149
LCL, *see* Lateral collateral ligament
Leg length discrepancy (LLD), 443
Lesser metatarsal osteotomy, 414; *see also* Foot surgery
  postoperative care, 415
  preoperative planning, 414–415
  surgical technique, 415
Lesser toe amputation, 488; *see also* Amputations
  postoperative instructions, 489
  preoperative planning, 488
  surgical technique, 488–489
  tennis racquet incision, 489
Lesser toe deformities, 409; *see also* Foot surgery
  distal interphalangeal joint arthrodesis, 411–412
  flexor tendon transfer, 412
  percutaneous flexor digitorum longus tenotomy, 411
  postoperative care and instructions, 414

preoperative planning, 409–410
proximal interphalangeal joint arthrodesis, 412
surgical techniques, 411–414
LHB, *see* Long head of the biceps
Limb reconstruction, 427
'near and far' fixation, 429
biomechanics, 427–428
completion of lengthening, 440
consolidation, 440
CORA, 430
corticotomy, 433
deformity correction principles, 436–438
femoral lengthening, 433
growth arrest in 12-year-old child, 439
half-pin insertion, 431–432
half-pin placement, 432
innovation in limb lengthening and reconstruction, 438–440
limb reconstruction principles, 427–428
mechanical axis deviation, 431
methods to improve stability, 428
precice lengthening nail, 438
preoperative planning, 428–431
radiograph of femoral LRS rail, 434
radiograph of tibial Ilizarov frame for lengthening, 435
surgical techniques, 428–433
'tension-stress' effect, 427
tibial Ilizarov frame for lengthening, 435
tibial lengthening, 434–435
viva questions, 441
wire insertion, 431
LLD, *see* Leg length discrepancy
Long head of the biceps (LHB), 88
Long radiolunate (LR), 190

LR, *see* Long radiolunate
LUCL, *see* Lateral ulnar collateral ligament
Lumbar spine, 53; *see also* Thoracolumbar spine surgery
anatomical levels in lumbar spine, 54
anterior lumbar interbody fusion, 59–60
anterior lumbar surgery, 59
knees-to-chest position for lumbar discectomy, 55
lumbar interbody fusion, 57–58
microdiscectomy, 53–55
minimally invasive spinal surgery, 58
posterior lumbar decompression, 55–57
posterior lumbar surgery, 53

MAD, *see* Mechanical axis deviation
Magnetic resonance (MR), 149, 374
Magnetic resonance imaging (MRI), 2, 47, 165, 269, 302
Malignant tumour principles, 20; *see also* Tumours
postoperative care, 22
preoperative planning, 20
surgical technique, 20–22
MC, *see* Mid-carpal
MCL, *see* Medial collateral ligament
MCP, *see* Metacarpophalangeal
MDT, *see* Multidisciplinary team
Mechanical axis deviation (MAD), 431
Medial collateral ligament (MCL), 283, 324; *see also* Soft tissue surgery of knee
completed, 363
landmarks on medial side of knee and attachment of, 362
multi-ligament injuries, 363–364
osteotomy and soft tissue surgery of knee, 364–365

postoperative care and instructions, 363
preoperative planning, 360
reconstruction, 360
surgical technique, 361–362
Medial patellofemoral ligament (MPFL), 334; *see also* Patellofemoral instability
postoperative care, 337
reconstruction, 334–337
Schoettle point, 336
Medical Research Council (MRC), 225
Metacarpophalangeal (MCP), 194
Metatarsophalangeal joint (MTPJ), 388
MI, *see* Myocardial infarction
Mid-carpal (MC), 161
MPFL, *see* Medial patellofemoral ligament
MR, *see* Magnetic resonance
MRC, *see* Medical Research Council
MRI, *see* Magnetic resonance imaging
MTPJ, *see* Metatarsophalangeal joint
Multidisciplinary team (MDT), 11
Myocardial infarction (MI), 2

National Institute for Health and Care Excellence (NICE), 339
Needle biopsy of bone, 11; *see also* Tumours
Jamshidi needle, 13
position of biopsy for proximal humeral tumour, 14
postoperative instructions, 14
preoperative planning, 11–12
surgical technique, 12–14
NICE, *see* National Institute for Health and Care Excellence
Non-steroidal anti-inflammatory drugs (NSAIDs), 209

NSAIDs, *see* Non-steroidal anti-inflammatory drugs

Open biopsy of bone, 14; *see also* Tumours
 postoperative instructions, 16
 preoperative planning, 14–15
 surgical technique, 15–16
Open elbow arthrolysis, 137; *see also* Elbow surgery
 anterior approach, 138–141
 arthroscopic arthrolysis, 141–142
 column procedure, 140
 distal lateral humerus, 139
 operative planning, 137
 Outerbridge-Kashiwagi procedure, 140
 postoperative care, 142
 preoperative planning, 137
 surgical technique, 138
Open reduction, 449; *see also* Developmental dysplasia of the hip; Paediatric orthopaedic surgery
 anterior approach, 451–452
 medial approach, 450–451
 postoperative instructions, 452
 preoperative planning, 449–450
 surgical technique, 450
Open shoulder procedures, 98; *see also* Shoulder surgery
 acromioclavicular joint excision, 99–100
 acromioclavicular joint reconstruction, 101–103
 acromioplasty, 98–99
 anterior stabilization, 104–105
 bony stabilizations, 107–108
 medially based inferior capsular shift, 106
 medial 'T'-shaped capsular incision, 105
 posterior stabilization, 106–107
 rotator cuff repair, 100–101
 soft tissue stabilization, 103–104
 subdeltoid bursa and axillary nerve, 101
Opiates, 7

Oral opiates, 7
Os peroneum syndrome, 381
Osteotomy, 462; *see also* Paediatric orthopaedic surgery
 postoperative instructions, 464
 preoperative planning, 463
 surgical technique, 463–464
Outerbridge-Kashiwagi procedure, 140
Oxygen therapy, 7–8

Paediatric orthopaedic surgery, 443
 cerebral palsy surgery principles, 476–479
 congenital talipes equinovarus correction, 469–473
 developmental dysplasia of hip, 446–459
 epiphysiodesis, 443–446
 slipped upper femoral epiphysis, 459–464
 surgical treatment of Perthes disease, 473–476
 temporary hemiepiphysiodesis, 479–480
 tendo-Achilles lengthening, 464–469
 viva questions, 481
Palmaris longus (PL), 226
Patellofemoral instability, 334; *see also* Soft tissue surgery of knee
 ligament reconstruction, 334–337
 Schoettle point, 336
 tibial tubercle transfer, 337–339
Patellofemoral replacement, 302; *see also* Knee surgery
 postoperative instructions, 305
 preoperative planning, 302–303
 surgical technique, 303–305
Patient-controlled analgesia (PCA), 7
PCA, *see* Patient-controlled analgesia
PCL, *see* Posterior cruciate ligament

PE, *see* Pulmonary embolism
Pelvic osteotomy, 452; *see also* Developmental dysplasia of the hip; Paediatric orthopaedic surgery
 Pemberton osteotomy, 455–456
 Salter osteotomy, 452–455
Pelvic osteotomy, 452–456; *see also* Developmental dysplasia of the hip
Pemberton osteotomy, 455–456; *see also* Pelvic osteotomy
Peripheral nerve surgery, 63
 brachial plexus surgery principles, 80
 cable nerve grafting, 79
 carpal tunnel decompression, 63–68
 epineural repair, 77, 78
 fascicular nerve repair, 77, 78
 methods of repair, 77–80
 nerve grafting, 79
 nerve transfers, 80
 peripheral nerve surgery principles, 76–80
 postoperative care, 80
 preoperative planning, 76–77
 surgical technique, 77
 ulnar nerve decompression at elbow, 72–75
 ulnar nerve decompression at wrist, 68–72
 viva questions, 84
Peroneal tendinopathy, 381; *see also* Ankle surgery
 bone block procedures, 383
 postoperative care, 382–383
 preoperative planning, 381–382
 surgical technique, 382
Perthes disease, 473; *see also* Paediatric orthopaedic surgery
 hip arthrogram, 474
 postoperative instructions, 476
 preoperative planning, 474–475
 surgical technique, 476
PIN, *see* Posterior interosseous nerve

Index

Pinning, 459; *see also*
  Paediatric orthopaedic surgery
  billings lateral radiograph showing slip, 461
  positioning for billings lateral radiograph, 460
  postoperative instructions, 462
  preoperative planning, 459–460
  surgical technique, 460–462
PIP, *see* Proximal interphalangeal
PIPJ, *see* Proximal IPJ
PL, *see* Palmaris longus
Plaster of Paris (POP), 213
PLIF, *see* Posterior lumbar interbody fusion
PMMA, *see* Polymethylmethacrylate
POL, *see* Posterior oblique ligament
Polymethylmethacrylate (PMMA), 291
Ponseti technique, 469–471
POP, *see* Plaster of Paris
Posterior cruciate ligament (PCL), 282, 324
Posterior cruciate ligament reconstruction, 356; *see also* Soft tissue surgery of knee
  footprint on medial wall of notch, 358
  postoperative care, 359–360
  preoperative planning, 356–357
  surgical technique, 357–359
  tibial attachment of, 359
Posterior interosseous nerve (PIN), 115
Posterior lumbar interbody fusion (PLIF), 57
Posterior oblique ligament (POL), 360
Posterior stabilised (PS), 282
Posterolateral corner reconstruction, 353; *see also* Soft tissue surgery of knee
  modified larson, 356
  postoperative care, 355
  preoperative planning, 353
  surgical technique, 354–355
Primary total hip arthroplasty, 239; *see also* Hip surgery
  acetabular reaming, 248
  box chisel 'starting point' in femoral preparation, 251
  lateral approach, 246
  lateral approach to hip, 245
  lateral position for hip surgery, 241
  path of sciatic nerve, 243
  position of drill holes, 254
  posterior approach, 243
  posterior approach to hip, 242
  postoperative care, 255
  preoperative planning, 239–241
  quadrants of acetabular screw positioning, 249
  skin incision for lateral approach to hip, 245
  skin incision for posterior approach to hip, 242
  surgical technique, 241–254
  typical neck cut, 247
Primary total knee replacement, 279; *see also* Knee surgery
  anterior femoral cut, 287
  distal femoral resection, 286
  flexion and extension gaps, 289
  gap balancing, 284
  measured resection, 284
  mechanical and tibiofemoral axes, 281
  medial parapatellar approach, 284
  postoperative care, 292–293
  preoperative planning, 279–282
  surgical technique, 282–292
  tibial cut, 288
Pronator teres (PT), 226
Proximal femoral osteotomy, 456; *see also* Developmental dysplasia of the hip; Paediatric orthopaedic surgery
  postoperative instructions, 459
  preoperative planning, 456–457
  stages in varus derotation osteotomy, 458
  surgical technique, 457–459
Proximal interphalangeal (PIP), 193
Proximal IPJ (PIPJ), 410
Proximal metatarsal osteotomy, 400–401; *see also* Hallux valgus correction
Proximal row carpectomy, 178; *see also* Wrist surgery
  postoperative care, 180
  preoperative planning, 178–179
  proximal row carpectomy, 180
  surgical technique, 179
Proximal tibial osteotomy, 313; *see also* Knee surgery
  medial opening wedge, 315
  postoperative care, 316
  preoperative planning, 313–314
  step cut to avoid tibial tuberosity, 317
  surgical technique, 314–316
PS, *see* Posterior stabilised
PT, *see* Pronator teres
Pulmonary embolism (PE), 280

Radial head replacement, 113; *see also* Elbow surgery
  dynamic position of posterior interosseous nerve, 120
  elbow, 117
  Kaplan approach, 119
  Kocher approach, 116, 117, 118
  lateral capsule incision, 120
  operative planning, 114–115
  patient position, 115
  postoperative care, 122–123
  preoperative planning, 113–114
  radial head replacement, 122
  radial neck cut, 121
  surgical technique, 115–122
  trial reduction to test range of motion, 122
Radioscaphocapitate (RSC), 190

Ray amputations, *see* Foot amputations
Revision total hip arthroplasty, 255; *see also* Hip surgery
　AAOS classification of acetabular bone loss, 261
　closure and postoperative care, 261
　extended trochanteric osteotomy, 257
　Paprosky classification of femoral defects, 259
　preoperative planning, 255–257
　revision of infected implants, 260
　surgical technique, 257–260
Revision total knee replacement, 293; *see also* Knee surgery
　ladder of constraint, 296
　postoperative care, 301
　preoperative planning, 293–296
　quadriceps snip, 298
　quadriceps turndown, 298
　reconstructive options for bone loss, 300
　surgical technique, 296–301
　tibial tubercle osteotomy, 299
RSC, *see* Radioscaphocapitate

Salter osteotomy, 452–455; *see also* Pelvic osteotomy
Sarcomas, 11
Sauve-Kapandji procedure, 182–183; *see also* Distal radio ulnar joint arthrodesis
Scaphoid non-union advanced collapse (SNAC), 174
Scaphoid non-union surgery, 189; *see also* Wrist surgery
　postoperative care, 191
　preoperative planning, 189
　surgical technique, 190–191
Scapholunate advanced collapse (SLAC), 174
Scapholunate ligament (SLL), 165
Scapho-trapezium-trapezoid (STT), 186

Scarf osteotomy, 393–396; *see also* Hallux valgus correction
Shoulder arthroplasty, 108; *see also* Shoulder surgery
　contraindications, 108
　indications, 108
　procedure, 109–112
　risks, 108–109
Shoulder surgery, 85
　arthroscopic procedures, 90–97
　diagnostic shoulder arthroscopy, 85
　open shoulder procedures, 98–108
　shoulder arthroplasty, 108–112
　viva questions, 112
SLAC, *see* Scapholunate advanced collapse
Slipped upper femoral epiphysis; *see also* Paediatric orthopaedic surgery
　osteotomy, 462–464
　pinning, 459–462
SLL, *see* Scapholunate ligament
sMCL, *see* Superficial MCL
SNAC, *see* Scaphoid non-union advanced collapse
Soft tissue reconstruction, 228; *see also* Hand surgery
　air-powered dermatome, 231
　burns, 229
　postoperative care, 233
　preoperative planning, 228–230
　skin loss after sepsis, 229
　surgical technique, 230–233
　volar scar, 229
　Watson hand knife, 231
Soft tissue surgery of knee, 321; *see also* Knee surgery
　anterior cruciate ligament reconstruction, 342–352
　arthroscopic meniscal knee surgery, 328–331
　cartilage reconstruction surgery, 339–342
　knee arthroscopy, 321–328

　lateral patellar retinaculum release, 332–334
　medial collateral ligament reconstruction, 360–365
　patellofemoral instability, 334–339
　posterior cruciate ligament reconstruction, 356–360
　posterolateral corner reconstruction, 353–356
　viva questions, 365–366
SONK, *see* Spontaneous osteonecrosis of the knee
Spontaneous osteonecrosis of the knee (SONK), 279
SRN, *see* Superficial radial nerve
STT, *see* Scapho-trapezium-trapezoid
Superficial MCL (sMCL), 361
Superficial radial nerve (SRN), 164
Synovial cyst treatment, 201; *see also* Hand surgery
　mucous cyst, 202
　postoperative care, 203
　preoperative planning, 201
　surgical technique, 201–203

Table-top test, 193
TAL, *see* Tendo-Achilles lengthening; Transverse acetabular ligament
Tarsometatarsal joint (TMTJ), 388
Taylor spatial frame (TSF), 436
TEA, *see* Total elbow arthroplasty
Temporary hemiepiphysiodesis, 479; *see also* Paediatric orthopaedic surgery
　postoperative instructions, 480
　preoperative planning, 479–480
　surgical technique, 480
Tendinosis, 381
Tendo-Achilles lengthening (TAL), 464; *see also* Paediatric orthopaedic surgery
　Baker slide procedure, 465, 468
　DAMP procedure, 465

Hoke percutaneous
  tenotomy, 465
open techniques, 467–468
postoperative instructions,
  468
preoperative planning,
  464–467
surgical technique, 467
techniques of
  gastrocnemius recession,
  465
vulpius procedure, 465, 468
Tendon transfers, 224; *see also*
  Hand surgery
nerve transfers, 228
planning for anterior
  interosseous nerve injury,
  225
postoperative care and
  instructions, 227
preoperative planning,
  224–226
surgical techniques,
  226–227
Tennis/golfer's elbow release,
  142; *see also* Elbow
  surgery
flexor origin debridement, 148
golfer's elbow skin incision,
  147
operative planning, 143–144
preoperative planning,
  142–143
surgical technique, 144
tennis elbow debridement
  and decortications,
  145–146
Tenosynovitis, 381
'Tension-stress' effect, 427
TFCC, *see* Triangular
  fibrocartilage complex
THA, *see* Total hip
  arthroplasty
Thoracic spine, 43; *see also*
  Thoracolumbar spine
  surgery
anterior thoracic surgery, 48
posterior thoracic
  decompression and
  fusion, 46–48
posterior thoracic surgery,
  43
scoliosis, 48–50

scoliosis correction, 43–46
selection of rib level in
  anterior scoliosis surgery,
  48
stabilised with posterior
  thoracic rods and screws,
  46
thoracic discectomy +/−
  corpectomy, 50–53
thoracic flexion
  compression fracture
  with kyphosis, 44
thoracic structures at
  various vertebral levels,
  47
thoracic vertebrectomy, 45
Thoracolumbar spine surgery,
  43
lumbar spine, 53–60
thoracic spine, 43–53
viva questions, 60–61
Tibial tubercle transfer, 337;
  see also Patellofemoral
  instability
postoperative care, 339
surgical technique, 338–339
tibial tubercle
  anteromedialisation, 338
Tibial tubercle-trochlear
  groove (TT-TG), 337
TKR, *see* Total knee
  replacement
TLIF, *see* Transforaminal
  lumbar interbody fusion
TMTJ, *see* Tarsometatarsal
  joint
Total elbow arthroplasty
  (TEA), 123; *see also* Elbow
  surgery
cortical bone graft
  placement, 135
creation of fascial flap, 131
division of tricipital
  intermuscular septum,
  133
high-speed burr, 134
implanted components,
  136
modular distal humeral
  replacement, 124
operative planning, 124–125
posterior approach to elbow,
  127

postoperative care and
  instructions, 136
preoperative planning,
  123–124
radial head and tip of
  olecranon excised, 133
rasping humeral canal, 134
rasping of ulnar metaphysic,
  135
retraction of lateral head of
  triceps, 132
surgical technique, 126–136
trial of humeral component,
  134
triceps-reflecting approach,
  130
triceps-splitting approach,
  129
use of guide, fossa reamer
  and oscillating saw, 134
Total hip arthroplasty (THA),
  239
Total knee replacement (TKR),
  279
Total wrist arthroplasty
  (TWA), 176; *see also* Wrist
  surgery
postoperative care, 178
postoperative radiographs
  of total wrist arthroplasty,
  177
preoperative planning,
  176–177
surgical technique, 177–178
Transforaminal lumbar
  interbody fusion (TLIF), 57
Transverse acetabular
  ligament (TAL), 247
Trapeziectomy, 186; *see also*
  Wrist surgery
postoperative care, 188
preoperative planning, 187
surgical technique, 187–188
Triangular fibrocartilage
  complex (TFCC), 159
Trigger finger surgery, 234; *see
  also* Hand surgery
postoperative care, 235
preoperative planning, 234
surgical technique, 234–235
Trigger thumb surgery, 235;
  see also Hand surgery
postoperative care, 236

Trigger thumb surgery (*Continued*)
  preoperative planning, 235–236
TSF, *see* Taylor spatial frame
TT-TG, *see* Tibial tubercle-trochlear groove
Tumours, 11
  biopsy principle, 11
  bone cyst curettage, 17–19
  excision of benign bone tumour, 16–17
  malignant tumour principles, 20–22
  needle biopsy of bone, 11–14
  open biopsy of bone, 14–16
  viva questions, 22–23
TWA, *see* Total wrist arthroplasty

UKR, *see* Unicompartmental knee replacement
Ulnar nerve decompression at elbow, 72; *see also* Peripheral nerve surgery
  postoperative care, 75
  preoperative planning, 72–73
  relations of ulnar nerve, 73
  surgical technique, 73–75
Ulnar nerve decompression at wrist, 68; *see also* Peripheral nerve surgery
  boundaries of Guyon's canal, 69
  incision for, 70
  incision of volar carpal ligament, 71
  postoperative care, 72
  preoperative planning, 68–69
  relations of Guyon's canal, 70
  surgical technique, 69–72
Ulnar shortening osteotomy, 183; *see also* Wrist surgery
  approach between extensor and flexor carpi ulnaris, 185
  postoperative care, 186
  preoperative planning, 183–184
  surgical technique, 184, 186
Unicompartmental knee replacement (UKR), 305; *see also* Knee surgery
  anteromedial arthritis, 306–307
  component alignment in, 309
  postoperative care, 308
  preoperative planning, 305
  surgical technique, 307–308

Valgus extension osteotomy (VGEO), 474
Varus derotation osteotomy (VDRO), 456, 458
VDRO, *see* Varus derotation osteotomy
VGEO, *see* Valgus extension osteotomy
Vulpius procedure, 465, 468; *see also* Tendo-Achilles lengthening

WALANT, *see* Wide awake local anaesthesia no tourniquet
Weil's osteotomy, 414–415; *see also* Foot surgery
White slide, *see* Distal anterior, medial proximal
WHO, *see* World Health Organization
Wide awake local anaesthesia no tourniquet (WALANT), 166
World Health Organization (WHO), 6
Wrist arthrodesis, 169; *see also* Wrist surgery
  AO wrist fusion plate, 173
  approach between third and fourth compartments, 171
  approach to wrist joint, 171
  dorsal approach to wrist, 170–174
  dorsal skin incision for, 171
  exposure of carpal bones, 174
  partial fusion, 174–176
  preoperative planning, 169–170
  spider plate, 175
Wrist arthroscopy, 159; *see also* Wrist surgery
  patient setup, 160
  postoperative care, 162
  preoperative planning, 159–162
  radiocarpal and mid-carpal portals, 162
Wrist surgery, 159
  distal radio ulnar joint arthrodesis, 182–183
  distal ulna excision, 180–182
  distal ulna hemi-resection, 183
  first extensor compartment release, 162–165
  ganglion excision, 165–168
  proximal row carpectomy, 178–180
  surgery for scaphoid non-union, 189
  total wrist arthroplasty, 176–178
  trapeziectomy, 186–188
  ulnar shortening osteotomy, 183–186
  viva questions, 191–192
  wrist arthrodesis, 169–176
  wrist arthroscopy, 159–162